Guided Endodontics

Niraj Kinariwala · Lakshman Samaranayake
Editors

Guided Endodontics

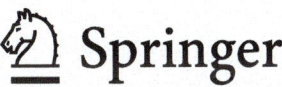 Springer

Editors
Niraj Kinariwala
Karnavati School of Dentistry
Karnavati University
Gandhinagar
Gujarat
India

Lakshman Samaranayake
Faculty of Dentistry
University of Hong Kong
Hong Kong
China

ISBN 978-3-030-55283-1   ISBN 978-3-030-55281-7   (eBook)
https://doi.org/10.1007/978-3-030-55281-7

This Springer imprint is published by the registered company Springer Nature Switzerland AG
The registered company address is: Gewerbestrasse 11, 6330 Cham, Switzerland

Foreword

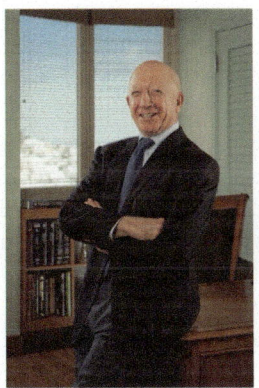

With X-Rays, *Z* Is the New Dimension!

We are all familiar with the *X*- and *Y*-planes when we view X-ray digital images. Now be prepared to step-up and embrace the third dimension which will dramatically improve the accuracy of our diagnostic interpretations and treatment planning.

Dr. Kinariwala and his colleagues describe a paradigm shift in endodontic therapy that provides an accurate insight and step-by-step planning on the usage of static and dynamic navigation for difficult root canal treatments. This state-of-the-art technology is quite remarkable in enabling the dentists to view any portion of the jaws in three dimensions on a screen or to create a 3D printed life-sized model for more sophisticated diagnosis and/or treatment planning.

3D-guided endodontics is a technology-driven treatment protocol, which provides safe and predictable solution in cases of partial and complete root canal calcifications and root end surgeries. With the advancement of CBCT and software, assessment of root canal anatomy, canal projection and tentative working length can be easily analysed, which allows clinicians to actually plan endodontic treatments beforehand.

Static guided endodontic approach has proven to be a safe, clinically feasible method to locate root canals and prevent root perforations. Special software aligned with CBCT and 3D scan allows virtual planning of the root canal access cavity. Subsequently, a 3D template can be developed to guide the drill into calcified canal. This virtual planning can help to preserve the tooth structure and avoid any procedural errors.

Dynamic navigation can also be an efficient tool for predictable treatments. These are state-of-the-art devices that allow virtual real-time navigation intraorally. This book is the first to describe a paradigm shift in endodontic therapy that provides an accurate insight and step-by-step planning on the usage of static and dynamic navigation for difficult root canal treatments.

When this technology is adopted, it will also enable the dentist to make a very accurate model of the jaws without resorting to the distortions and the messiness of impressions. Additionally, this book will illuminate the importance of STL files for 3D printing.

It will be hard for some seasoned clinicians to adopt this technology because they are too invested in more conventional ways of diagnosing and treatment planning. But if we look in the rear-view mirror, we would see how so many clinicians struggled to let go of X-ray films and adopt digital X-ray imaging. Ultimately, those dentists did embrace digital X-ray technology once they could reach beyond their fears. *The same holds true for 3D guided endodontics; it is not whether a clinician will adopt 3D guided endodontics, it is only a matter of when.*

San Francisco, CA, USA   Stephen Cohen
31 March 2020

Preface

Books may look like nothing more than words on a page, but they are actually an infinitely complex imaginotransference technology that translates odd, inky squiggles into pictures inside your head. —*Jasper Fforde*

Quantum leap advances in technology are currently transforming dentistry beyond recognition, and endodontics is no exception. *Guided Endodontics* is a novel, exciting and tech-savvy sub-domain of this subject. Here, we provide the reader the first-ever tome to delve into *Guided Endodontics*, explaining its fascinating intricacies in detail.

I began adapting this technology many moons ago, and eventually, I realized about the scarcity of literature on the science of navigation in endodontics. This realization dawned on me when I was invited to the *ConsAsia* Conference at the University of Sharjah, UAE in 2018, as a guest speaker. I was truly surprised by the immense interest generated by my presentation and clinical cases and many post-conference queries I received from colleagues and students. That implied a lack of general awareness and the true potential of *Guided Endodontics* in clinical dentistry. Immediately afterwards, I took steps to gather like minds and expert clinicians across the world and drafted the first book ever on this science; *Guided Endodontics* that you are now reading was the outcome.

This book addresses in depth the intricacies of cone-beam computed tomography, digital impression systems, three-dimensional printing technology, template designing software and dynamic navigation, which are the core attributes of *Guided Endodontics*. Clinical application of concepts of guided endodontics by renowned experts in the field is a distinctive feature of this book. The detailed, proven and practical instructions provided in this book will guide the novice and the specialist alike to predictably accomplish challenging clinical cases such as preserving teeth with calcified canals and management of root-end resection surgeries efficiently.

At the same time, I would like to remind our readers that efficient irrigation is the heart of successful root canal treatment as endodontic diseases are of microbiological origin. Biomechanical preparation of the root canal system has always been at the centre of the management strategy. To conclude, we trust that *Guided Endodontics* will help you to achieve this goal more effectively and efficiently.

Gandhinagar, Gujarat, India   Niraj Kinariwala
June 2020

Acknowledgements

I extend my gratitude to my co-editor, Prof. Samaranayake, and all the authors for spending tireless hours and hundreds of emails and phone calls to make this dream into reality. I want to acknowledge Dr Sverre Klemp, Markus Bartels and Alison Wolf from Springer Nature for believing in our team. Can't thank enough Niveka Somasundaram for coordinating this project tirelessly. I am indebted to my gurus (teachers), Dr Shraddha Chokshi and Dr Rupal Vaidya, for cultivating my interest and skills in the field of endodontics. I want to thank Dr Vaishali Parekh for her constant encouragement and words of wisdom. My parents, Jyoti Kinariwala and Bharat Kinariwala, and family are my pillars of strength. They are my guide and give me the courage to battle all obstacles in life. My wife, Dr Zeal Patel, and beloved daughter, Kiara, have been my support system. I must acknowledge the pieces of advice and counselling I received from my co-editor and mentor, Prof. Samaranayake. I would also like to acknowledge Dr Aneri Chokshi and Dr Ankita P. Sahal for their help in the compilation of this book. Last but not the least, I extend my gratitude to all my students, colleagues, family and friends for believing in me and supporting me throughout my professional journey.

Niraj Kinariwala

Contents

Navigation in Dentistry and Minimally Invasive Endodontics

1

Niraj Kinariwala

Breathtaking technological advancements over the last few decades have significantly impacted our lives. From computers to smartphones, single purpose to multipurpose devices, technology has become an intrinsic part of our daily routine. There are numerous examples of technological advances in the fields of both medicine and dentistry, where the benefits to patients have been clearly evident and hence rapidly adopted and integrated into our daily clinical routine. Examples range from those introduced in the nineteenth century, such as the introduction of anesthesia to deliver safer surgical care, and more recent adoption of robotic surgery as well as microscopy-enabled microsurgery and microdentistry. So, what will be the next most impactful technical development in dentistry? It is now generally accepted that guided surgery or navigation in surgical dentistry will be the next to join this list.

"Navigation in surgery" encompasses a broad arena, which, depending on the specific clinical challenge, may have various interpretations. So, what is navigation surgery? The concept is most accurately defined by the questions posed: "Where is my (anatomical) target?", "How do I reach my target safely," "Where am I (anatomically)?," or "Where and how shall I position my drill or implant?" Apart from these important anatomical orientation questions, surgical navigation could also be used as a quantitative tool, and in the fullness of time, an information archive and a database to provide right information at the right time.

Navigation in dentistry is an important example of technological advancements applied to medicine and health science. Navigation in dentistry is also known as guided dentistry. It is emerging as one of the most reliable representatives of digital technology as it continues to transform surgical interventions into safer, predictable, and less invasive procedures.

N. Kinariwala (✉)
Karnavati School of Dentistry, Karnavati University, Gandhinagar, Gujarat, India
e-mail: niraj@ksd.ac.in

© Springer Nature Switzerland AG 2021
N. Kinariwala, L. Samaranayake (eds.), *Guided Endodontics*,
https://doi.org/10.1007/978-3-030-55281-7_1

1.1   Inception of Navigation (Guidance) in Medical Science

The first serious experiments to precisely localize specific anatomical structures within the human body can be traced back to the late nineteenth century. Much has happened since then, but the main challenge to specifically target an anatomical structure in a safe and less invasive manner is still the paramount guiding principle. It was only with the advent of medical imaging in connection with the exponential growth of computer-processing capabilities that made precise and safe targeting of anatomy a reality. Medical imaging was an important prerequisite to enable navigation. However, pioneering surgeons remain the driving force behind the development of surgical navigation. These clinicians pushed for the development of new technology to solve their surgical challenges. In essence, three key factors pushed the development of navigation in surgery as we know it today: neurosurgery, stereotaxy, and medical imaging.

1.1.1   Neurosurgery

The symbioses of technology and surgery seem to be the strongest when faced with the challenge to operate on the most delicate organ of the human body, the brain. The entire history of neurosurgery reflects an epic quest to conduct brain surgery as minimally invasive as possible. The reason being that neurosurgery is the art of surgery on and in an organ abundant with sensitive or eloquent areas, which directly affect a patient's mental and physical state. The brain is confined in a tight space, packed together with other vital structures, like vessels and cranial nerves, which themselves can cause major functional deficits if damaged. Due to the abundance of risk structures, eloquent cortical and subcortical areas, surgical access can be limited. The intraoperative view of the target area is often constrained and lacks anatomical landmarks for orientation. Therefore, neurosurgeons are often early adopters of new technology, which holds the promise of mitigating surgical risks and enhancing patient outcome.

1.1.2   Stereotaxy

The name, stereotaxy, stems from Greek for "stereo" (solid) and "taxis" (arrangement, order). Stereotaxy is a neurosurgical procedure, which requires the exact localization and targeting of intracranial structures for the placement of electrodes, needles, or catheters. Initially, this problem was addressed using anatomical drawings as an atlas for intracranial target planning and with the help of mechanical head frames attached to the patient's skull. The planned target could then be transferred onto the actual intraoperative patient setup. This was most advantageous, as once the surgical trajectory was defined, only a bur hole was required and an electrode or a needle could be advanced with minimal brain trauma.

This type of minimally invasive procedure was termed stereotaxy. Other surgical interventions, which utilize the concept of stereotaxy, are ablation, biopsy, injection, stimulation, implantation, and radiosurgery. In the 1950s, E.A. Spiegel and H.T. Wycis invented the first stereotactic instruments for clinical use for humans and initiated the modern era of stereotactic neurosurgery. However, using the anatomical atlases to plan surgeries spawned many inaccuracies as one could not take into account a patient's individual anatomy. Such issues were further exacerbated when anatomy was altered due to pathology like a growing or infiltrating tumor. This is where medical imaging was able to bridge the gap and enables the use of patient-specific anatomy for stereotactical planning.

1.1.3   Medical Imaging

The discovery of the X-ray by Wilhelm Roentgen in 1895 opened the path for an entirely new era of medical diagnosis and treatment. It was the first time that surgeons were able to see inside a patient's body without opening it. This constituted a revolution for medical technology starting in the military section to locate bullets in extremities followed by radiography of the stomach. Shortly thereafter, the first radiographs of the skull were made to support stereotactic targeting. However, radiographs, which are simple X-ray images, could not display any intracranial soft tissue; therefore, clinicians experimented with other methods to overcome this problem. Walter Dandy, for example, fortuitously discovered ventriculography in 1918, when he was performing a radiograph on a patient with an open, penetrating head injury and the ventricles were filled up with air. Based on the idea of ventriculography, pneumoencephalography was developed where most of the cerebrospinal fluid (CSF) was drained from around the brain and replaced with air or other gases. This enabled a better image of structures in the brain on an X-ray image and allowed the calculation of stereotactic coordinates for targets in the basal ganglia and thalamus because of their definite and stable relationship to the third ventricle.

With the advent of computers, it was possible to calculate a three-dimensional (3D) image from a set of two-dimensional (2D) X-ray images. In the 1970s, Sir Hounsfield introduced the very first computer tomography (CT) imaging device, which he called "computerized axial tomography." As CT images allowed 3D targeting, it evoked a developmental leap in stereotactic head frame design. Stereotactic procedures using rigid head frames fixed to the skull proved to be extremely accurate and are still currently used in clinical practice.

The CT remains an important workhorse for the neurosurgeon and the initial patient assessment, but it was the introduction of the magnetic resonance imaging (MRI) in the 1980s, which not only allowed the imaging of soft tissue in greater detail, but also enabled the imaging of functional brain areas, like motoric or speech regions.

The introduction of the MRI marked another important milestone toward navigation in surgery. MRI images not only show more soft tissue detail, but also allow

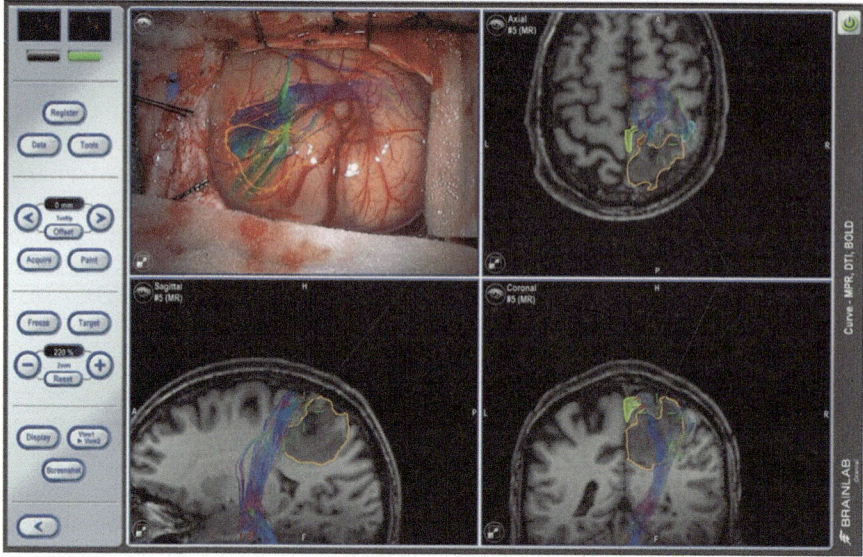

Fig. 1.1 Exemplary neuronavigation screenshot showing microscope-based navigation and the overlay of functional information: eloquent cortical areas (light blue outline), subcortical fibers (colorful fibers) in relation to the tumor (yellow outline) allowing to navigate to the tumor avoiding critical risk structures. (Copyright: Brainlab AG)

visualizing a lesion in relation to other risk structures, enabling the preoperative planning of an optimal surgical route or radiosurgery plan. Modern planning systems allow the surgeon to outline the tumor and use multimodal images, like CT for bone and MRI for soft tissue (Fig. 1.1).

1.1.4 From Frame-Based Static Stereotaxy to Frameless Dynamic Navigation

Frame-based stereotactical procedures in neurosurgery had a limited application. Only bur-hole procedures such as biopsies, electrode placements, or the resection of small intracranial tumors were possible. Other disadvantages of frame-based procedures include significant patient discomfort from scanning to surgery, the inability to visualize the biopsy needle pass, a very limited view of the surgical field through the bur hole, and no intraoperative control over the stereotactic pathway or awareness of complications, like rupturing a vessel [1].

In 1990, David Roberts developed the concept of frameless stereotaxy for neurosurgery to overcome the limitations of frame-based stereotaxy [2]. The biggest advantage of frameless stereotaxy is the capability to track a surgical instrument in "real time" and constantly visualize its position on the preoperative CT or MRI. This marked the inception of dynamic navigation in surgery as we know it today. Dynamic navigation is a successor or natural evolution of frame-based stereotaxy. It is not only used to guide the surgeon to find a specific anatomical target, avoid areas of risk, and offer intraoperative orientation in the absence of anatomical landmarks, but it can also support the optimal alignment of drill or implants and act as a 3D measurement system.

1.2 Evolution of Digital Dentistry

The digital revolution is changing the world, and dentistry is no exception. The introduction of digital devices and processing software together with new aesthetic materials and powerful manufacturing tools are radically transforming the dental profession. Quest for safer, less invasive, and predictable treatments has transformed dentistry as well.

Today, the digital revolution is changing the workflow and consequently changing operating procedures. In modern digital dentistry, the four basic phases of work are image acquisition, data preparation/processing, the production, and the clinical application on patients.

Classically, case history and physical examination, along with X-ray data from two-dimensional radiology (periapical, panoramic, and cephalometric radiographs), represented the necessary preparatory stages for formulating a treatment plan and for carrying out the therapy. With only two-dimensional X-ray data available, making a correct diagnosis and an appropriate treatment plan could be difficult; therapies essentially depended on the manual skills and experience of the operator. *3D guided endodontics* helps not only in diagnosis and treatment planning but can also be used as an efficient tool in executing the treatment.

Digital dentistry involves use of digital devices, processing softwares, and manufacturing tools (Fig. 1.2). Data or image acquisition is the first operational phase of digital dentistry (Fig. 1.3). It employs digital devices such as digital cameras,

Fig. 1.2 Triad of digital dentistry

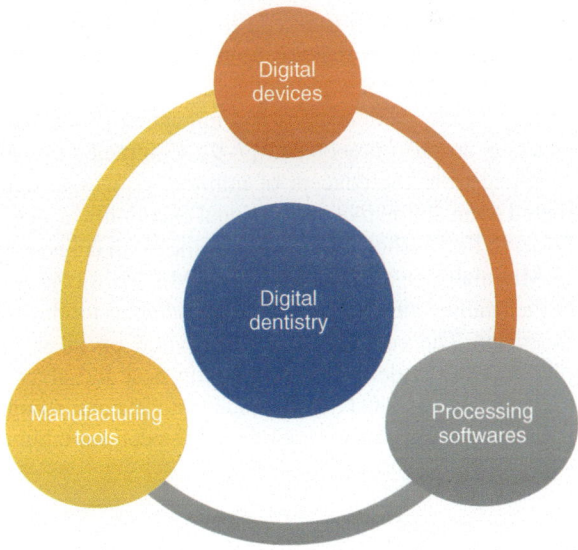

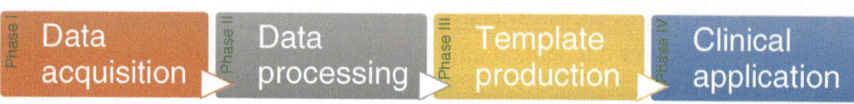

Fig. 1.3 Phases of work in digital dentistry

intraoral scanners, extraoral scanners, face scanners, CBCT, and micro-CT with low radiation dose.

Digital photography, combined with the use of appropriate software for image processing, allows us to design a patient's smile virtually. It is called digital smile design, a valuable tool for previsualization and communication in modern aesthetic and cosmetic dentistry.

Intraoral scanners allow us to take accurate optical impression of the dental arches, using only a beam of light. The optical impression is now replacing the classic method with tray and impression materials. The information on dentogingival tissues acquired from an optical impression can be used not only to make a diagnosis and for communication, but also to design prosthetic restorations. Indeed, optical impression data (e.g., the scanning of prosthetic preparations) is easily imported into processing software for designing/planning prosthetic restorations; the models created in this way are then physically produced with materials of high esthetic value, with powerful milling machines. In this book, data acquisition, processing, template production, and its clinical applications have been explained, in detail, with clinical case reports.

1.3   Concept of Minimally Invasive Endodontics

Access cavity preparation is considered a fundamental step in orthograde endodontic treatment. The first step to gain access to root canal treatment is to prepare a coronal cavity, which is crucial for the results, stability, and longevity of the tooth [3]. An access cavity that has been prepared improperly in terms of position, depth, or extent hinders the achievement of optimal results [4]. Straight-line access to the orifices of the root canals is recommended [5, 6], but, recently, minimal invasive concepts are also preconized [7–9]. Contracted endodontic cavities (CECs) have stemmed from the concept of minimally invasive dentistry. They have been presented as an alternative to traditional endodontic access cavities (TECs) designed to preserve the mechanical stability of the tooth (Figs. 1.4 and 1.5).

Minimally invasive endodontics (MIE) is a concept for maximum preservation of the healthy coronal, cervical, and radicular tooth structure during the endodontic treatment. The concept of CEC is based on preservation of pericervical dentin (PCD). PCD is defined as the dentin near the alveolar crest. This critical zone, roughly 4 mm coronal to the crestal bone and extending 4 mm apical to crestal bone, is crucial to transferring load from the occlusal table to the root, and much of the

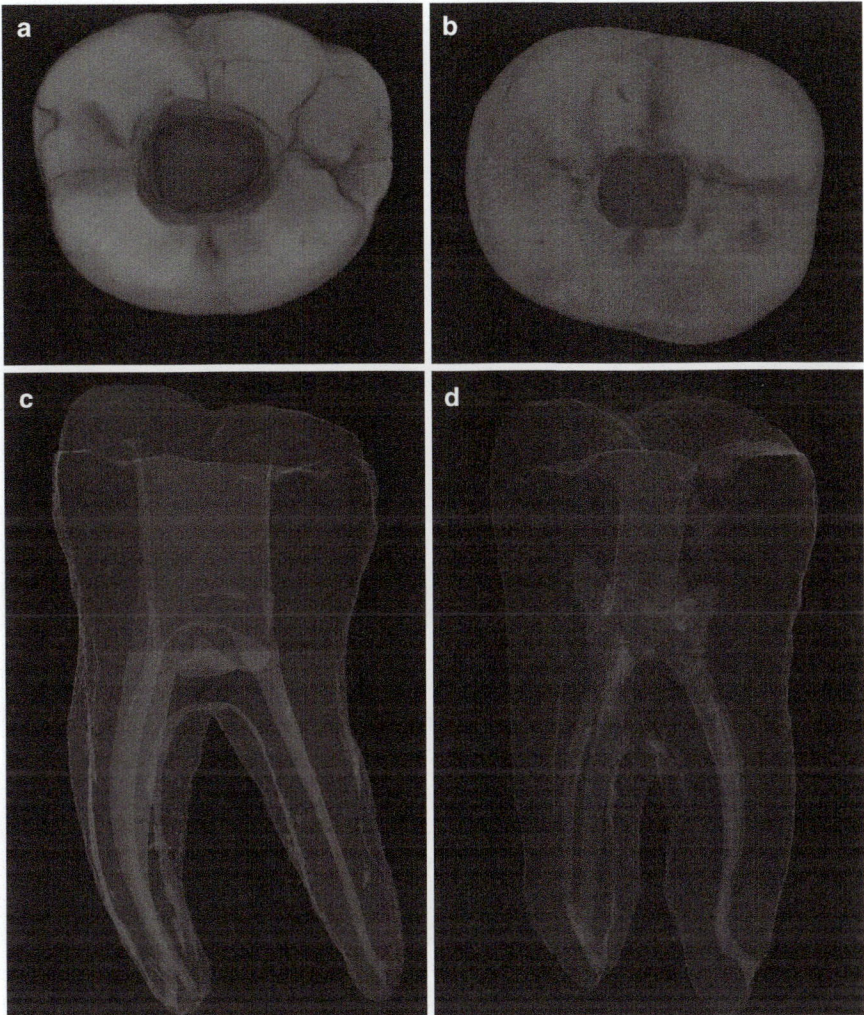

Fig. 1.4 TEC and CEC in mandibular molars. The occlusal view from micro-CT cross sections perpendicular to the occlusal plane of (**a**) the TEC and (**b**) CEC. A sagittal view of (**c**) the TEC and (**d**) CEC from 3D volumetric representations. (License no: 4787041186027; [10])

PCD is irreplaceable. In conventional deroofing process, much of PCD is lost, which reduces fracture resistance of the tooth (Fig. 1.4). More conservative approach can help in preservation of PCD (Figs. 1.5, 1.6, and 1.7). Guided endodontics helps in preservation of PCD and offers the most conservative approach for cases with high difficulty level: calcified canals.

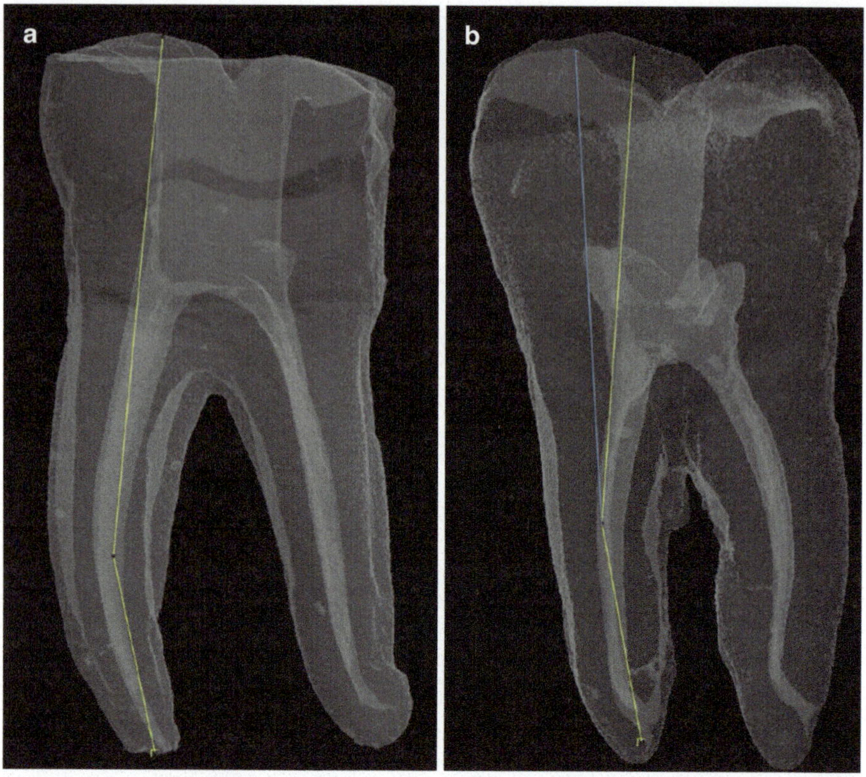

Fig. 1.5 3D volumetric representation of micro-CT data showing the angle of file access in the MB canals in the maximum curvature view for the (**a**) TEC and (**b**) CEC groups. The blue line in (**b**) shows the different access angle after a complete removal of the pulp chamber roof and coronal interferences. (License no: 4787041186027; [10])

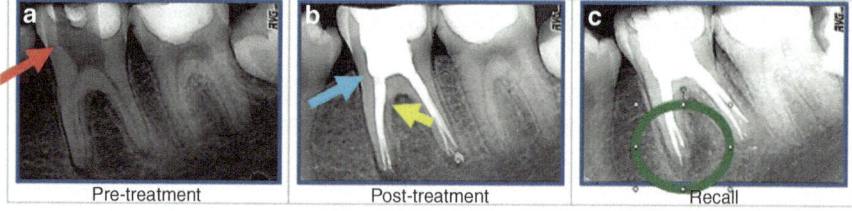

Pre-treatment   Post-treatment   Recall

Fig. 1.6 (**a**) The deroofing problem. The likely bur used by the referring general dentist is a 56 carbide; one of the most popular burs in dentistry, it is possibly the most iatrogenic instrument in modern medicine. Red arrow delineates the typical gouging. (**b**) Postoperative view provided by the endodontist. Blue arrow indicates the grossly excessive dentin removal of pericervical dentin (PCD). This serious gouging is typical of round bur access. Yellow arrow indicates the large canal flaring with unacceptable dentin removal (blind funneling). (**c**) Green circle highlights worsening lesion on mesial root ends. (License no: 4787071066122; [3])

Fig. 1.7 A more appropriate access shape is overlayed. Partial deroofing and maintenance of a robust amount of PCD is demonstrated. A soffit that includes pulp horns on mesial and distal is depicted. Soffit is a small piece of roof around the entire coronal portion of the pulp chamber. (License no: 4787071066122; [3])

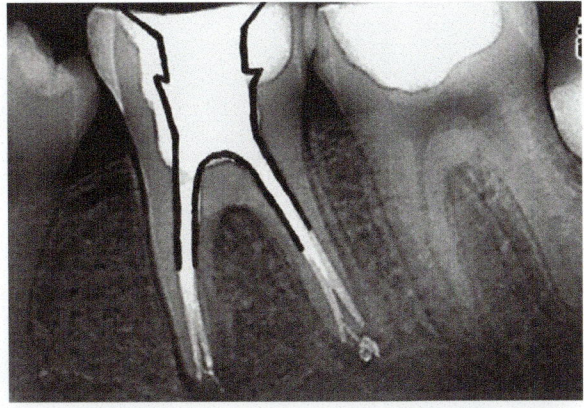

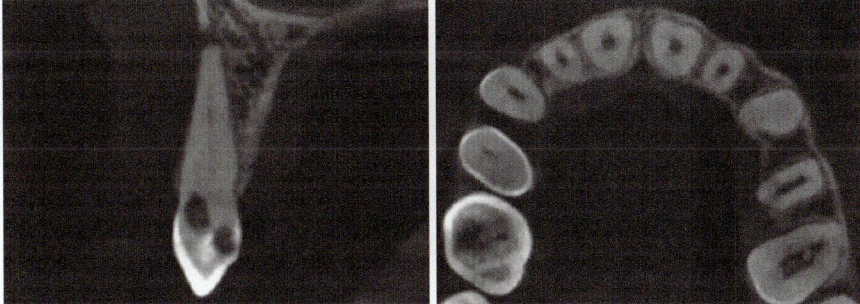

Fig. 1.8 Main indication for endoguide: root canal calcification or obstruction

1.4 Need for 3D Guided Endodontics

Guided Endodontics is also known as Targeted Endodontic Treatment (TET). In cases of calcified canals and endodontic microsurgery, Guided endodontics can deliver more predictable treatment outcomes compared to conventional treatment strategies. Guided approach can be static or dynamic. "Static guided Endodontics" is a way to use CBCT merged with an optical impression, creating the platform for the design of a virtual drill path subsequent to the clinical procedure of drilling using a guide.

Pulp canal obliteration or calcification is characterized by the deposition of hard tissue within the root canal space (Fig. 1.8). When a young person with a vital tooth and an open apex is exposed to a trauma, the pulp response may result in a narrowing of the pulp cavity by deposition of hard tissue. In anterior teeth, it occurs commonly as a result of concussion, subluxation, or luxation injuries [11, 12]. In elderly patients, the ongoing deposition of both secondary and potential tertiary dentin may reduce the root canal space as well. External injuries resulting in tertiary dentin can be caused by caries, wear, irritation from preparations, and/or subsequent filling materials [13, 14]. In these cases, even the most experienced clinicians can

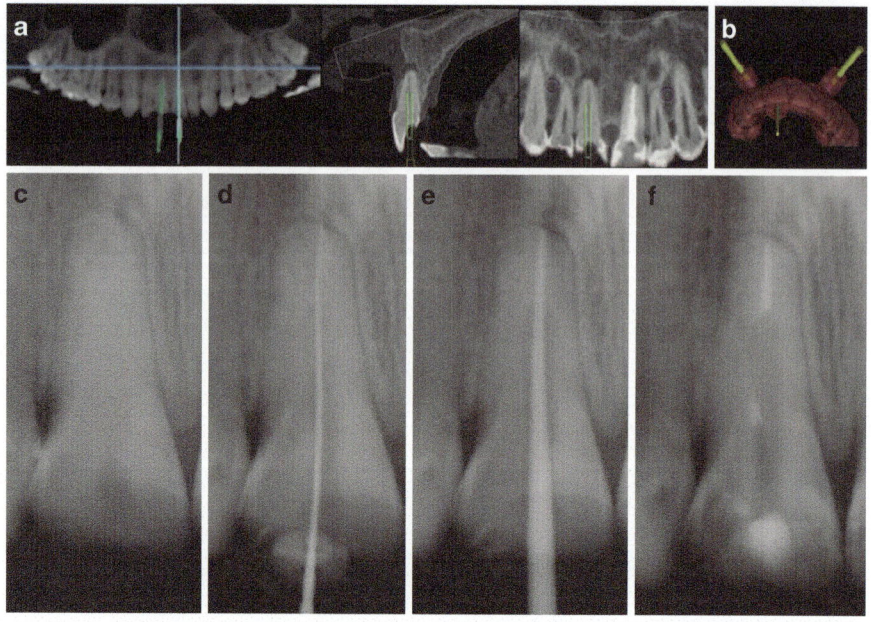

Fig. 1.9 (**a**) CBCT image with virtual drill path designed to reach the center of the target point (patent canal); (**b**) Design of Endodontic guide before 3D printing; (**c**) Radiograph of symptomatic maxillary central incisor root canal with calcific metamorphosis; (**d**) Radiograph taken after localization of canal with guided endodontics; (**e**) Radiograph of master cone fit; and (**f**) Obturated canal with postspace preparation. (Courtesy: Antônio Paulino Ribeiro Sobrinho, Warley Luciano Tavares, Lucas Moreira Maia)

encounter difficulties to prepare an adequate access cavity. Guided endodontics is extremely helpful for predictable, minimally invasive, and successful endodontic treatment of such cases (Fig. 1.9).

A CBCT scan is an excellent measure for localizing the root canals in order to make an orthograde root canal treatment of seemingly obliterated root canals (Fig. 1.9). In particular, the axial view gives the placement of a canal in relation other landmarks of the tooth: the circumference and the position of the potential other neighboring root canals. These relations can be measured at the CBCT scan, but may be difficult to apply directly with accuracy into the clinical scenario.

In contrast, a virtual drill path can be made at the scan with the use of appropriate software. If this virtual drill path shall be converted into a real drill path, some kind of surface guiding based on the CBCT scan is necessary. It could be a dynamic guiding or a static guiding. A static guiding is made by using a guide made from a combination of a CBCT scan and a surface scan, whereas the dynamic guiding uses the CBCT data in combination with recordings of the drill movements running real time. Navigation can support several aspects of endodontic treatment, from localization of calcified canals to guiding the osteotomy for apicoectomy.

The surgeon's quest for safer, less invasive, and more cost-efficient procedures has come a long way and continues to move forward at an unprecedented pace. What started as basic localization technique has followed the growth of modern technology beyond specialized uses. We have explained all the aspects of 3D guided endodontics, in detail, in subsequent chapters.

References

1. Mezger U. Navigation in surgery. Langenbeck's Arch Surg. 2013;398:501–14.
2. Enchev Y. Neuronavigation: geneology, reality, and prospects. Neurosurg Focus. 2009;27(3):E11.
3. Clark D, Khademi J. Modern molar endodontic access and directed dentin conservation. Dent Clin N Am. 2010;54:249–73.
4. Weine FS. Endodontic therapy. 3rd ed. St. Louis, MO: Mosby Company; 1982.
5. Patel S, Rhodes J. A practical guide to endodontic access cavity preparation in molar teeth. Br Dent J. 2007;203:133–40.
6. Johnson BR. Endodontic access. Gen Dent. 2009;57:570–7.
7. Gutmann JL. Minimally invasive dentistry (Endodontics). J Conserv Dent. 2013;16(4):282–3.
8. Krishan R, Paque F, Ossareh A, et al. Impacts of conservative endodontic cavity on root canal instrumentation efficacy and resistance to fracture assessed in incisors, premolars, and molars. J Endod. 2014;40:1160–6.
9. Gluskin AH, Peters CI, Peters OA. Minimally invasive endodontics: challenging prevailing paradigms. Br Dent J. 2014;216:347–53.
10. Alovisi M, et al. Influence of contracted endodontic access on root canal geometry: an *in vitro* study. J Endod. 2018;44(4):614–20.
11. Andreasen FM, Zhijie Y, Thomsen BL, Andersen PK. Occurrence of pulp canal obliteration after luxation injuries in the permanent dentition. Endod Dent Traumatol. 1987;3:103–15.
12. Flores MT, Andersson L, Andreasen JO, et al. Guidelines for the management of traumatic dental injuries. I. Fractures and luxations of permanent teeth. Dent Traumatol. 2007;23:66–71.
13. Bjørndal L, Darvann T. A light microscopic study of odontoblastic and non-odontoblastic cells involved in tertiary dentinogenesis in well-defined cavitated carious lesions. Caries Res. 1999;33:50–60.
14. Fleig S, Attin T, Jungbluth H. Narrowing of the radicular pulp space in coronally restored teeth. Clin Oral Investig. 2017;21:1251–7.

CBCT in Endodontics

Niraj Kinariwala

Medical computed tomography (CT) was first developed by Sir Godfrey Hounsfield in 1967, and since then, many advancements have been made involving detectors, beam source, and movement patterns of the detectors and beam sources [1]. Cone beam computed tomography (CBCT) was first introduced in Europe in 1996 and in the United States in 2001 (Fig. 2.1). By 1998, Mozzo et al. [2] had laid the foundation for the new revolution in three-dimensional (3D) imaging by describing how a volumetric CT machine would be useful for dental imaging. For decades, clinicians have relied on standard two-dimensional (2D) images that offered little useful information about the third dimension, z-axis, which denotes depth of the anatomical volume. In last decade, CBCT has become an integral part of dental practices.

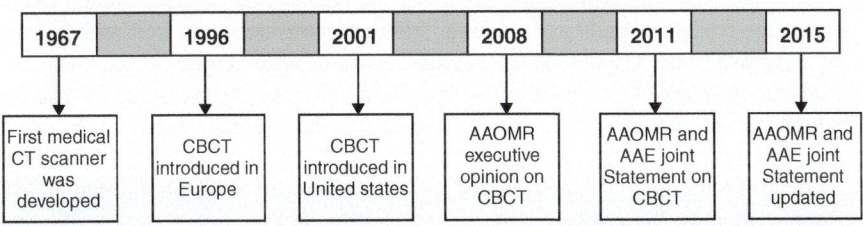

Fig. 2.1 Timeline of evolution of CBCT and development of guidelines for endodontics. *CT* computed tomography, *CBCT* cone beam computed tomography, *AAOMR* American Academy of Oral and Maxillofacial Radiology, *AAE* American Association of Endodontists

N. Kinariwala (✉)
Karnavati School of Dentistry, Karnavati University, Gandhinagar, Gujarat, India
e-mail: niraj@ksd.ac.in

© Springer Nature Switzerland AG 2021
N. Kinariwala, L. Samaranayake (eds.), *Guided Endodontics*,
https://doi.org/10.1007/978-3-030-55281-7_2

2.1   Important Aspects of CBCT Imaging

CBCT is accomplished by using a rotating gantry to which an X-ray source and detector are fixed. A divergent pyramidal- or cone-shaped source of ionizing radiation is directed through the middle of the head and neck, with X-ray detector on the opposite side of the patient. The X-ray source and detector rotate around a fixed fulcrum within the region of interest (ROI). During the exposure sequence, hundreds of planar projection 2D images are acquired of the field of view (FOV) in an arc of at least 180°. The images are then reconstructed to visualize 3D data set, using a variation of the algorithm developed by Feldkamp et al. in 1994 [3]. This technique allows clinicians to obtain 2D reconstructed images in all planes, and reconstructions in 3 dimensions with low level exposure to X-radiation [4].

Patient Positioning Depending on the system employed, maxillofacial CBCT can be performed with the patient in three possible positions: (1) sitting, (2) standing, and (3) supine. Equipment that requires the patient to be supine has a larger physical footprint and may not be readily accessible for patients with physical disabilities. It may not be possible to adjust standing units to a height to accommodate wheelchair-bound patients. Seated units are the most comfortable; however, fixed seats may not allow ready scanning of physically disabled or wheelchair-bound patients.

2.1.1   Field of View (FOV)

The size of the FOV describes the scan volume of a particular CBCT machine and depends on the detector's size and shape, the beam projection geometry, and the ability to collimate the beam, which differs from one manufacturer to another. Beam collimation limits the patients' ionizing radiation exposure to the ROI and ensures that an appropriate FOV can be selected based on the specific case.

Based on available or selected scan volume height, the use of units can be designed as follows:

1. Localized region (also referred to as focused, small field or, limited field): approximately 5 cm or less
2. Single arch: 5–7 cm
3. Interarch: 7–10 cm
4. Maxillofacial: 10–15 cm
5. Craniofacial: greater than 15 cm

CBCT units can be classified into small, medium, and large volume based on the size of their FOV (Fig. 2.2). Small-volume CBCT machines are used to scan a range from a sextant or a quadrant to one jaw only. They generally offer higher image

Fig. 2.2 Area covered by small, medium, and large FOVs. (License no: 4793551439602; [5])

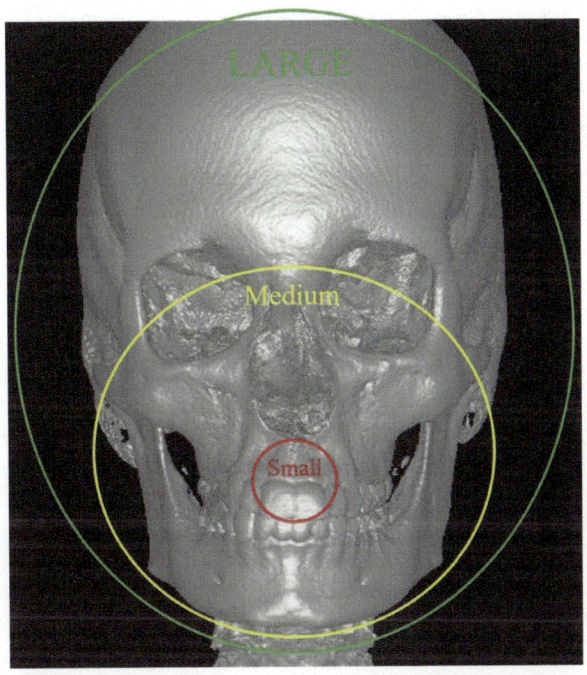

resolution, because X-ray scattering (noise) is reduced as the FOV decreases. Noise is false grey scale level of a single pixel, which influences the quality of the image generated.[1] Medium-volume CBCT machines are used to scan both jaws, whereas large FOV machines allow the visualization of the entire head commonly used in orthodontic and orthognathic surgery treatment planning. The main limitation of large FOV CBCT units is the size of the field irradiated [5]. Unless the smallest voxel size is selected in the larger FOV machines, there is also a reduction in image resolution as compared with intraoral radiographs or small FOV CBCT machines with inherent small voxel sizes [5].

In endodontics, the area of interest is limited, and small-volume CBCT machines are preferred, because there is less radiation dose to the patient, higher spatial resolution, and shorter volumes to be interpreted.

As the earliest sign of periapical pathology is discontinuity in the lamina dura and widening of the periodontal ligament space, it is desirable that the optimal resolution of any CBCT imaging system used in endodontics does not exceed 200 µm, which is the average width of the periodontal ligament space.

---

[1] Too low tube current (mA) causes noise in the image. Higher mA decreases amount of noise, which comes at an increased radiation dose to the patient.

2.1.2   Cone Beam Computed Tomography Image Formation

The image formation process consists of three stages:

1. Acquisition stage
2. Reconstruction stage
3. Image display

2.1.2.1 Acquisition Stage

Cone beam acquisition techniques mostly use a single $180°$ rotation or more in which the X-ray source and a reciprocating X-ray detector are attached by an arm and they rotate around patients' heads. The FOV determined by the area of interest depends primarily on the detector's size, beam projection geometry, and selected collimation, whenever available. The primary images captured during a CBCT scan consist of a sequence of 2D projection images, also known as projection data, raw data, basis projections, or basis frames. Projection data are promptly reconstructed into what constitutes the real outcome of CBCT: a volumetric data set [6, 7].

In some cases, multiple consecutive scans are acquired, which are then merged (i.e. stitched) into one image. This merger can be carried out to combine two or more small-diameter FOVs (Fig. 2.3) or two small-height FOVs. Between the scans, the chair or C-arm moves along a preset path, leaving a small overlap between the images. Stitching of the image volume could be carried out through a simple overlap (as the relative movement of patients between the scans is known exactly) or through automatic matching of the images using image registration [8].

2.1.2.2 Reconstruction Stage

The projection data images are processed in the workstation computer, not only visually but also geometrically. It gets processed by application of reconstruction algorithm. On completion of slice-by-slice reconstruction, data is compiled as a single volume for visualization. The restructured CBCT image consists of voxels (volumetric pixels), which are analogous to a pixel in 2D image.

Reconstruction times vary depending on the acquisition parameters (voxel size, FOV, image noise), hardware (processing speed, data throughput from the acquisition computer to the workstation), and software (reconstruction algorithms) used. Reconstruction should be accomplished in an acceptable time (less than 5 min) to complement patient flow.

2.1.2.3 Image Display and Manipulation

Reconstruction phase is followed by image display, which has mainly three functions. The main functions are

- Multiplanar reformatting (MPR) (Fig. 2.4)
- Panoramic or curvilinear and cross-sectional reconstructions
- Maximum intensity projection (MIP) and volume rendering (Fig. 2.5)

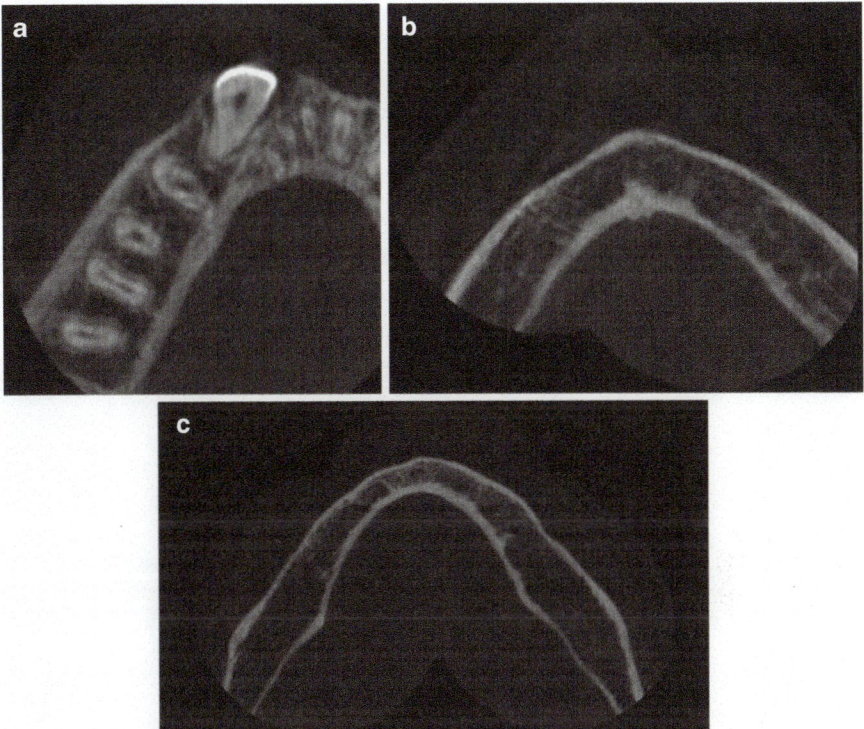

Fig. 2.3 Image stitching in CBCT. (**a**) Small FOV covering the right mandible. (**b**) Stitching of two FOVs. (**c**) Stitching of three FOVs, covering a larger area of the mandible. (License no: 4793551439602; [5])

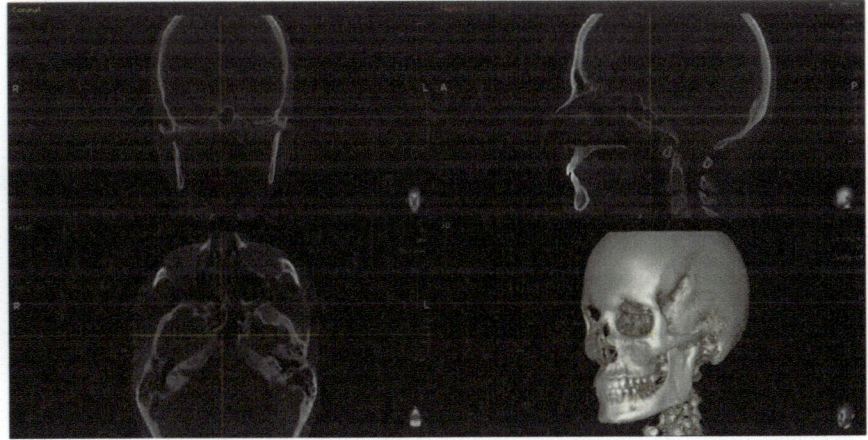

Fig. 2.4 MPR screen, with the coronal, sagittal, axial, and 3D rendering views. (License no: 4793551439602; [5])

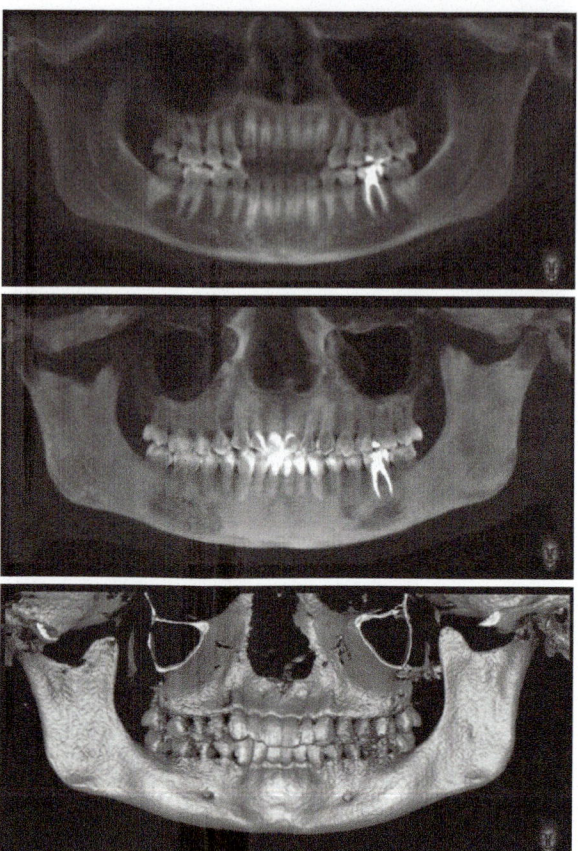

Fig. 2.5 Panoramic reconstruction (upper), transformed with an MIP (middle), and volume rendering (lower). (License no: 4797030409216; [5])

2.1.3   Artifact Reduction

An image artifact is a visualized structure in the reconstructed data that is not present in the object under investigation. Artifacts can significantly affect the quality of CBCT images by decreasing the contrast between adjacent objects and ultimately lead to an inaccurate or false diagnosis [9]. Among different kinds of artifacts (such as scatter, noise artifacts, and others), beam-hardening artifacts are considered to be the most prominent artifacts induced by dental implants and metallic restorations [10]. "Beam hardening is the process by which low-energy photons in a polychromatic beam are attenuated after passing through metallic objects, such as dental implants, leading to an increase in beam average energy level, that is, the beam becomes harder." Metallic restorations or objects and endodontic materials such as root canal filling are the main causes of beam hardening in CBCT data volumes. Due to the high density of these materials, it creates an area effect. Beam hardening artifacts reduce the image quality in the axial plane; it presents as white and black

Fig. 2.6 Beam
hardening effect

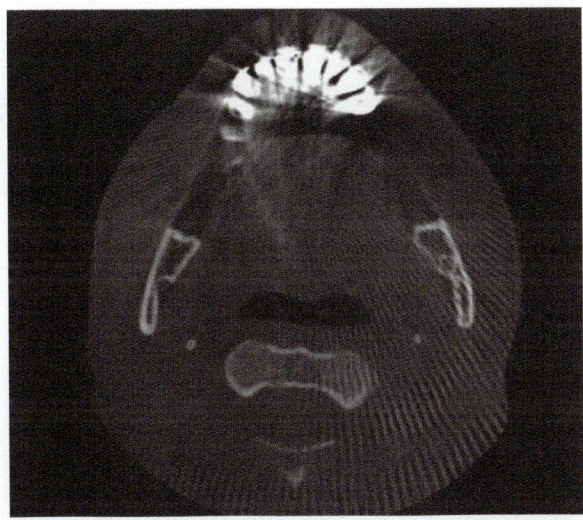

lines and may be "sun ray" in appearance (Fig. 2.6). Metal artifact reduction can be carried out by adaptive scanning technique, processing technique, or postprocessing technique [11].

2.2   Recommendations of CBCT in Endodontics

In 2015, American Association of Endodontics (AAE) and American Academy of Oral and Maxillofacial Radiology (AAOMR) have updated their recommendations for use of CBCT in Endodontics.

2.2.1   Diagnosis

Endodontic diagnosis is dependent upon thorough evaluation of the patient's chief complaint, history, and clinical and radiographic examination. Preoperative radiographs are an essential part of the diagnostic phase of endodontic therapy. Accurate diagnostic imaging supports the clinical diagnosis.

Recommendation 1: Intraoral radiographs should be considered the first imaging modality of choice in the evaluation of the endodontic patient.

Recommendation 2: Limited FOV CBCT should be considered the imaging modality of choice for diagnosis in patients who present with contradictory or non-specific clinical signs and symptoms associated with untreated or previously endodontically treated teeth.

In some cases, the clinical and planar radiographic examinations are inconclusive. Inability to confidently determine the etiology of endodontic pathosis may be attributed to limitations in both clinical vitality testing and intraoral radiographs to

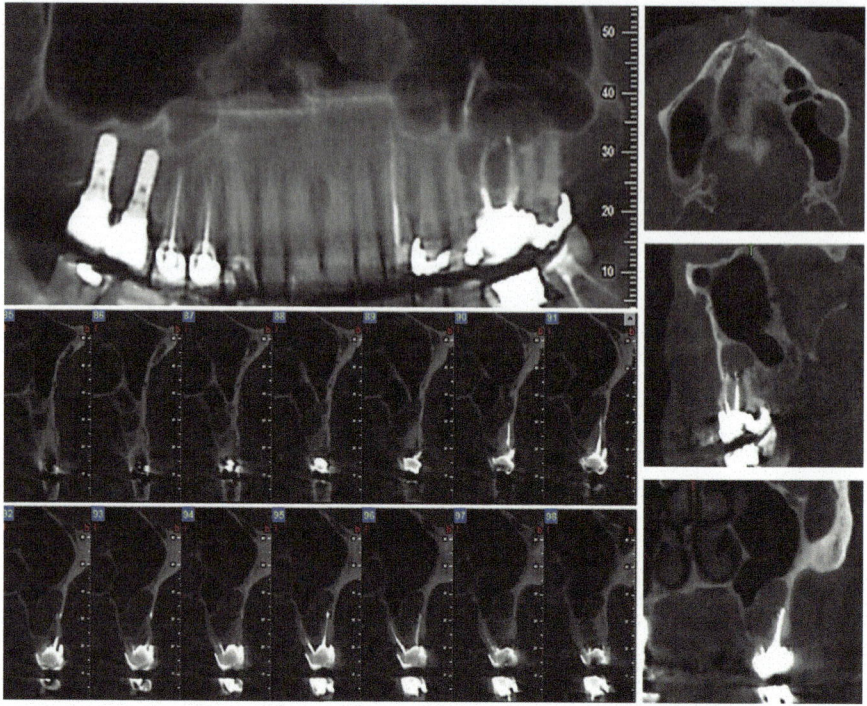

Fig. 2.7 A 3D representation of a periapical pathology. (License no: 4793551310168)

detect odontogenic pathoses. CBCT imaging has the ability to detect periapical pathosis before it is apparent on 2D radiographs [7].

Preoperative factors such as the presence and true size of a periapical lesion play an important role in endodontic treatment outcome. Success, when measured by radiographic criteria, is higher when teeth are endodontically treated before radiographic signs of periapical disease are detected [8] (Fig. 2.7).

Previous findings have been validated in clinical studies in which primary endodontic disease detected with intraoral radiographs and CBCT was 20% and 48%, respectively. Several clinical studies had similar findings, although with slightly different percentages [9, 10]. Ex vivo experiments in which simulated periapical lesions were created yielded similar results (11, 12). Results of in vivo animal studies, using histologic assessments as the gold standard, also showed similar results observed in human clinical and ex vivo studies (13).

Persistent intraoral pain following root canal therapy often presents a diagnostic challenge. An example is persistent dentoalveolar pain also known as atypical odontalgia (14). The diagnostic yield of conventional intraoral radiographs and CBCT scans was evaluated in the differentiation between patients presenting with suspected atypical odontalgia versus symptomatic apical periodontitis, without radiographic evidence of periapical bone destruction (15). CBCT imaging detected 17% more teeth with periapical bone loss than conventional radiography.

2.2.2   Initial Treatment

2.2.2.1 Preoperative

Recommendation 3: Limited FOV CBCT should be considered the imaging modality of choice for initial treatment of teeth with the potential for extra canals and suspected complex morphology, such as mandibular anterior teeth, and maxillary and mandibular premolars and molars, and dental anomalies (Figs. 2.8 and 2.9).

2.2.2.2 Intraoperative

Recommendation 4: If a preoperative CBCT has not been taken, limited FOV CBCT should be considered as the imaging modality of choice for intra-appointment identification and localization of calcified canals (Fig. 2.10).

2.2.2.3 Postoperative

Recommendation 5: Intraoral radiographs should be considered the imaging modality of choice for immediate postoperative imaging.

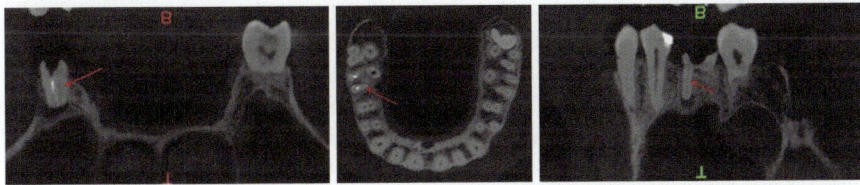

Fig. 2.8   The arrows point to an untreated canal in the three planes. (License no: 4793551310168)

Fig. 2.9   Visualization of molars' root canal morphology on the axial view (circles). (License no: 4793551310168)

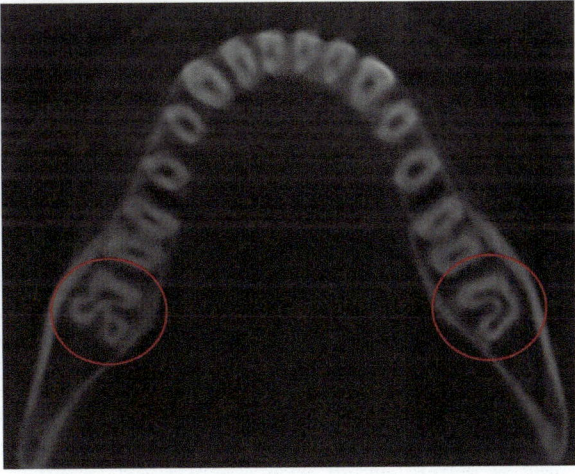

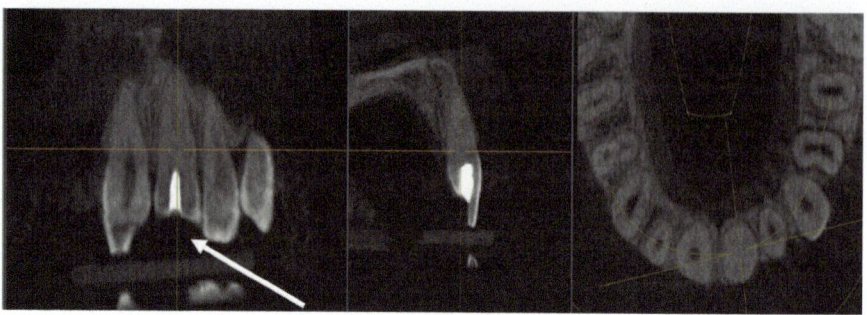

Fig. 2.10 Calcified canal in central incisor. CBCT helps in localization of calcified canal in different planes. (Courtesy: Jørgen Buchgreitz and Lars Bjørndal)

2.2.3 Nonsurgical Retreatment

Recommendation 6: Limited FOV CBCT should be considered the imaging modality of choice if clinical examination and 2-D intraoral radiography are inconclusive in the detection of vertical root fracture.

Recommendation 7: Limited FOV CBCT should be the imaging modality of choice when evaluating the nonhealing of previous endodontic treatment to help determine the need for further treatment, such as nonsurgical, surgical, or extraction.

Recommendation 8: Limited FOV CBCT should be the imaging modality of choice for nonsurgical re-treatment to assess endodontic treatment complications, such as overextended root canal obturation material, separated endodontic instruments, and localization of perforations (Fig. 2.11).

2.2.4 Surgical Retreatment

Recommendation 9: Limited FOV CBCT should be considered as the imaging modality of choice for presurgical treatment planning to localize root apex/apices and to evaluate the proximity to adjacent anatomical structures.

2.2.5 Special Conditions

Recommendation 10: Limited FOV CBCT should be considered as the imaging modality of choice for surgical placement of implants (26).

Recommendation 11: Limited FOV CBCT should be considered the imaging modality of choice for diagnosis and management of limited dentoalveolar trauma, root fractures, luxation, and/or displacement of teeth and localized alveolar fractures, in the absence of other maxillofacial or soft tissue injury that may require other advanced imaging modalities (27).

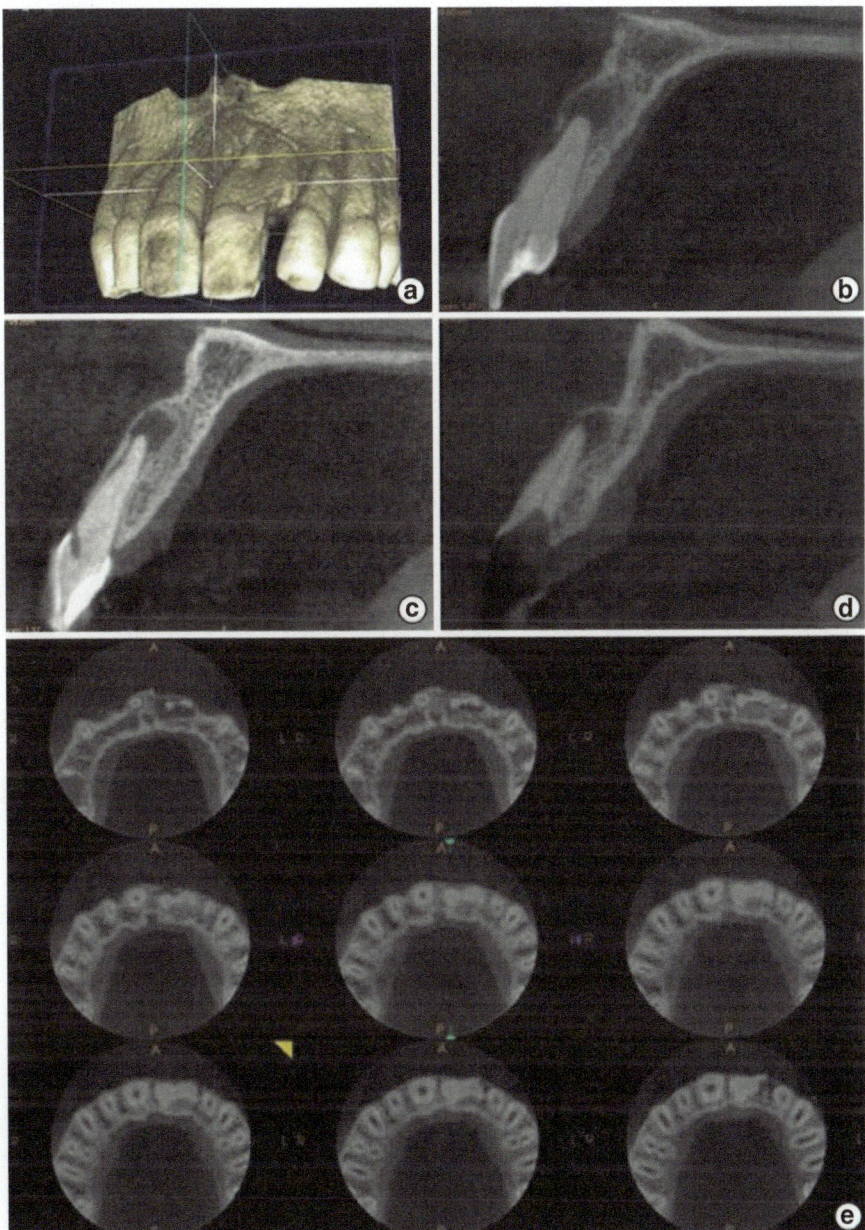

Fig. 2.11 (**a**) Reconstruction of CBCT images shows the presence of extra root fused with the root of the tooth #21. (**b**) Periapical lesion of tooth #21. (**c**) Perforation area extended to labial surface. (**d**) Presence of canal in supernumerary root. (**e**) Axial sections of CBCT images showing unusual root anatomy of tooth #21 from cervical area to apical area of the tooth. (Courtesy: Badole GP, Shenoi PR, Parlikar A. *Restor Dent Endod*. 2018;43(4): e44. Published 2018 Oct 26. doi: https://doi.org/10.5395/rde.2018.43.e44)

Recommendation 12: Limited FOV CBCT is the imaging modality of choice in the localization and differentiation of external and internal resorptive defects and the determination of appropriate treatment and prognosis (28, 29).

Recommendation 13: In the absence of clinical signs or symptoms, intraoral radiographs should be considered the imaging modality of choice for the evaluation of healing following nonsurgical and surgical endodontic treatment.

Recommendation 14: In the absence of signs and symptoms, if limited FOV CBCT was the imaging modality of choice at the time of evaluation and treatment, it may be the modality of choice for follow-up evaluation. In the presence of signs and symptoms, refer to Recommendation 7.

Based on these recommendations, CBCT can be used in endodontic diagnosis, treatment, and posttreatment phases. Following are few examples of use of CBCT in endodontics. These recommendations and various guidelines can be summarized as below:

- CBCT is a new and emerging technology that has the potential for use and application in a variety of clinical tasks, both diagnostic and prognostic.
- 2D radiography or plain radiography is the first choice of imaging in many clinical scenarios, and CBCT should be used when 2D imaging alone cannot answer the question on hand. When using CBCT, published criteria should be used for selection of the appropriate FOV.
- A thorough clinical examination must precede the use of CBCT, as is the case with any other radiation-based examination. CBCT is a higher X-ray dose modality, and hence, caution should be exercised while selecting the FOV to be scanned.
- For endodontic purpose, always small field of view CBCT should be opted. If possible, depending upon the CBCT device, image should be recorded in high-definition mode for better visualization of canals. Open mouth CBCT are advised for guided treatments for better evaluation of anatomy and avoid any superimpositions. Bite plate or cotton roles can be used for this purpose.
- Clinicians who own and operate CBCT machines need to have sufficient training about best practices on how to operate their CBCT and the measures needed to acquire the best image quality scans, while at the same time lowering the radiation dose for their patients.
- The effective doses for dentoalveolar CBCT range from 11 to 674 μSv. The effective doses for craniofacial CBCT range from 30 to 1073 μSv. Clinicians are encouraged to provide adequate training for their staff; maintain proper imaging, radiation shielding, radiation records; and detect problems early on to make sure that their patients receive the best care in their practice (ALARA [As Low As Reasonably Achievable]).

References

1. Beckmann EC. CT scanning the early days. Br J Radiol. 2006;79(937):5–8.
2. Mozzo P, Procacci C, Tacconi A, Martini PT, Andreis IA. A new volumetric CT machine for dental imaging based on the cone-beam technique: preliminary results. Eur Radiol. 1998;8:1558–64.
3. Feldkamp LA, Davis LC, Kress JW. Practical cone beam algorithm. J Opt Soc Am. 1994;1:612–9.
4. Scarfe WC, Farman AG. What is cone-beam CT and how does it work? Dent Clin N Am. 2008;52(4):707–30.
5. Nasseh I, Al-Rawi W. Cone beam computed tomography. Dent Clin N Am. 2018;62:361–91.
6. Abramovitch K, Rice DD. Basic principles of cone beam computed tomography. Dent Clin N Am. 2014;58(3):463–84.
7. Pauwels R, Araki K, Siewerdsen JH, et al. Technical aspects of dental CBCT: state of the art. Dentomaxillofac Radiol. 2015;44(1):20140224.
8. Kopp S, Ottl P. Dimensional stability in composite cone beam computed tomography. Dentomaxillofac Radiol. 2010;39:512–6.
9. Demirturk Kocasarac H, Helvacioglu Yigit D, Bechara B, et al. Contrast-to-noise ratio with different settings in a CBCT machine in presence of different root-end filling materials: an in vitro study. Dentomaxillofac Radiol. 2016;45(5):20160012.
10. Schulze RKW, Berndt D, d'Hoedt B. On cone-beam computed tomography artifacts induced by titanium implants. Clin Oral Implants Res. 2010;21:100–7.
11. Pauwels R, Stamatakis H, Bosmans H, et al. The SEDENTEXCT Project Consortium. Quantification of metal artifacts on cone beam computed tomography images. Clin Oral Implants Res. 2013;24(Suppl. A100):94–9.

Digital Impression Systems, CAD/CAM, and STL file

3

Bálint Vecsei, Alexandra Czigola, Ivett Róth, Peter Hermann, and Judit Borbély

3.1   Introduction

For successful oral therapy with the use of digital dentistry, it is necessary to have accurate virtual images [1]. Failures can arise if the scanned images are not accurate enough. Sufficient accuracy, in this context, means clinically acceptable accuracy. This, of course, can be different in each segment of dentistry. Facial tissue scanning accuracy ranges between 140 and 1330 μm, which is acceptable for a smile design project. When reconstructing the dataset of a cone-beam computer tomography (CBCT) scan, jawbone scanning accuracy will be around 100–700 μm. This deviation range is a bit wider than that achievable by CT, which can be as low as 100 μm but comes at a much higher radiation dose cost to the patient. Navigated implant placement seems to work appropriately within CBCT's deviation range. Intraoral optical impression accuracy ranges between 16 and 378 μm, but its trueness and precision highly depend on scanning strategy, scanning technology, scanned area size, and actual clinical situation [1–4]. Extraoral laboratory scanners work within a range of 20–55 μm; their accuracy depends not as much on the specific technology (whether it is a laser or a structured light scanner) as on certain dental parameters such as the shape and margin ends of the scanned abutment [5]. The clinically acceptable range for the marginal discrepancy of a crown ranges extensively between 30 and 140 μm based on different reports. The clinically acceptable level in most studies is ≤120 μm [6]. In digital dental treatment, accurate and precise work should aim to be close to 50 μm, which can be easily achieved with modern equipment.

Guided endodontics needs a highly accurate guiding sleeve position with an optimum approach angle for minimally invasive access cavity preparation or for microsurgical endodontic access to reduce the risk of damaging critical anatomical

B. Vecsei (✉) · A. Czigola · I. Róth · P. Hermann · J. Borbély
Department of Prosthodontics, Semmelweis University, Budapest, Hungary

© Springer Nature Switzerland AG 2021
N. Kinariwala, L. Samaranayake (eds.), *Guided Endodontics*,
https://doi.org/10.1007/978-3-030-55281-7_3

structures [7, 8]. A preoperative CBCT might be necessary in exceptional cases such as complicated endodontic anatomy, root resorption, or pulp canal calcification, even if this means a higher radiation dose for the patient. From the CBCT dataset (DICOM), it is possible to export the three-dimensional data as an STL file. These data can be combined with an STL generated using an intraoral digital impression system. With these three-dimensional data and adequate software, the dentist can design the treatment and fabricate a guide for better visualization and access during the operation [9].

3.2   Direct and Indirect CAD/CAM Approaches

Dental CAD/CAM systems consist of various hardware and software used for data acquisition as well as restoration design and manufacture. They serve three main functions: (1) three-dimensional digitization and generation of a digital data set; (2) a design manipulation process for generating the manufacturing data set; and (3) fabrication of dental restoration by a digitally controlled system [10].

The first step, acquisition from the oral cavity, can be done with one of two methods: direct and indirect scanning. Both use scanners, but different types for different purposes. A scanner is a digitizing tool to register the structural characteristics of the scanned object. If the object is a tooth or an implant, with the surrounding tissues in the oral cavity, we use direct intraoral scanners for acquisition. To digitize stone casts, molds, or dental impressions, we use extraoral laboratory/desktop scanners. As the latter do not capture information directly from the oral cavity, we use the term indirect data acquisition (Fig. 3.1).

Digital impression systems evolve quite remarkably. In recent years, many new intraoral scanners have been developed. Existing, well-functioning, accurate devices are continually being improved. With these devices, we can adapt to the challenges of modern times—faster, more precise, more productive work is possible.

3.3   Evolution of CAD/CAM and Digital Impression Systems

The history of digital impressions goes back to 1973. More than 50 years ago, Francois Duret took from the idea of a digital revolution that had already been a few decades long in the industry and wrote his thesis on digital impressions. The process, which was still a theory, was introduced officially in 1984 on a patient [11]. The essence of the procedure was that a unique device generated a signal from the oral cavity for the computer. After that, he was able to plan the crown for the abutment, which he was able to create with a computer numerical control (CNC) freezer attached to the machine—chairside same-day dentistry. This was the start of involving CAD/CAM in dentistry.

The term "CAD/CAM" is an acronym for computer-aided design (CAD) and computer-aided manufacturing. At first, CAD/CAM was used in aircraft and

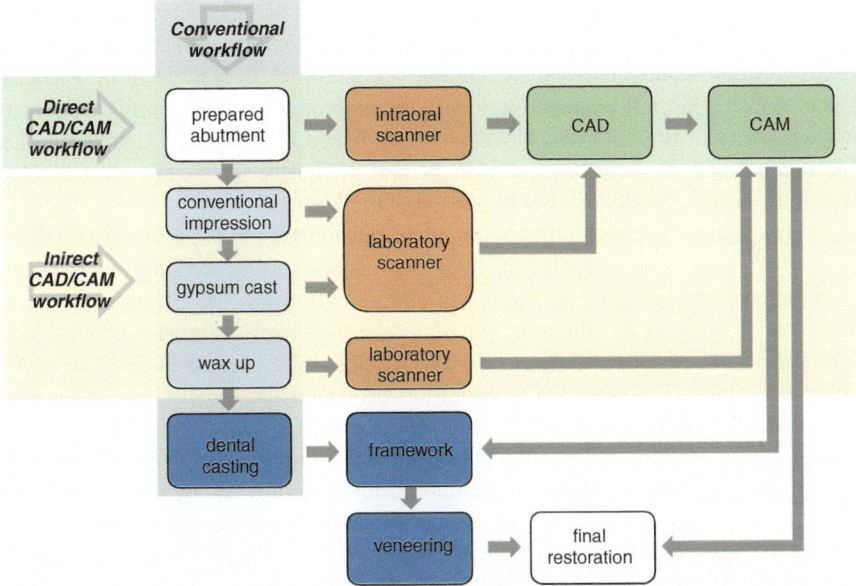

Fig. 3.1 Flowchart of the direct and indirect CAD/CAM workflow compared to the conventional workflow of processing a restoration. Orange shows the digitizing procedures

automotive industries; it was developed in the 1960s. The first application in dentistry was a decade later in 1971 [11, 12]. Dr. Francois Duret was the first person who wrote the basic principles of CAD/CAM technology. He graduated in 1971 from Claude Bernard University (Lyon, France) and Optical Impressions (Empreinte Optique) was the title of his thesis. Dr Duret created his first CAD/CAM restoration in 1983 and demonstrated his own system in 1985 at the France Dental Association's international congress when he created a posterior crown for his wife. The first CAD/CAM device (which was developed and built by Dr Duret) was patented in 1984 and named Sopha System. That was the first and most important milestone in the history of CAD/CAM technology. In 1989 at the Midwinter Meeting, Dr Duret made a crown in 4 h on the stage. The impression was made by an optical scanner and final restoration was designed on a computer screen and milled from a ceramic block with a numerically controlled milling machine [13]. The following thought is how Dr Edward McLaren remembered that historical moment.

> The room was filled with tension and excitement as the lights were slowly dimmed in the auditorium. The next 2 hours offered a glimpse of the future of dentistry. The topic was something out of a science-fiction novel, and it instilled in the audience a sense of awe, wonder, and just a touch of fear. As the auditorium lights came up, everyone sat in stunned silence as they contemplated all the possibilities offered by the presenter: dentistry going digital. [14]

Dr Duret's system was not spread commonly, but other studies were inspired by it. In parallel with his discovery, Mörmann also created a chairside CAD/CAM system—but focused on inlay cavities [15]. Dr Werner Mörmann from Switzerland and his electrical engineer Dr Marco Brandestini developed the first chairside CAD/CAM system named CEREC (Chairside Economical Restorations of Esthetic Ceramic). Dr Marco Brandestini was working on blood flow ultrasound scanners at his laboratory in Bothell (WA, USA) when his friend Dr Mörmann visited him. Dr Mörmann asked an interesting question: "could cavities be scanned by ultrasound?" Dr Brandestini was skeptical but he started to think about his friend's idea. Then he said: "It doesn't work with ultrasound; the wavelength is too large. It must be done optically." After this conversation, their interest was awakened, and they started working on a new project together. It was a long journey to develop the triangulation approach; nowadays, it is the principle of operation of many intraoral scanners. The first generation of CEREC (Siemens Corporation) was created in 1987 to make chairside inlays. The Siemens Corporation produced the CEREC 2 software in 1994, which enabled the user to create full crowns. CEREC 3 was developed by Sirona Dental System in 1999. According to the manufacturer's recommendation, inlays, onlays, crowns, and even three-unit bridges can be made by third-generation CEREC. Nowadays, CEREC 3 is the most common chairside system in the world (Fig. 3.2). The first CEREC chairside treatment was on 19 September 1985 at the University of Zurich when Dr Mörmann and Dr Brandestini created an inlay from a Vita Mark I feldspathic ceramic (Vita Zahnfabrik) block [16].

At the beginning of the 1980s, Dr Matts Andersson from Sweden also researched CAD/CAM technology. Due to a drastic increase in gold prices, nickel-chromium alloys were used commonly in dentistry. However, metal allergy became a problem, and an alternative material had to be used for dental frameworks: it was titanium. Precision casting of titanium alloy was difficult; Dr Andersson fabricated titanium copings by spark erosion and fused them with composite. Later, Dr Andersson developed the Procera system, which is a centralized milling center networked with numerous laboratory digitizers around the world for the fabrication of CAD/CAM restorations. Such networked production systems were adapted by a number of companies worldwide [15].

Fig. 3.2 Chairside fabricated onlay processed by the CEREC system

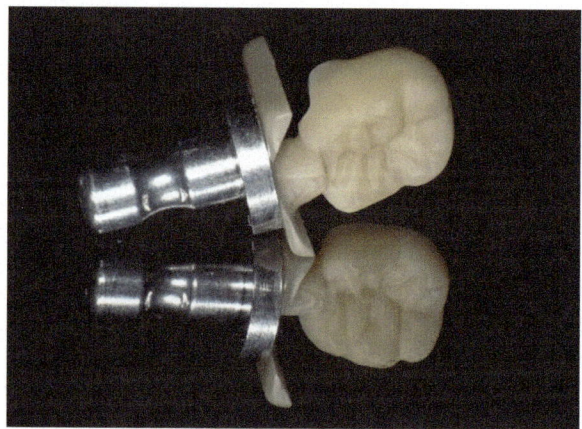

At first, the innovations of CAD/CAM technology were limited to the laboratory, but with the appearance of intraoral scanners, dentists became involved in the digital workflow. The first laboratory-connected intraoral scanner was developed in 2007 by Align Technology (San Jose, CA) and named the iTero Element intraoral scanner. The second was the Lava Chairside Intraoral Scanner (3M ESPE), which was demonstrated in February 2008 at the Midwinter Meeting [17].

Nowadays, we have scanners that provide wireless, real, colorful scans with HD quality images and can send much more practical and useful information to the dental laboratory, and much faster, than traditional impressions. Several intraoral scanning devices exist, and more software innovations have been recently presented at the International Dental Show 2019 in Cologne, Germany, and this tendency seems to be growing continuously.

Early CAD/CAM workflow permitted the creation of inlays, onlays, crowns, and short bridges. Lately, CAD/CAM systems have been able to make fixed partial dentures, implant abutments, removable partial dentures, and complete dentures. In dentistry, using computer-aided design and computer-aided manufacturing systems has become increasingly popular. More than 30,000 dentists worldwide have their own intraoral scanner and CNC milling machines; about a third, more than 10,000, of these are in the United States and Canada [12]. Nowadays, more than 20% of practices in the United States use digital imaging devices. However, of German laboratories, 75% use extraoral scanners, with only 15–20% of dentists using intraoral scanners, but their number is continuously rising. The number of newly installed intraoral scanners was more than 500 in Germany and almost 400 in France. More than 1140 devices were sold in Europe in 2017 [18]. In October 2009, Dr Christensen mentioned that digital impression taking would be leading dentistry in a few years. Although he was wrong with the timing of that spread, several recently presented intraoral scanners confirm the expansion of digital technology in dentistry. As more and more laboratory and dental offices invest in new systems, the price of new devices will decrease [19, 20].

3.4   STL File Extension

The STL file is a data file format for computers containing information of an object's geometry by describing it with connected triangles. The triangles' density depends on the initial resolution and mathematical algorithms.

The STL extension is a hard-disk data file for a computer. The acronym's origins are explained in several ways: standard tessellation language, standard triangle language, and stereolithography are all terms in use. Tessellation means to fragment the surface into smaller shapes to make it realizable and countable with computers. Possibly, the term standard triangle language describes most of the essence of the extension: a description of the geometry of a spatial object with related triangles. The number of triangles and their density depends mainly on the resolution and the mathematical algorithm that was used to create the data.

Therefore, the STL file is a commonly used format that translates the morphology of the surface and shape of three-dimensional objects into data interpretable by computers. In digital workflows, STL files that represent oral structures are available from multiple sources. The easiest and quickest way to create STL data of a jaw is to use an intraoral scanner. In an indirect CAD/CAM procedure, we can obtain STL data by digitizing the gypsum model based on conventional silicon impression using a laboratory scanner. At the same time, the DICOM data file of the more commonly used CBCT recordings can also generate the desired STL data. If STL files from the same case come from multiple sources, they can be aligned together with superimposition, and used for modeling or manufacturing numerous modern design processes and tools for more precise and less invasive treatment. These benefits are used by navigated implantology as well as guided endodontics.

The mathematical algorithm, which digitizes the surface, is a crucial point when creating the STL file. In digitization procedures, there is a mathematical conversion of the surface points measured by the device (matching, filtering, smoothing, weighing, and selective removal) [10]. The measured points in space (vertices, vertex) are not enough on their own to model the surface. It is also necessary to know the lines (edge) that connect these points. These edges define a surface. This surface is called a face, which is a flat surface surrounded by three edges (edge, straight) that connect a minimum of three vertices. That is, the polygon itself. The polygon can be a simple convex polygon, like a quadrilateral, but in dentistry, we usually deal with triangular polygons. These simple polygons can be easily manipulated and calculated by computer. The spatial body constructed from these polygons is known as the 3D digital data of a polyhedron and is referred to as the mesh. The mesh is a polyhedron-based set of 3D digital data consisting of points, edges, and (triangle) faces (Fig. 3.3).

The variation of the polygons basically determines the accuracy of the mesh. The density of the triangle polygons (resolution), the level of triangle regularity (tessellation), and the topography of the triangles (height variations) determine how well they approximate the actual surface of the spatial object [21]. The density of vertex points fundamentally determines the accuracy of the obtained point cloud [22].

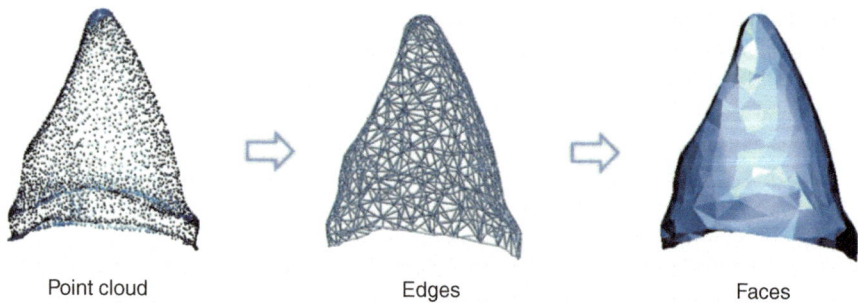

Point cloud   Edges   Faces

Fig. 3.3 Building tiles of the mesh: point cloud from vertices; edges, which connect the points; they determine the faces, which then represent the surface of the digitalized object

Mesh quality can vary across different areas of the virtual object. Sharp boundaries, precise designs can only be described with a large number of triangles, while average or quick mesh is sufficient for smooth surfaces. This allows optimizing the trade-off between quality and calculation time [23].

3.5   Digital Workflow

CAD/CAM means a digital workflow with scanning, designing, and milling as its phases. The scanning device converts the shape of the prepared teeth into three-dimensional units of information (voxels). The computer translates this information into a three-dimensional map (point cloud). The operator designs a restoration shape on computer interface. A cutting path is then generated for milling tools to create the restoration from a block of material [24, 25].

CAD/CAM technology was developed to make esthetic, tooth-colored, and strong restorations with an easier, faster, and more accurate production method. Dentists and laboratories have a wide variety of ways in which they can work with CAD/CAM technology [12]. Based on where the production is done, dental CAD/CAM systems provide chairside production with in-office milling for same-day dentistry, laboratory production with the dental laboratory milling the restorations, or centralized fabrication in a production center [26].

Based on the scanning method, CAD/CAM systems can be divided into direct or indirect systems. Indirect CAD/CAM workflow is based on scanning the gypsum cast made from conventional impression; indirect systems work with laboratory scanners. Direct CAD/CAM workflow starts with scanning the prepared teeth directly with intraoral scanners. Digital impression systems focus on the imaging process and rely on dental laboratories to complete the design and fabrication procedure, while chairside systems focus on integrating all three processes, that is, intraoral scanning, design, and milling, right in the dental office [27].

3.5.1   Digital Workflow with Indirect CAD/CAM Impression Systems

Indirect CAD/CAM methods are based on scanning the stone model made from conventional impressions with an extraoral (laboratory) scanner. The digital workflow starts with a PVS (polyvinylsiloxane) impression of prepared teeth; a sectioned gypsum model is then made, and a laboratory scanner creates a 3-dimensional set of points on the spatial information of the dies and the whole arch. Thus, the resulting virtual cast is a realistic digital model of patient's oral cavity. Design is done on computer screen using CAD software. Dental technicians can design frameworks/substructures or full-contour restorations. Finally, the virtual wax-up is processed by a milling machine. Following the milling process, substructures need to be veneered, and full-contour restorations stained and glazed. There are also systems where a complete conventional wax-up is made and then digitized to create a digital-wax pattern followed by automatic processing [15]. Applying CAM, the restorations are milled from solid blocks with dental milling CNC machines. Spurred on by Dr. Duret's developments, research and innovation has been actively ongoing to fabricate crowns and FPDs, matching the anatomical shape of the occlusal surface using CAD/CAM technologies [15]. At the beginning, only simple shapes of substructures could be milled, but as technology improved and machines became better, all complicated shapes of occlusal configurations are achievable.

The disadvantage of indirect impression systems is that they are highly dependent on impression and model material quality and processing methods; related issues include volumetric changes, distortions, and abrasion or fracture of the models.

3.5.1.1 Extraoral Scanners

Laboratory scanners are used to digitize cast models made from conventional impressions. Extraoral laboratory scanners are either tactile or optical. Tactile scanners, also known as contact scanners, capture surface details through mechanical contact between a detection unit and object to be scanned. Optical scanners, also known as noncontact scanners, capture 3D images using laser or structured light technologies [5, 28].

Contact scanners are highly accurate but very slow, because there is a need for mechanical contact between a moving probe and the entire surface of a model. Although they are rarely used for lab practice these days, they are still needed for some special indications in implants [29].

Optical scanners use some type of electromagnetic wave, typically light, to detect the surface details of the model. These scanners are very fast, but surface characteristics can affect the emitted light. Very bright surfaces and refraction from translucent surfaces can alter the measurement. There are different extraoral noncontact scanners: structured light scanners, laser light scanners, and confocal microscopy scanners [29]. Structured light scanners project a narrow band of light on a three-dimensional surface that produces a line of illumination that is distorted if viewed from a perspective other than that of the projector. Structured light scanners use that information to geometrically reconstruct the surfaces of a model [5].

Laser light scanners work by projecting a point of light or line of laser on the object and register its position with a set of cameras to triangulate the three-dimensional position of the point [30]. Confocal microscopy scanners are a subtype of structured light scanners or laser scanners. They are based on an optical technique used to increase the resolution and contrast by using a very small spatial pinhole lighting spot to eliminate out-of-focus light [29].

3.5.2   Digital Workflow with Direct CAD/CAM Impression Systems

Direct impression means taking an intraoral digital impression directly of the prepared and unprepared teeth by an intraoral scanner. Intraoral scanners create a

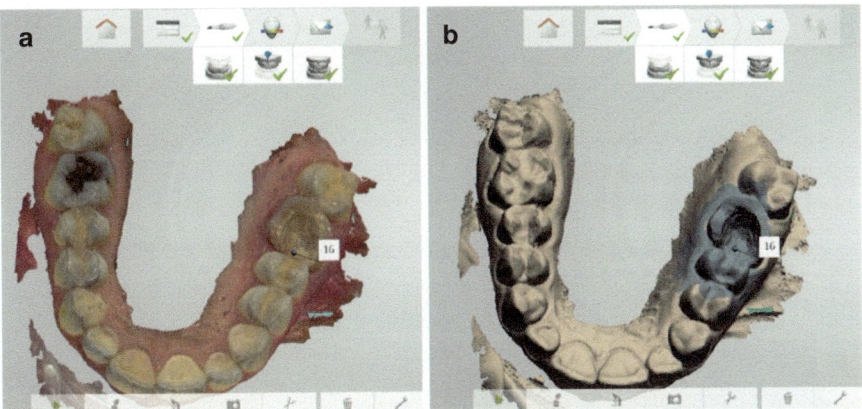

Fig. 3.4 (**a**) Intraoral scan of a patient's upper arch with the prepared onlay cavity, (**b**) the digital replica of the patient's dentition rendered on a computer screen. High-resolution scan images were added to the virtual cast to create a high-quality digital impression of the preparation margin

digital replica of the patient's dentition on computer screen (Fig. 3.4). The scan can be analyzed when magnified and additional scans may be added for perfection. After verification, the digital file is imported into a CAD software program to virtually design either a coping, a substructure, or full-contour restoration. Restorations are milled, and in case of a coping or substructure, a model may be printed to apply veneering ceramics. In case of full-contour restoration, non-model-based work is also possible [31].

3.5.2.1 Intraoral Scanners (IOS)

Intraoral scanners are intraoral digital devices for capturing direct optical impressions of the prepared teeth and oral cavity [32–34]. They are gaining popularity and improve rapidly. Older systems required powdering the scanning surface and were quite complicated to use. Newer powderless, wet scanning systems, which can also reach the posterior regions, are more convenient for scanning [35]. Initially, only quadrant scans were technically possible to digitize; nowadays, full arch scans are also available [36, 37].

Intraoral scanners are based on various data capture principles such as confocal laser technology, confocal microscopy, triangulation, wavefront sampling, multi-scan imaging, stereophotogrammetric video, and accordion fringe interferometry [17, 33]. A light source (laser or structured light) is projected onto the dental arch, prepared teeth, and implant scan bodies (i.e., cylinders screwed on the implants and used for transferring the 3D implant position to be scanned) [33, 34] (Fig. 3.5). The images of dentogingival tissues captured by imaging sensors are processed by the scanning software, which generates point clouds [34, 38]. These point clouds are then triangulated by the same software, creating a 3D surface model (mesh) [34, 38]. The 3D surface models of dentogingival tissues are the result of the optical impression and are the "virtual" alternative to traditional plaster models [38, 39]. In

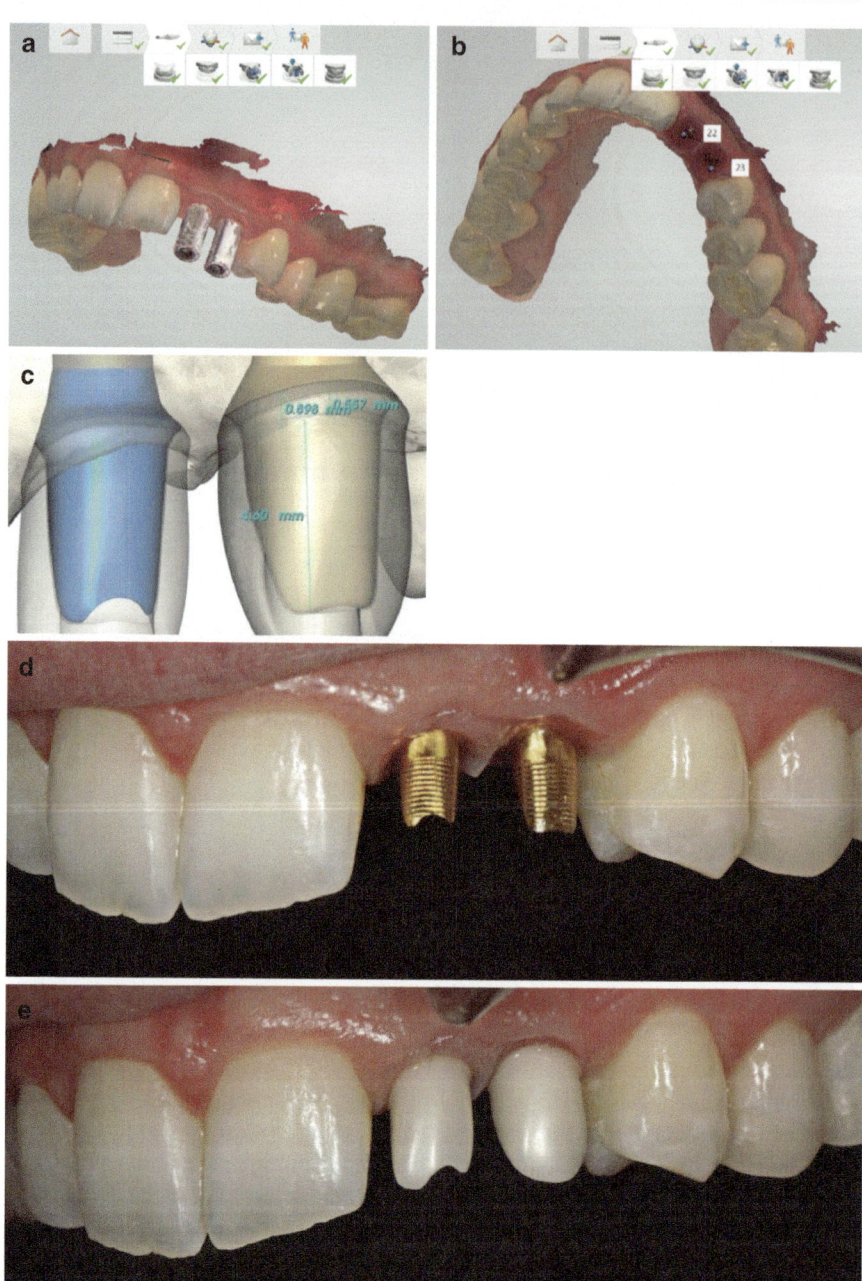

Fig. 3.5 (**a**–**e**) Digital impression (TRIOS, 3Shape) with the implant scan bodies and the emergence profile scan transform the 3-dimensional implant position and the supraimplant mucosa outline into the three-dimensional data set to design an individualized titanium nitride-coated implant abutment and a ZrO$_2$ substructure of cut-back crown. (Atlantis abutments, Dentsply Sirona)

particular, from the genesis of a "cloud of points," a polygonal mesh is derived, representing the scanned object; the scan is further processed to obtain the final 3D model [17, 32].

It is important to take digital impressions according to the manufacturer's instructions. Traditional principles of impression taking procedure also apply for intraoral scanning: soft tissue control and isolation remain basic principles. Intraoral scanners are time-efficient, simplify clinical procedures for the dentist, and eliminate plaster models. Intraoral scanning systems allow better communication with the dental technician and with patients [40]. Digital impressions are not susceptible to changes in accuracy once they are recorded and electronic transmission of the files to dental laboratories is completed efficiently with no loss of accuracy [27]. Disadvantages are that with IOS, it can be difficult to detect deep margin lines in prepared teeth, especially in case of bleeding; there is a learning curve; there are purchasing and managing costs [33, 40]. The current IOS are sufficiently accurate for capturing impressions for fabricating inlays/onlays, copings, frameworks, or full-contour restorations, single crowns and fixed partial denture on both natural teeth and implants; in addition, they can be used for smile design, and to fabricate posts and cores, removable partial prostheses, splints, obturators, and orthodontic aligners [33, 40].

The next step following the digital impression taking procedure is to evaluate the quality of the virtual cast. Inaccuracies can be eliminated by the dentist directly chairside within this step. Occlusal and axial reduction, insertion direction can be monitored on computer screen with built-in software tools. Margin line can also be checked enlarged by the software. Any imperfections of the virtual cast can be corrected without the need to retake the entire impression. Additional images of the areas of interest can be added to a previous scan. When satisfied with the impression and resulting virtual cast, it is sent to the laboratory along with the digital worksheet via e-mail.

There are open and closed dental CAD/CAM systems. Closed systems' files can be opened by the manufacturer's CAD software only. Most intraoral scanners work with open systems and are compatible with several types of CAD software and milling machines (3Shape TRIOS, Planmeca Planscan, CEREC Omnicam, iTero Element, Carestream CS 3500, 3M True Definition, GC AADVA, DWIO Dentalwings, KaVo Lythos, Dentium Rainbow, Zfx Intrascan, MFI Condor IOS, etc.) [33].

3.5.2.2 Labside System
Labside CAD/CAM workflow of direct impression systems means that data from the intraoral scanner are sent to the dental laboratory for the dental technician to process. The technician designs the restoration with CAD software in lab. The technician outlines the preparation margin, insertion direction, and sets the cementation gap. Several automatic functions are built in the software, but there is also a great variety of tools to individualize the design. After designing the framework or the full-contour restoration, the right colored block of material needs to be selected for the milling. The main purpose for which most laboratories to use CAD/CAM is to

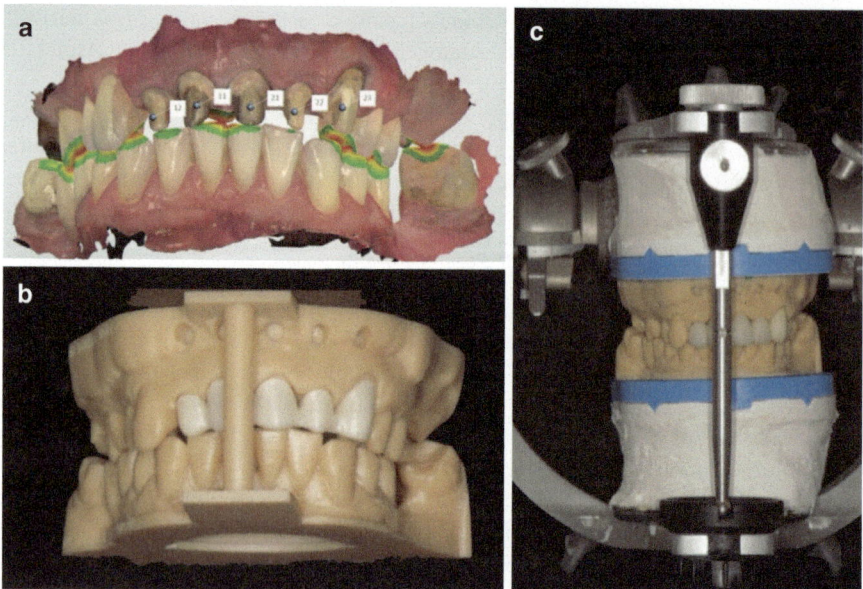

Fig. 3.6 (**a–c**) Zirconium-dioxide substructure of a 5-unit fixed partial denture created by labside CAD/CAM workflow in a direct impression system (3Shape, TRIOS). The data from the intraoral scanner were sent to the dental laboratory to design the restoration with CAD software and to mill a zirconium-dioxide substructure. Based on the digital data, the lab technician designed the model for 3D printing. Veneering of zirconium-dioxide substructure was done on this model

create zirconium-dioxide restorations. CAD/CAM technology is able to adjust precisely for zirconia shrinkage caused by sintering [12]. Based on the digital data, the lab technician designs the model for 3D printing. Veneering or zirconium-dioxide frameworks are done on this model (Fig. 3.6). Monolithic zirconia restorations can also be produced; they eliminate the problems of porcelain chipping. CAD/CAM systems offer long-time temporary restorations made of resin materials. There is also the possibility of copying provisionals. Centralized fabrication in a production center offers the option for laboratories to process CAD/CAM restorations of technique-sensitive materials like high strength ceramics and titanium. Dental technicians of local laboratories can do the CAD design and send the data to a milling center.

With all types of CAD/CAM systems, there is a need for skilled dental technicians who know how to work with the computer, even though a dental technician still finishes each restoration by hand (Fig. 3.7). CAD/CAM technology does not eliminate the need for skilled dental laboratory technicians [12].

3.5.2.3 Chairside Systems

At first, intraoral scanners were developed for chairside solutions. Dr Mörmann succeeded in his efforts to develop a Chairside Economical Restoration of Esthetic Ceramics (CEREC®) system that would simply produce a ceramic inlay restoration

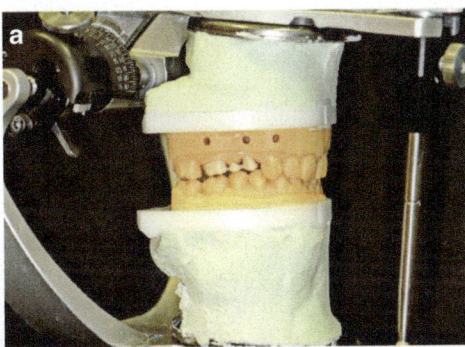

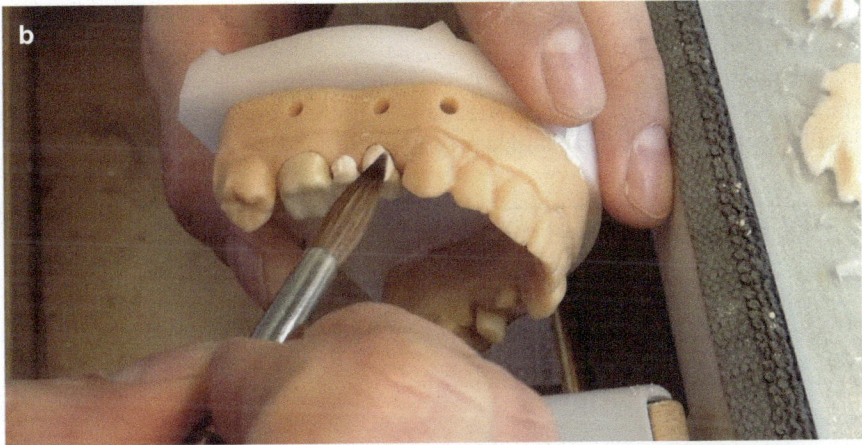

Fig. 3.7 (**a, b**) With all types of CAD/CAM systems, there is a need for skilled dental technicians. Dental technicians work with computers to design zirconium-dioxide frameworks and models for 3D printing, and then veneer the restoration by hand

at the dental chairside in a short time [15]. The main idea was to make esthetic ceramic restorations without the need for a dental laboratory, to make the procedure economic and offer Same Day Dentistry. A chairside system means that each step of the workflow is in the dental office. An intraoral scan is taken of the prepared tooth in the dental office and the designing of the restoration is done chairside. In-office dental CAD/CAM systems consist of a handheld scanner and a cart that houses a personal computer and a monitor. The intraoral scan data appear on the monitor as 3-dimensional (3-D) images. Design work is done on the monitor by the dentist, and data are sent over to the milling machine. Milling and finishing is done in the office. Inlays, onlays, solo crown monoblock restorations are milled with the CAM unit within a few hours from prefabricated blocks of ceramics. Final adjustments of staining, polishing, or sintering are done before cementation. Options include feldspathic, leucite, or lithium disilicate materials as well as blocks of composite [12]. Having a milling machine on site means that patients can receive their permanent restoration the same day they come in, without making a second appointment. There is no need for a temporary restoration [41].

The main difference between restorations milled by labside and chairside systems is the extension and the materials used. Chairside systems are made for solo restorations and short span bridges of the esthetic region; labside milling in dental laboratory or in milling centers offers a wide variety of extended restoration of high-strength materials.

3.6 Tooth Preparation Considerations

Dentists must understand how CAD/CAM systems work and have to adopt their preparation forms to milling technology to achieve exact fitting. Scannable tooth preparations are required with continuous chamfer margins. Sharp edges should be rounded, because they cannot be milled exactly. No irregularities of surface should be present; thinly extending edges are inadequate, because they might chip during milling. The diameter of the smallest grinder is 1 mm in most systems, so structures smaller than 1 mm cannot be milled precisely [26].

3.7 Computer-Aided Design (CAD)

As hardware and software systems improve, digital dentistry is more widely used by dentists and dental technicians [42]. Intraoral scans and CBCT images can be processed with specialized design software to virtually plan treatments and design prosthetic restorations [43].

3.7.1 Digital Smile Design

Predictable functional and esthetic results of dental treatments require a systematic approach for diagnosis, communication, and treatment planning. Digital smile design (DSD) is a conceptual tool that allows esthetic rehabilitative planning from a facial perspective, improving communication between specialists and increasing treatment predictability [44]. Esthetic analysis of the patient's facial and dental proportions is integrated in treatment planning. DSD as originally proposed by Coachman and Calamita is based on two-dimensional analysis of the patient's smile through intraoral and extraoral videos and photographs; however, as digital techniques improve, two-dimensional analysis is being replaced by three-dimensional smile analysis [43]. Digital smile design is a concept that requires learning, training, and understanding its fundamentals, objectives, and sequence [45, 46].

3.7.2 Design Software

Design software packages have different tools for designing and editing the 3D model of the final restorations [43]. Standard versions of design software are capable of designing crown or fixed partial denture frameworks, full-contour resto-rations, inlays, onlays, and common implant restorations. Indications and design capabilities can be widened with add-on modules. While many systems emphasize an indication spectrum that is as broad as possible, other manufacturers place emphasis on intuitive use and user-friendliness [26]. Digital technology improves fast; updates play an important role in keeping latest construction possibilities con-tinuously available to the users. The most commonly used data format with design software is the standard triangle language (STL) format. Many manufacturers, how-ever, use their own data formats specific to that particular manufacturer, with the result that data of various construction programs are not compatible with each other [26]. To keep the design process simple and fast, CAD software systems have sev-eral tools for design automation. CAD software can automatically detect the prepa-ration margins or the path of insertion (Fig. 3.8a, b). Depending on the material selected, the thickness of the final restoration can be verified [43]. For implant-supported prostheses, the CAD software can control the path of insertion across multiple implants and manage difficult screw access [43]. Most widely used dental CAD softwares include Dental System (3Shape, Copenhagen, Denmark), DentalCAD (Exocad, Germany), and inLab and CEREC (Dentsply-Sirona, Germany).

Fig. 3.8 (**a**, **b**) Design software packages have different tools for designing and editing 3D models of final restorations. To keep the design process simple and fast, CAD softwares have several automatic functions built in (detection of preparation margins, setting the path of insertion, etc.), but there is also a great variety of tools to individualize the design

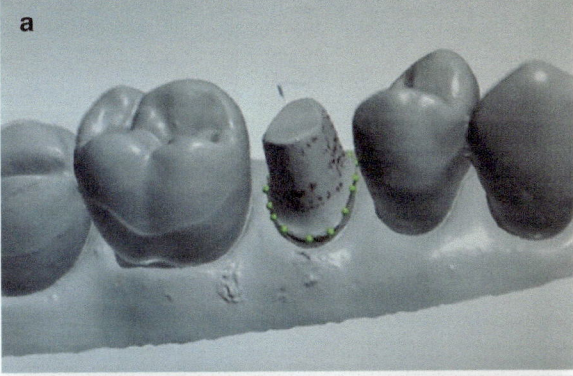

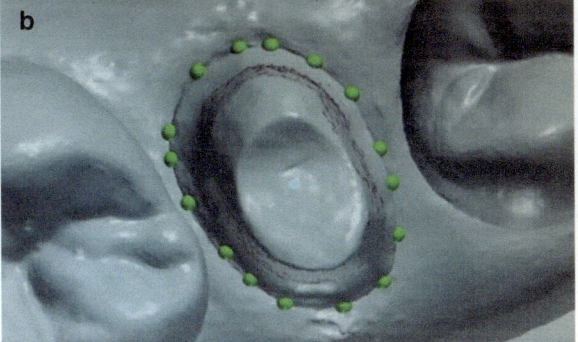

3.8   Computer-Aided Manufacturing (CAM)

Restorations designed by CAD software are fabricated by direct digital manufacturing devices. These devices can be divided into two main categories: subtractive and additive manufacturing technologies [47]. Subtractive manufacturing is the more common technology. This technique utilizes burs to mill the restoration (frameworks, copings, full-contour restorations) from a block of material. Cutting paths are generated by computer [48]. Production is based on conventional computer numerical control (CNC) milling (Fig. 3.9). Subtractive technologies are generally limited by geometric complexity and are not suitable for producing all shapes; additive manufacturing can fabricate far more complex organic forms [49]. Additive manufacturing technologies originate from the area of Rapid Prototyping (RP) adapted to the needs of dental technology. They generally slice the 3D model into

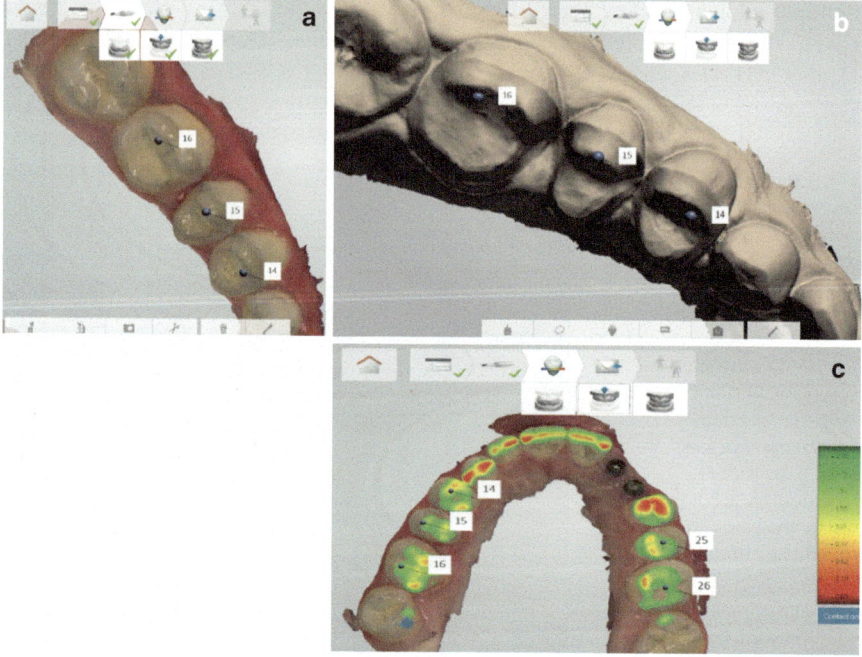

Fig. 3.9 (**a–c**) Intraoral scan was taken of premolar and molar teeth prepared for table tops (**a**); high-resolution scans were added to improve the quality of digital impression (**b**); color-scale helped to verify occlusal clearance (**c**). (**d–f**) Virtual articulation function of the CAD software adjusted the design of occlusal morphology (**d**). Subtractive manufacturing utilizes burs to mill the restoration from a block of material. Cutting paths are generated by computer. Production is based on computer numerical control (CNC) milling following CAD design; blocks of the right color were inserted in a milling machine (**e**); complicated shapes of occlusal configurations were achievable (**f**). (**g**) Adhesively cemented hybrid ceramic table-top restorations (Eanmic, Vita, Bad Sackingen) serve as natural tooth replacement

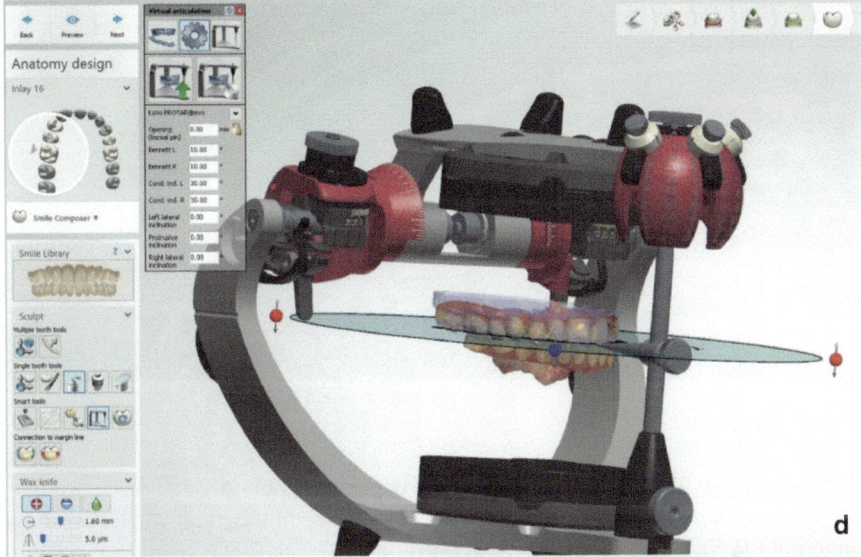

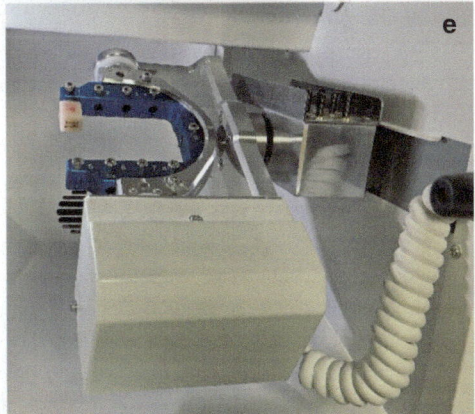

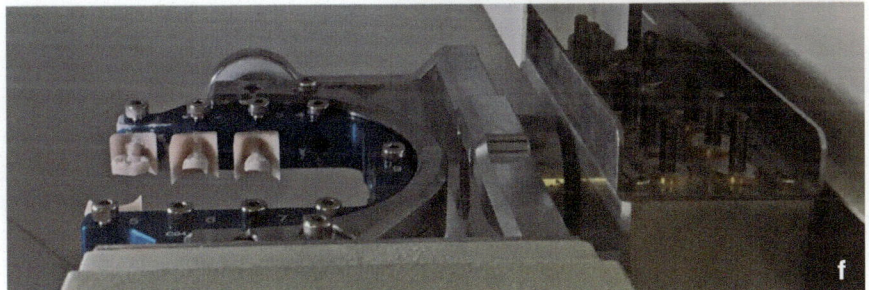

Fig. 3.9 (continued)

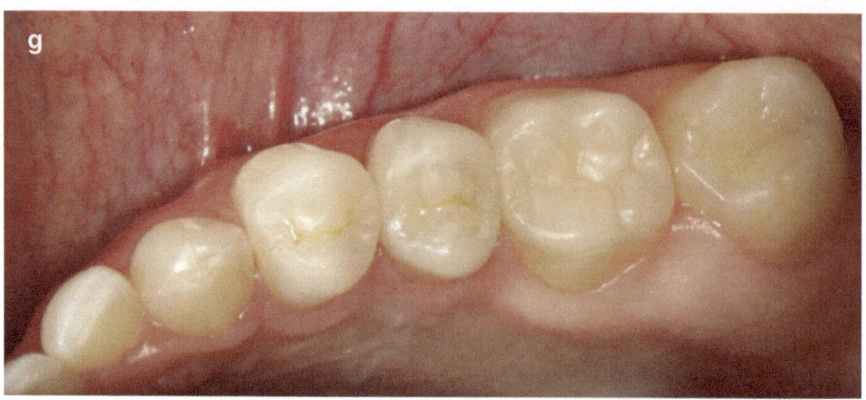

Fig. 3.9 (continued)

regular planes with instructions for material deposition, polymerization, or fusing in each plane. New additive technologies include: stereolithography, selective laser sintering (SLS), 3-D printing, fused deposition modeling (FDM), solid ground curing, and laminated object manufacturing (LOM) [48].

CNC milling systems have been the predominant approach; however, the advancement of additive technology will provide flexibility in design, fabrication, and economy [49].

3.9 Materials for CAD/CAM

Advances in CAD/CAM technology software and hardware have facilitated the development of new improved ceramic materials. Early generations of materials were monochromatic, but that was not the main problem associated with CAD/CAM restorations [42]. Restorations had poor marginal fit, anatomy and morphology, and a general lack of internal adaptation to the die because of low resolution scans, inadequate design software, and machining shortcomings. Technological advances in new systems and software development, coupled with specific clinical and laboratory techniques, have minimized or eliminated these problems so that marginal integrity and internal adaptation can be excellent [50]. The precision of fit that can be achieved with the assistance of CAD/CAM systems is reported to be 10–50 μm in the marginal area [51–54]. Under controlled industrial processing techniques, better-quality materials are produced with increased microstructural uniformity, higher density, lower porosity, and decreased residual stress. In the beginning, the labside system indication area was limited to mainly zirconium-dioxide framework design to replace metal casting. Chairside systems were limited to the molar region with inlay and onlay restorations. The introduction of multilayered translucent materials coupled with the possibility to mill sophisticated anatomy and morphology widened the indication area of CAD/CAM restorations.

There is a great variety of ceramic, metal, and resin materials to process with CAD/CAM technology. Zirconium-dioxide materials are widely used because of their strength, while glass ceramics are popular because of their esthetic properties. Individualized zirconia and titanium abutments are an important area of CAD/CAM production.

Glass ceramic materials offer excellent translucency but moderate strength. Adhesive cementation strengthens the material, increasing its flexural strength when the glass component is etched with hydrofluoric acid and adhesively bonded to the tooth [55]. The first esthetic ceramic blocks were made of feldspathic ceramic for in-office milling (Vitablocs Mark I (Vita, Bad Sackingen), later to be replaced by next-generation Vitablocs Mark II and CEREC Blocs). Early blocks were monochromatic. Later developments of multilayered, translucent blocks give even better esthetics mimicking the transition from dentin to enamel (Vitablocs Trilux, Reallife (Vita, Bad Sackingen)) (Fig. 3.10). Shade characterization and glazing can further improve the esthetic result [55]. The indication area covers solo restorations: inlays, onlays, and veneers.

Leucite-reinforced ceramic blocks have higher flexural strength than feldspathic ceramics because of the leucite crystal phase they contain (IPS Empress CAD, Ivoclar Vivadent, Paradigm C, 3M ESPE) (Fig. 3.11). Customization can be

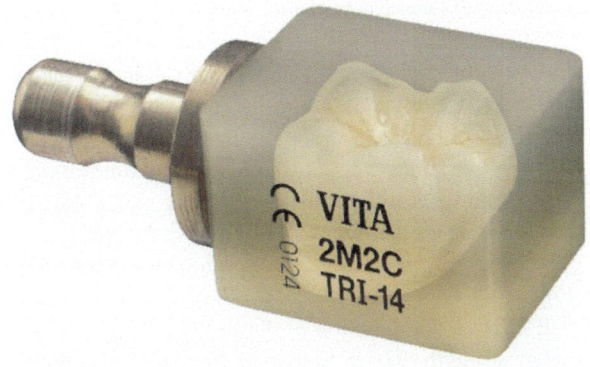

Fig. 3.10 Multilayered, translucent ceramic blocks give superior esthetics mimicking the transition from dentin to the enamel layer. Vita Trilux (Vita, Bad Sackingen) polychromatic, tooth-colored feldspathic ceramic blank with integrated shade gradient reproduces the natural play of colors

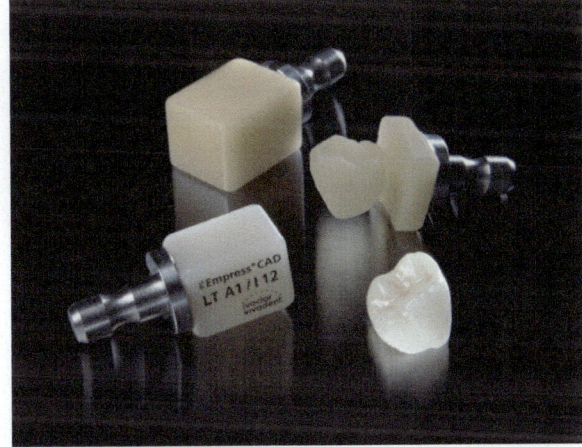

Fig. 3.11 IPS Empress CAD (Ivoclar Vivadent) leucite-reinforced ceramic blocks have higher flexural strength than feldspathic ceramics because of the leucite crystal phase. With homogeneity and light scattering behavior, they provide a balanced chameleon effect and true-to-nature translucency

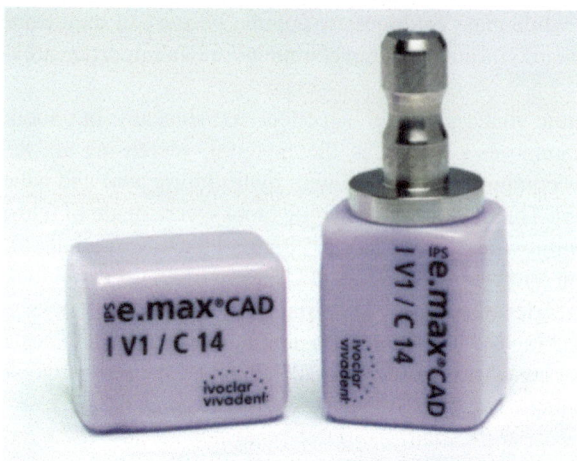

Fig. 3.12 IPS e.max CAD (Ivoclar Vivadent) lithium disilicate blocks are characterized by outstanding esthetics, exceptional light-optical properties, and great stability. They are manufactured as blue violet partially crystallized blocks that are easy to mill. A firing process is required to complete the crystallization of the restoration and to reach its final flexural strength and tooth color. A wide range of translucency levels, shades, and block sizes are available for various restorations

achieved through staining and glazing, and further strengthening achieved with bonding to tooth structure through adhesive cementation. They are commonly used for inlays, onlays, veneers, partial crowns, and crowns [56].

Lithium disilicate ceramics present 2–3 times the flexural strength of feldspathic glass ceramics. Lithium disilicate (IPS e.max CAD, Ivoclar Vivadent) was initially developed as a substructure material that offered greater translucency, and it gained popularity as monolithic restoration for chairside CAD/CAM systems [57] (Fig. 3.12).

It offers a combination of durability and beauty, as well as the ability to bond at higher strength. The CAD/CAM blocks are available in four translucency levels (high translucency, medium translucency, low translucency, medium opacity) and in different shades for each category [57]. It is manufactured in blue violet partially crystallized blocks that are easy to mill. A firing process is required to complete the crystallization of the restoration and to reach its final flexural strength and tooth color [57, 58]. The indication area covers inlays, onlays, veneers, partial crowns, single crowns, three-unit fixed partial dentures in the esthetic zone, and implant superstructures, as well as hybrid abutments and hybrid abutment crowns (Fig. 3.13).

Vita Suprinity is a recent glass ceramic material enriched with zirconia (approx. 10% by weight) that offers a high-strength, zirconia-reinforced lithium silicate ceramic (Fig. 3.14).

The list of various materials for processing by CAD/CAM devices depends on the respective production system. Dry milling devices are designed for the production of ZrO_2 substructures and resin materials, while wet milling covers the complete palette of materials from resins to glass ceramics and highly presintered ZrO_2

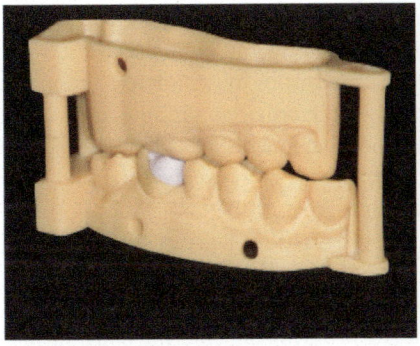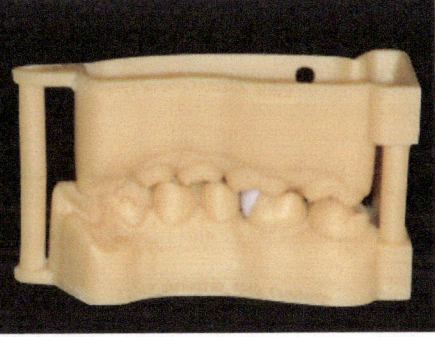

Fig. 3.13 IPS e.max CAD (Ivoclar Vivadent) lithium disilicate onlay on a 3D-printed model before sintering. Models help to check the occlusion, adjust the interproximal contact, and finish restorations; model-based work is also possible with inlays, onlays, or solo crowns

Fig. 3.14 (**a–c**) An individual crown was designed with buccal cut-back for esthetic veneering. Zirconia-reinforced lithium-silicate crown was milled in a pre-sintered phase. Accurate shade selection is the key to success. Outstanding esthetics were a achieved with veneering to mimic individual characteristics of adjacent natural teeth

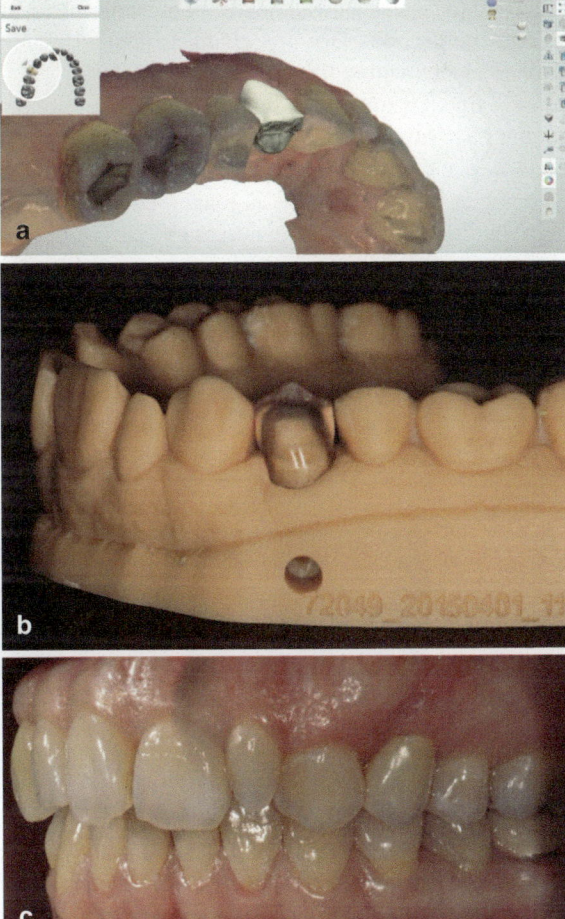

[26]. During a wet milling process, the milling diamond or carbide cutter is protected by a spray of cool liquid against overheating of the milled material.

Zirconium-dioxide restorations can be fabricated from fully sintered zirconium dioxide (HIP, hot isostatic pressed) or partially sintered zirconium dioxide blanks (white-stage). Zirconia blanks can be manufactured in green stage. Green blanks are pressed from ceramic powder and binding agents with no presintering. Blocks are soft as chalk with a low degree of stability and great problems in transport and application. At present, zirconium oxide is not processed as a green stage in any of the CAD/CAM systems on the market.

White stage means presintered blanks with adequate stability. A white body has already undergone shrinkage of approximately 5% during presintering and a shrinkage of some 20% (linear) is to be expected when milled restorations are sintered. Processing of white stage can be either with carbide metal grinders without water cooling or with diamond grinders with liquid cooling [51, 59]. The advantage of the method is a shorter milling time and reduced wear of the cutters, since the material is less rigid and hard. There is a minimal investment cost for the milling device. The disadvantage is that a lower degree of presintering results in higher shrinkage values for the frameworks. Dry processing is applied mainly with respect to zirconium dioxide blanks with a low degree of presintering [26]. Some systems also process densely sintered zirconium dioxide in a HIP condition with diamond tools and water cooling. There is no sinter shrinkage and sinter distortions. No sinter furnace is necessary, and no additional time is needed for a sintering procedure. The disadvantage is that the milling time is longer, cutters wear-off quickly, and devices with high rigidity and stability are necessary [26, 54, 60].

Zirconium-dioxide was first used as replacement for metal substructures. Material advancements led first to colored and later to translucent and multilayered materials. These improvements made monolithic zirconia popular. There is no chipping with monolithic zirconium-dioxide restorations, they have high flexural strength, and require minimum tooth preparation (Fig. 3.15). Monolithic zirconia crowns may be fabricated with as little as 0.5 mm of occlusal reduction [61]. The color of the restoration is homogeneous, and there is no need for concern about

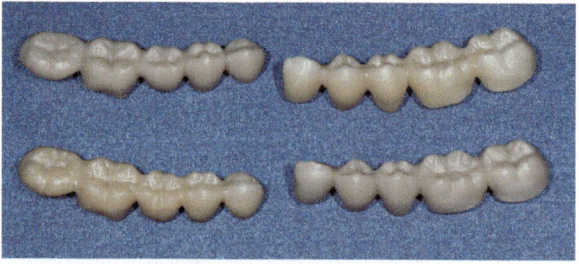

Fig. 3.15 Monolithic zirconium-dioxide fixed partial dentures milled from monochromatic and multilayered blocks. There is no chipping with monolithic zirconium-dioxide restorations; they have high flexural strength and require minimum tooth preparation. Multilayered, translucent blocks have made monolithic restorations popular

opaque show-through during adjustment of the occlusion. Polished surfaces are very important, because wear on the opposing dentition depends on surface characteristics. It is easy to polish the material using porcelain-polishing equipment. Monolithic zirconia is emerging as a promising option [62].

3.10   Extraoral Laboratory Scanners

The main advantage of CAD/CAM systems is that industrially fabricated materials produce advanced quality restorations through a consistent manufacturing process [5]. In the first two decades of the dental CAD/CAM workflow, extraoral laboratory scanners had a higher significance during the procedures. The dentist took conventional impressions and sent them to the laboratory where technicians made a cast from gypsum. This cast was scanned in the laboratory by an extraoral scanner.

Extraoral scanners are devices that can capture, transform, and process the information of an object's surface geometry to a digital interpretation. Most of them use some light source to obtain data of the casts or conventional PVS impressions. These are noncontact scanners.

Noncontact scanners have three main types based on image acquisition technology. There are laser light scanners, which project a point or a line of laser on the object and detect the reflected light with cameras. Based on triangulation, the computer calculates the projected point's distance and position in three-dimensional space. Another type of extraoral noncontact scanners uses structured light for optical three-dimensional shape measurement. The scanner projects a light pattern (lines or a mesh) on the object. In line with the shape of the scanned surface, the light pattern will be distorted—the detectors capture the image and the computer calculates the morphology of the object. These scanners use a particular color of light, and for best results, they are closed-case-type scanners to eliminate disturbances caused by ambient light [23, 29].

The third noncontact scanner group uses confocal microscopy. The required large optics and the stability of the scanned object allow these types to work properly in nonclinical situations. This imaging technique is grounded in the recognition of focused and defocused images from selected depths.

The scanners mainly capture a compilation of images in a second or record a length of video footage. The captured image or video determines the x and y coordinates of surface points, and the distance of the detector determines the z coordinate [23]. Thus, all recorded points can be identified in three-dimensional space.

Few scanners in dental laboratory use contact probes touching the object during the scanning procedure [29]. However, these are the most accurate devices: they can reach an accuracy of 1–2 μm and are mainly used in industrial environments rather than dental treatment. It is probably their time requirement and cost issues that make them less than ideal for dental treatment; furthermore, such high accuracy is unnecessary in dental practice as the clinically accepted range is more than 10 times greater than the accuracy of these scanners.

Some of the available extraoral laboratory scanners will be described below:

3.10.1 Straumann CARES Scan CS2

The Straumann CARES Scan CS2 is an in-lab scanner and is the central hardware component of the Straumann CARES CAD/CAM system. Accurate scans (which is the first step of the CAD/CAM workflow) are obtained using advanced 3D laser technology. Master models and sectioned models can also be scanned with Straumann CARES Scan CS2 in a short time (30 s for master models and 3 min for single dies). Calibration is not needed in the laboratory, because the laser technology is calibrated for a lifetime due to a fixed mounted optical measurement unit on a moveable plate.

This closed-case-type scanner is compatible with the Straumann CARES Visual software and the Straumann CARES milling process. The laboratory scanner works with ten moving axes for scanning models or dies and uses multiple scanning angles (from 35° to 75°). Maximum die height is 22.3 mm, maximum jaw height is 30 mm, and the measuring accuracy is 10 μm. The delivery package includes the scanner, computer box, monitor box, and accessory kit.

3.10.2 Identica Hybrid

Identica Hybrid is a laboratory scanner produced by Medit (Medit Company, Seoul, Korea). Identica Hybrid uses triple camera scanning technology, which helps to enhance the quality and accuracy of scan data and is capable of color scanning. It can scan gypsum casts or impressions at the same accuracy in both. Identica Hybrid has a 3-axis impression arm that helps automatically scan two sides of the impression. This is the autodouble impression scan mode, which allows scanning the impression in one step.

In the conventional method, the technician can only scan the upper and lower gypsum casts and dies separately. Identica Hybrid has a special method, which allows scanning the casts and dies together. The dental technician can scan a full model, multiple dies together, or up to eight dies separately. The full arch can be scanned within 16 s, 41 s are enough for scanning eight dies, and the processing time is 11 s. Using blue LED light scanning technology, Identica Hybrid can capture the highest-quality scans with accuracy within 7 μm according to international and industry standards for accuracy and precision. Identica Hybrid is compatible with multiple articulator types such as Artex, Sam, Kavo. New Identica Software (v2.0) upgrade is color-coded, which facilitates its use. The scanning area is 80 × 60 × 60 (mm) and the instrument's dimensions are 290 × 290 × 342 (mm) (Fig. 3.16). The scanner is distributed to more than 60 countries.

3.10.3 3Shape D2000

The 3Shape D2000 is a closed-case-type laboratory desktop scanner. It is working with blue LED multiline technology. Four cameras with 5 MP acquire the data from

Fig. 3.16 Extraoral
scanning with
Identica Hybrid

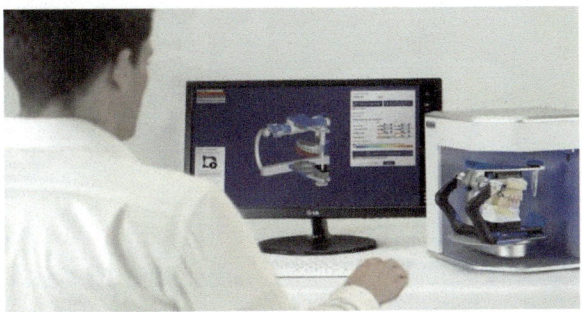

models and dies quickly, accurately, and with real colors. There is no need to section
the dies. There is a possibility to simultaneously scan the models of both jaws. This
option speeds up the normal workflow and can be a time-saving alternative for dental laboratories. Auto-Occlusion technology makes it faster than other desktop scanners. This extraoral scanner is also able to scan conventional impressions with
highly accurate results. The scanning software can instantly invert the impression's
scan. The scans are saved as industry standard open STL. According to the ISO
12836 standard, the scanner can reach an accuracy of 5 μm for crowns and bridges
and 8 μm for implant bars. A full arch scan takes 25 s, while the dies scanning time
ranges between 15 and 19 s.

3.11   Intraoral Scanners

Some of the available intraoral scanners are described below:

3.11.1 TRIOS Intraoral Scanner (3Shape, Copenhagen, Denmark)

In the year 2000, two graduate students, Tais Clausen and Nikolaj Deichmann,
founded 3Shape in Denmark's capital Copenhagen. 3Shape is a developer and manufacturer of 3D scanners and CAD/CAM software solutions for the dental and audio
industries. Their first intraoral scanner, the monochromatic **TRIOS standard,** was
introduced to the market in 2011. Its data capture process uses a video sequence
based on confocal laser technology.

In 2013, the **TRIOS Color** was presented at the International Dental Show (IDS)
in Cologne. It is able to scan the intraoral situation in realistic-looking color and it
was available in a cart-and-pod version like the TRIOS standard at that time. At IDS
2015, **TRIOS 3** was released by the company. The third generation of its intraoral
scanner was available in both a pen-grip and a handle-grip design. It can be incorporated into a dental unit and is also available in a cart version with a touch screen,
or as an USB version, which can be connected to a high-performance laptop
(Fig. 3.17). An intraoral camera comes included with the intraoral scanner, which

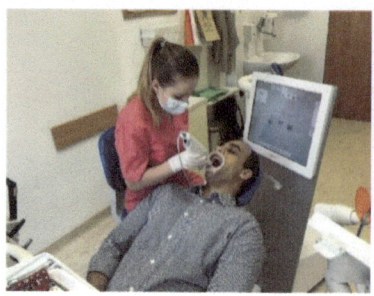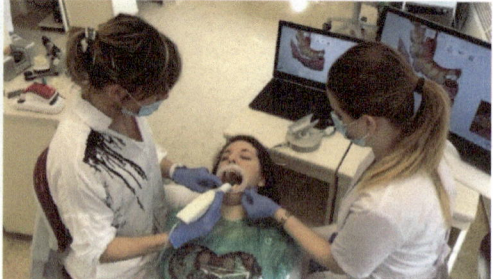

Fig. 3.17 TRIOS cart-and-pod version in use at Semmelweis University, Budapest

Fig. 3.18 Tooth shade
measurement with TRIOS 3

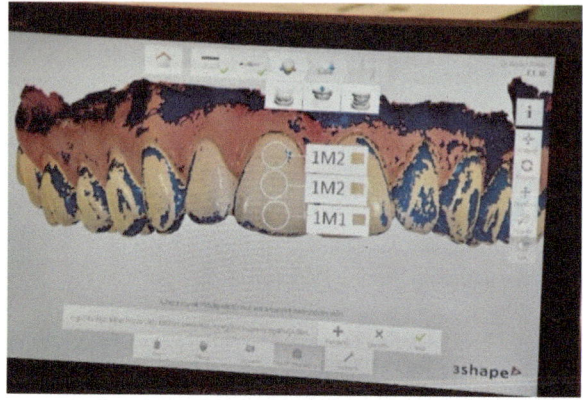

means there is no need to purchase one separately. Using it to take HD photos, communication with patients is made easier.

As a brand-new feature, an automatic tooth shade measurement tool was also incorporated into the scanner, and tooth shades are automatically determined during scanning. It was one of the first scanners with a built-in shade measurement tool on the market; therefore, there are only a few studies about its reliability, but these agree that it can be an alternative means of tooth shade measurement besides spectrophotometers (Fig. 3.18) [63–65]. In 2017, the **TRIOS 3 wireless** version (Fig. 3.19) was also demonstrated at IDS. It connects wirelessly to laptops as well as the TRIOS cart. The operator enjoys free movement without any cables during scanning. On the other hand, it is necessary to change the rechargeable battery of the scanner between scans when using this wireless version. Another feature is remote control: the dentist can manage the steps of scanning in the software without touching the screen.

In 2019 at IDS, the **TRIOS 4** was also introduced to the market. Again, it is a wireless scanner with instant-heat smart tips that enable 30% longer battery life. It features a new special caries diagnostics tool with built-in fluorescent technology, but this requires a second scan that is overlaid on the digital model. Another scanning tip detects interproximal caries via transillumination. Like the previous scanners, it too offers powder-free scanning. Monochrome and color scanning are both

Fig. 3.19 Wireless TRIOS 3

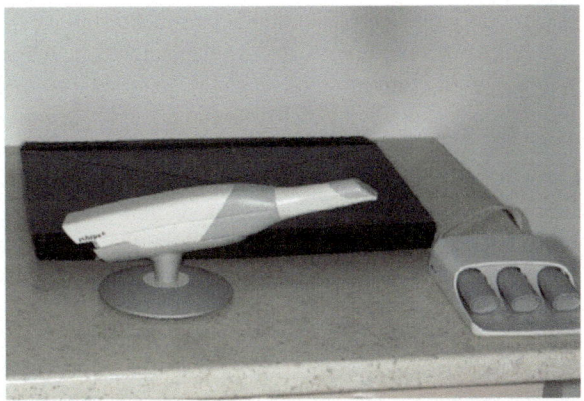

available. Similarly, to previous versions, the scanner can take HD pictures or record videos. Earlier-generation special functions such as shade determination or blocking surfaces are also available. In the scanning software, it is possible to choose the insertion direction of the prosthetic work or place the margin line. Distances from antagonistic teeth can be measured in millimeters.

With this scanner, it is possible to scan a whole arch and there is a wide range of indications. For prosthetic use, there are the software packages: TRIOS Design Studio or Dental System. With a new software called Splint Studio, one can make splints, night guards, etc. For orthodontic treatment, there are several types of software too, such as Ortho System or Clear Aligner Studio. TRIOS treatment simulator helps the communication with patients as it shows them their present dentition and then compares that to the expected results. With Implant Studio, the user can plan the implant's ideal position after planning the prosthetic treatment. This program can merge CBCT and intraoral scans together, and the dentist can plan the implant guide for the surgery. Despite the lack of a fully equipped chairside system, 3Shape has developed chairside software for same-day dentistry: TRIOS Design Studio. For laboratory use, 3Shape CAMbridge is available, with the open system data being transmitted through a cloud-based platform (TRIOS Inbox). TRIOS Patient Monitoring is also a new development, which allows clinicians to easily compare intraoral scans taken over time. The software tracks and quantifies gingival retraction, bruxism, and teeth movement, and highlights changes that may need attention.

3.11.2 iTero Element (Align technology, Inc., San Jose, California)

Founded in March 1997 and now the leader in modern clear aligner orthodontics, Align Technology designs, manufactures, and markets the Invisalign® system. It provides dental treatment options for orthodontic malformations. They started to market the Invisalign system in 1998. iTero launched their first intraoral scanner in 2007; this system employs a parallel confocal imaging technique and it works by highly accurate 3D laser scanning. It is also a powder-free, color-capable scanner. It is especially made for orthodontic treatments, but it can be used for restorative work including crowns, veneers, and implants. In 2011, Align Technology started to work together with iTero intraoral scanners and they also offer the iTero 3D digital scanning system and services for orthodontic and restorative dentistry.

In 2015, the next-generation **iTero Element** Intraoral Scanner was introduced to the market at the 36th International Dental Show in Cologne, Germany. With the new 40% smaller and lighter wand, doctors can scan 20× faster than before. With iTero Element, dentists are able to show the final result of ortho treatment to the patients upon scanning the initial situation. If the dentist scans their patients regularly during treatment, they can follow the results compared to the expected treatment. This intraoral scanner has an open architecture, which makes it compatible with the Invisalign system. It is a color scanner to distinguish between gingival and tooth structures. iTero Element has two different configurations: a custom wheel stand option and iTero Element Flex (available as of 2018), which is a wand-only system connectable to a laptop via USB.

In 2018, Align Technology expanded their iTero Element portfolio with the launch of the **iTero Element 2**. It enables faster start-up and offers faster scan-processing times. They changed the wand placement from the left side of the monitor into a center-mounted wand cradle for easy ergonomics during scanning (Fig. 3.20).

In 2019, **iTero Element 5D** was showcased at IDS, with a new caries detector feature via NIRI (Near-Infrared Imaging) technology [66]. This is the first scanner with this technology, and it can be used for interproximal caries screening. It may be used with a laptop too. All iTero Element scanners generate full-color and high-definition 3D scans. This system is compatible with Invisalign Outcome Simulator,

OrthoCAD®, and OrthoCAD Viewer software. It is also designed to connect to restorative as well as orthodontic labs and also third-party treatment planning, custom implant abutment, chairside milling, and lab CAD/CAM systems. The Timelapse technology feature takes historical scan data and compares them to the current scan in a visual manner, allowing patients to see changes in their tooth wear, tooth movement, and changes in gingiva over time. It works as an intraoral camera too.

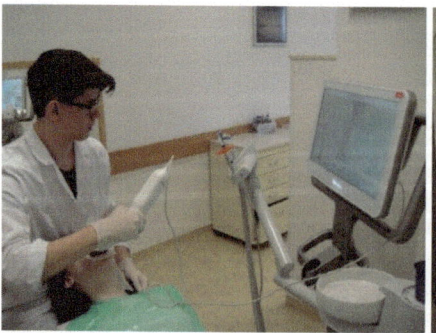
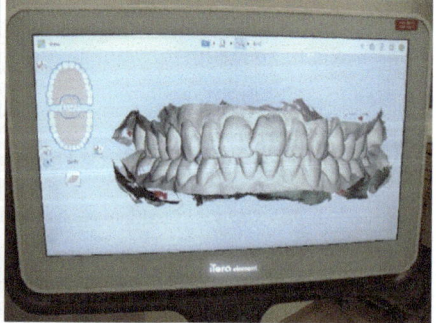

Fig. 3.20 A dental student using iTero Element 2; scanned upper and lower jaws on the display screen of iTero element 2

3.11.3 CEREC Primescan (DENTSPLY Sirona, York, Pennsylvania, United States)

DENTSPLY International was founded as Dentists' Supply Company in 1899 in New York City and the company that became Sirona Dental Systems was founded in 1877 in Erlangen, Germany. In 2016, these two companies merged and created DENTSPLY Sirona, which became one of the world's largest manufacturers of professional dental solutions. In the early 1980s, on the foundations of Werner H. Mörmann's idea, CEREC's first intraoral scanner and chair-side CAD/CAM unit was developed [16]. In 1985, **CEREC 1** was especially made for planning inlay restorations (marginal discrepancy was 140–256 μm [67]) and it was the first commercially available digital impression system for use in the field of dentistry. The triangulation scanning technique was first introduced into dentistry in 1987 through CEREC by Sirona Dental Systems LLC. In 1988, onlay and veneer capabilities were added to the unit [68]. In 1994, the **CEREC 2** was introduced to the market. Making full or partial crowns and copings was possible with this system (marginal fit of 50–150 μm [67]). All these systems generated 2-dimensional (2D) images [67]. In 2000, the **CEREC 3** was introduced and by 2003 it had 3-dimensional capability. A new software was added in 2005 that enabled automatic virtual occlusal adjustment. The **CEREC Bluecam** cart intraoral scanner was introduced in 2009 as a monochromatic scanner. Before scanning, dentists had to use titanium powder as a contrast agent on tooth surfaces to create a matte surface for different materials. The system provides a marginal crown fit of 39.2 μm [67]. It works by triangulation with the help of a Blue Light Emitting Diode (LED) Camera and Automatic Capture. Built-in "shake control" eliminates blurry images and produces significantly more detailed images.

From 2013 on, Dentsply Sirona has distributed the **CEREC Omnicam** intraoral scanner. This scanner can be used powder-free and it provides 3D images in realistic color; tooth shade determination is also available. Three different variants are marketed: CEREC AC (Acquisition Center)—The mobile cart version; CEREC AF (Acquisition Flex)—The flexible tabletop unit; CEREC AI (Acquisition Integrated)—The dental-unit-integrated, economic version, and CEREC AI for Rear, which can be attached to the rear cabinetry at the 12 o'clock position. Omnicam has a special doctor-patient communication method: doctors can show a lifelike video to the patient about his or her dentition. For implant and orthodontic purposes, the Galileos Implant and Ortho software are available. Galileos Implant is also useful in prosthetic and surgical planning. Cerec Ortho allows dentists to design ortho devices.

In 2019, **CEREC Primescan** was introduced at IDS. The Primescan kept the same cart design as Omnicam, but the mouse cursor is now controlled with a touch pad and the keyboard has been removed as well (Fig. 3.21). The scanner remains wired to the cart, but the cart itself is wireless (60-min battery buffer). The new touch screen is bigger than before (16:9 instead of 4:3). The scanner head is substantially larger; it means a large imaging area can be recorded with fewer movements. The company says that this scanner is able to capture an increased depth of

Fig. 3.21 Scanning a model with Cerec Primescan

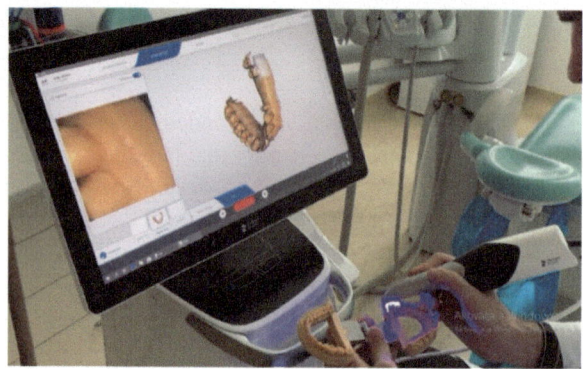

Fig. 3.22 Designing in chairside software of CEREC

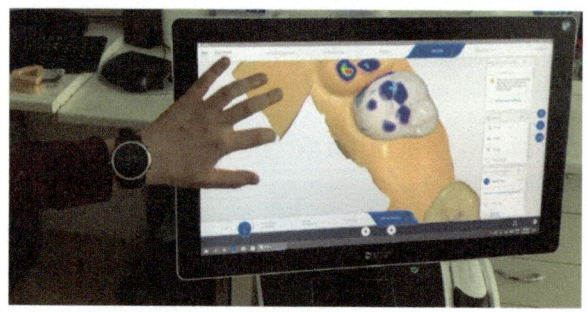

field up to 20 mm. Autoclavable stainless steel sleeves and single-use disposable sleeves are also available. The CEREC solution spectrum covers three important areas: restorative field, implants, and orthodontics, both for chairside (Fig. 3.22) and clinic-to-laboratory workflows. It can be used chairside for guided implant dentistry, too, so that we can create the fastest surgical guide on the market after scanning the patient. For chairside restorative solutions, CEREC has its own grinding and milling units and ceramic furnace (called CEREC SpeedFire). Besides their certified material partners, Dentsply Sirona offers a wide range of its own materials for CAD/CAM restorations (e.g., Celtra Duo, CEREC Zirconia). The files can be sent to the Lab via Connect Case Center; alternatively, because it is an open system, STL files can be exported as well. DENTSPLY Sirona makes data transfer easier with the help of a solution called Hub. On Hub, the patient's information and CAD/CAM data can be kept synchronized everywhere in the practice and in the lab. Right after the patient has been scanned, the technician can start designing the restoration without any manual file transfer being required. This device is ideal for practices with multiple scanners. It duplicates all data to provide protection against data loss. It makes lab-office communication easier. It is one of the most accurate intraoral scanners available currently with an accuracy of almost 20 μm [4, 69].

3.11.4 Planmeca Emerald (Planmeca OY, Helsinki, Finland)

Planmeca Oy was founded in 1971 by Mr Heikki Kyöstilä in Helsinki, Finland. In the beginning, Planmeca manufactured dental units, and later, X-ray units and digital imaging systems. In the 2000s, they produced the CBCT system for 3D dental imaging and the **Planmeca Romexis** software platform for processing X-Ray images. In 2011, the **Planmeca ProMax** 3D family was introduced, which brings together a CBCT image, a 3D face photo, and a 3D model scan into a three-dimensional virtual patient.

Planmeca's **PlanScan**, the world's first intraoral scanner integrated into a dental unit, was first introduced to the market in 2014. In addition to a cart version, a Portable solution is also available, which can be easily connected to a laptop via an USB port. If connected to a dental unit, the scanner can also be operated with wireless foot control, leaving the user's hands free during scanning. It has autoclavable and changeable tips in different sizes to make scanning easier in every clinical situation. In the tips, there are built-in heated mirrors to avoid fogging. It is a powder-free intraoral scanner that uses blue laser technology with real-time laser video-streaming to capture accurate monochromatic digital images. The Planmeca Planscan® is an open system, since it allows conversion of the acquired proprietary files into STL files, readable by all CAD systems. On the other hand, the Planscan is an important part of Planmeca FIT, which is the company's own chairside system that combines all steps of the CAD/CAM workflow from scanning to designing and milling (Fig. 3.23).

The color-capable **Planmeca Emerald** was first introduced to the market in 2017. The scanner is available in a pod version and can also be integrated into a dental unit. The handpiece has two controlling buttons for more ergonomic scanning and tips of two different sizes (Standard Tip, Slim Line tip). Optical mirrors in the handpiece can be heated to prevent fogging. The Emerald also operates on the principle of triangulation, does not require powder on tooth surfaces, and captures video sequences. While scanning, the operator can also take 2D images, which can help in designing the restoration. The scanner can be used as an intraoral camera.

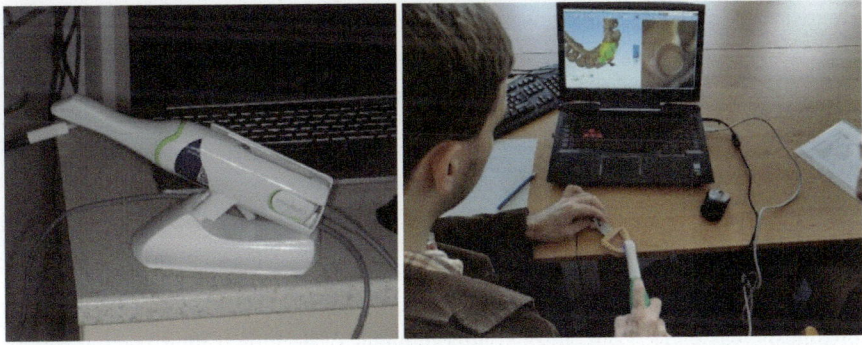

Fig. 3.23 The Planmeca PlanScan and scanning with the Planmeca Emerald

There is a fully built chairside and labside system with milling units. Design software can be used with chairside milling units (Planmill 40S, 30S) and laboratory (Planmill 50) milling units. They have their own 3D printer called Planmeca Creo 3D. For a completely digital chairside CAD/CAM workflow, dentists can design restorations in just a few steps with the Planmeca PlanCAD Easy design software, which is also part of Planmeca Romexis. A wide range of possible indications are covered in implantology, orthodontics, and prosthodontics. Users can use the scanned data for maxillofacial surgeries as well, by combining scans with CBCT datasets.

In 2019 at IDS, a new faster scanner, the **Planmeca S** was showcased with a new Cariosity transillumination tip, which is a tool for detecting caries, and a shade assistant feature for determining tooth shade. The software component has not changed significantly compared to the previous versions.

3.11.5 Medit i500 (Medit, Seoul, South Korea)

The Medit company was founded in 2000 in Seoul, South Korea. They specialized in CAD/CAM solutions for dental clinics and labs, including intraoral and 3D scanners, as well as software for the industrial market. In 2018, they introduced their first intraoral scanner, the Medit i500. Equipped with two high-speed LED cameras, this color scanner uses 3D-in-motion video technology and triangulation. Dentists do not need to use powder on intraoral surfaces. The very lightweight handpiece has only one button to start scanning. This is a plug-in scanner and can be connected to a high-performance laptop via USB. A special and unique function of the scanner is impression scanning. Oral scan data can be merged with impression scan data. If the preparation is subgingival, we can complete the scanned data with a scan of the conventional impression to make the preparation margins more visible. Occlusion analysis and high-resolution scans for prepared tooth are also available. Dentists can take HD pictures and make their case more detailed for the lab. Users can adjust the maximum scan depth between 12 and 21 mm using the scan depth selector in the software. Scanning can be recorded in the software, and users can replay the whole scanning process. This can be helpful in improving the user's scanning technique. Dentists can manage everything in a single software package named Medit Link (Fig. 3.24). It is an open software with cloud-based storage. STL files can be used in several other types of design software, allowing a wide range of treatments in the fields of prosthodontics, implantology, or orthodontics.

A Case Report Highlighting Digital Technology Advancements
Figure 3.24 shows photographs of patient with missing teeth in lower arch. Even with orthodontic brackets on, accurate digital impressions were obtained. Digital tooth shade was measured while taking impression with an intraoral scanner. Prosthesis designing was carried out on a software and 3D printing of temporary prosthesis was carried out. In next appointment, CNC milled multilayered monolithic final restoration was delivered (Figs. 3.25 and 3.26).

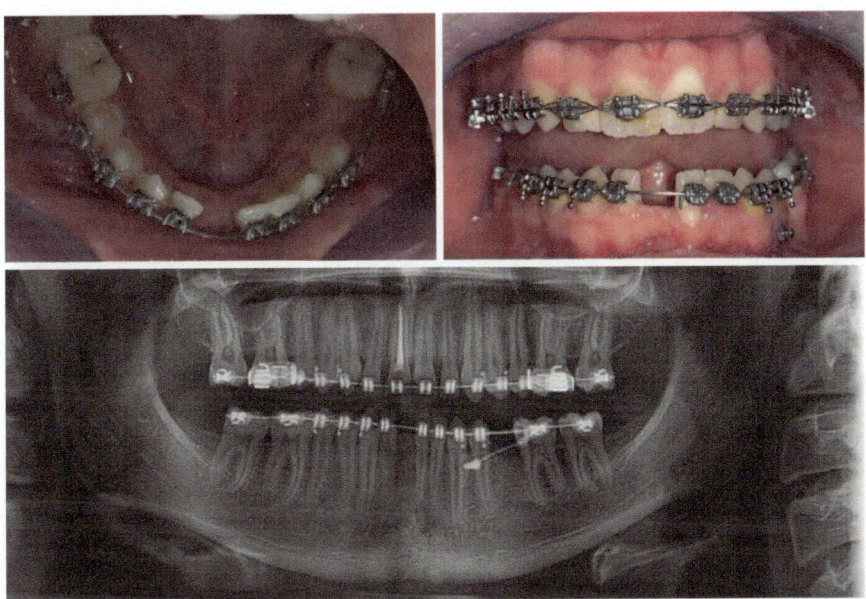

Fig. 3.24 Photographs of patient with orthodontic brackets and wire. Lower right central incisor is missing

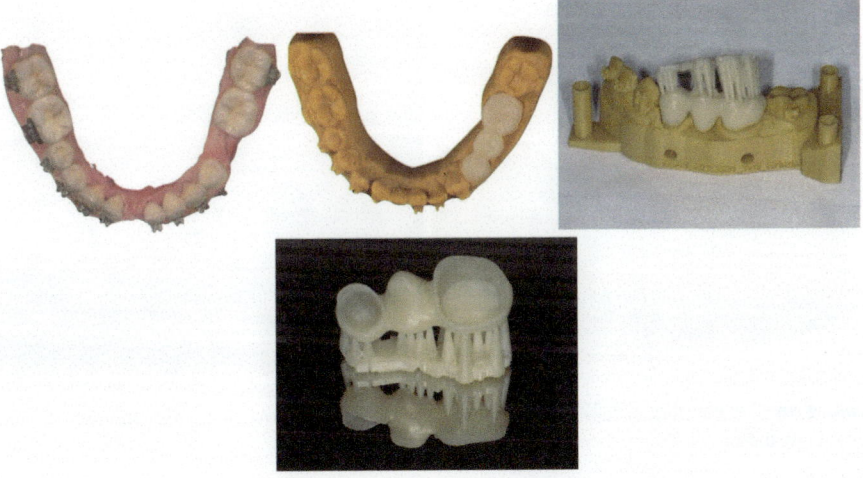

Fig. 3.25 3D printed temporary restoration

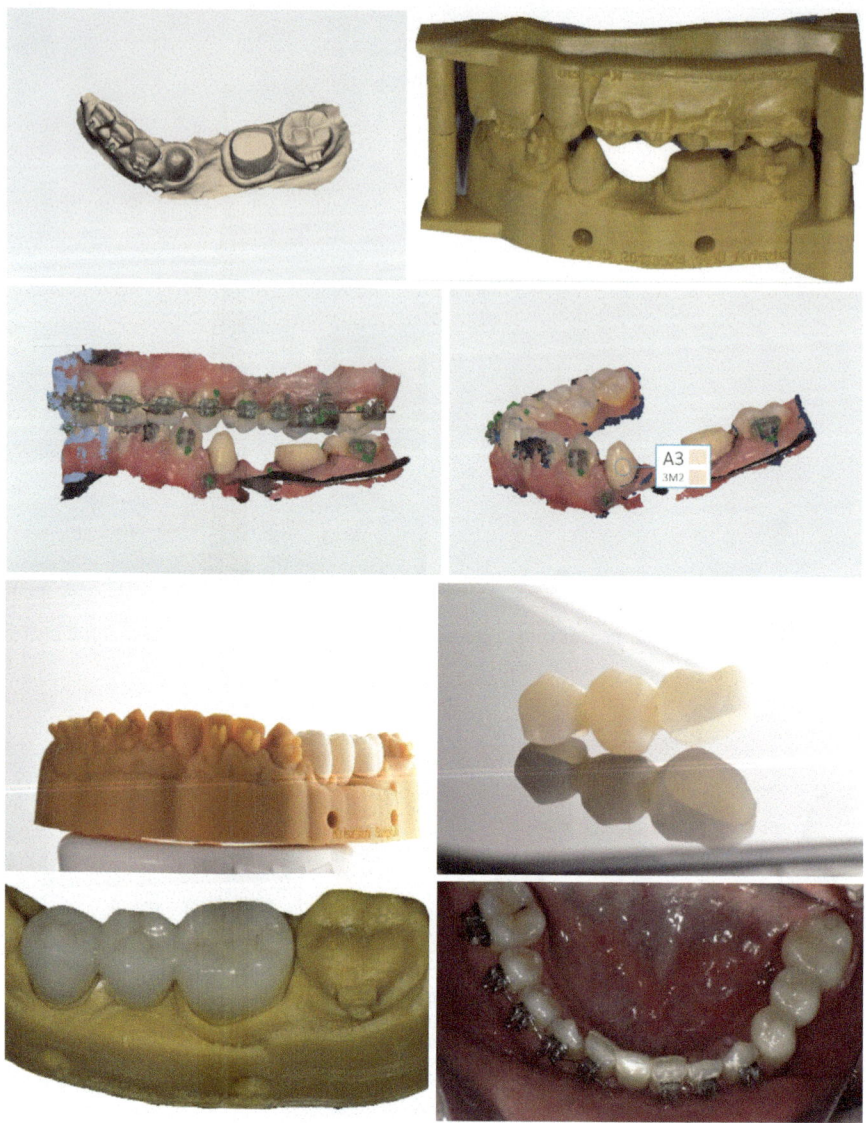

Fig. 3.26 Case workflow depicting digital scanner, digital shade matching, 3D printing cast, and final prosthesis

References

1. Bohner L, et al. Accuracy of digital technologies for the scanning of facial, skeletal, and intra-oral tissues: a systematic review. J Prosthet Dent. 2019;121(2):246–51.
2. Vecsei B, et al. Comparison of the accuracy of direct and indirect three-dimensional digitizing processes for CAD/CAM systems - an in vitro study. J Prosthod Res. 2017;61(2):177–84.

3. Kim RJ, Park JM, Shim JS. Accuracy of 9 intraoral scanners for complete-arch image acquisition: a qualitative and quantitative evaluation. J Prosthet Dent. 2018;120(6):895–903.e1.
4. Ender A, Zimmermann M, Mehl A. Accuracy of complete- and partial-arch impressions of actual intraoral scanning systems in vitro. Int J Comput Dent. 2019;22(1):11–9.
5. Gonzalez de Villaumbrosia P, et al. In vitro comparison of the accuracy (trueness and precision) of six extraoral dental scanners with different scanning technologies. J Prosthet Dent. 2016;116(4):543–550.e1.
6. Jang Y, et al. Evaluation of the marginal and internal fit of a single crown fabricated based on a three-dimensional printed model. J Adv Prosthod. 2018;10(5):367–73.
7. Gaudin A, Pérez F, Galicia J. Digital technology in endodontics. In: Tamimi F, Hirayama H, editors. Digital restorative dentistry: a guide to materials, equipment, and clinical procedures. Cham: Springer International Publishing; 2019. p. 229–47.
8. Connert T, et al. Guided endodontics versus conventional access cavity preparation: a comparative study on substance loss using 3-dimensional-printed teeth. J Endod. 2019;45(3):327–31.
9. van der Meer WJ, et al. 3D Computer aided treatment planning in endodontics. J Dent. 2016;45:67–72.
10. International Organization for Standardization. Dentistry—digitizing devices for CAD/CAM systems for indirect dental restorations - test methods for assessing accuracy. Geneva: International Organization for Standardization; 2012.
11. Birnbaum NS, Aaronson HB. Dental impressions using 3D digital scanners: virtual becomes reality. Compend Contin Educ Dent. 2008;29(8):494–6, 498–505.
12. Davidowitz G, Kotick PG. The use of CAD/CAM in dentistry. Dent Clin N Am. 2011;55(3):559–70, ix.
13. Péter H, Péter K, András K. Fogpótlástani anyagtan és odontotechnológia. Budapest: Semmelweis Kiadó; 2015.
14. McLaren EA, Culp L, White S. The evolution of digital dentistry and the digital dental team. Dent Today. 2008;27(9):112–4, 116–7.
15. Miyazaki T, et al. A review of dental CAD/CAM: current status and future perspectives from 20 years of experience. Dent Mater J. 2009;28(1):44–56.
16. Mormann WH. The evolution of the CEREC system. J Am Dent Assoc. 2006;137(Suppl):7S–13S.
17. Logozzo S, et al. Recent advances in dental optics – Part I: 3D intraoral scanners for restorative dentistry. Opt Lasers Eng. 2014;54:203–21.
18. Research R. ATLAS DENTAL European Markets///structures, challenges and scenarios. Köln: GFDI; 2019.
19. Ferencz JL. Today's CAD/CAM: flexible digital technologies expanding workflow options. Compend Contin Educ Dent. 2015;36(3):222–3.
20. Christensen GJ. Impressions are changing: deciding on conventional, digital or digital plus in-office milling. J Am Dent Assoc. 2009;140(10):1301–4.
21. Nedelcu R, et al. Finish line distinctness and accuracy in 7 intraoral scanners versus conventional impression: an in vitro descriptive comparison. BMC Oral Health. 2018;18(1):27.
22. Lee JJ, et al. Accuracy of single-abutment digital cast obtained using intraoral and cast scanners. J Prosthet Dent. 2017;117(2):253–9.
23. Richert R, et al. Intraoral scanner technologies: a review to make a successful impression. J Healthc Eng. 2017;2017:8427595.
24. Freedman M, Quinn F, O'Sullivan M. Single unit CAD/CAM restorations: a literature review. J Ir Dent Assoc. 2007;53(1):38–45.
25. Luthardt R, et al. Design and production of dental prosthetic restorations: basic research on dental CAD/CAM technology. Int J Comput Dent. 2002;5(2–3):165.
26. Beuer F, Schweiger J, Edelhoff D. Digital dentistry: an overview of recent developments for CAD/CAM generated restorations. Br Dent J. 2008;204(9):505–11.
27. Fasbinder DJ. Computerized technology for restorative dentistry. Am J Dent. 2013;26(3):115–20.
28. Vlaar ST, van der Zel JM. Accuracy of dental digitizers. Int Dent J. 2006;56(5):301–9.

29. Ramiro GP, et al. Digitalization in restorative dentistry. In: Tamimi F, Hirayama H, editors. Digital restorative dentistry: a guide to materials, equipment, and clinical procedures. Cham: Springer International Publishing; 2019. p. 7–39.
30. Kusnoto B, Evans CA. Reliability of a 3D surface laser scanner for orthodontic applications. Am J Orthod Dentofac Orthop. 2002;122(4):342–8.
31. Fasbinder DJ. Digital dentistry: innovation for restorative treatment. Compend Contin Educ Dent. 2010;31(4):2–11, quiz 12.
32. Ting-shu S, Jian S. Intraoral digital impression technique: a review. J Prosthod. 2015;24(4):313–21.
33. Zimmermann M, et al. Intraoral scanning systems - a current overview. Int J Comput Dent. 2015;18(2):101–29.
34. Martin CB, et al. Orthodontic scanners: what's available? J Orthod. 2015;42(2):136–43.
35. Flugge TV, et al. Precision of intraoral digital dental impressions with iTero and extraoral digitization with the iTero and a model scanner. Am J Orthod Dentofac Orthop. 2013;144(3):471–8.
36. Ender A, Mehl A. Influence of scanning strategies on the accuracy of digital intraoral scanning systems. Int J Comput Dent. 2013;16(1):11–21.
37. Kattadiyil MT, et al. Intraoral scanning of hard and soft tissues for partial removable dental prosthesis fabrication. J Prosthet Dent. 2014;112(3):444–8.
38. Imburgia M, et al. Accuracy of four intraoral scanners in oral implantology: a comparative in vitro study. BMC Oral Health. 2017;17(1):92.
39. Aragon ML, et al. Validity and reliability of intraoral scanners compared to conventional gypsum models measurements: a systematic review. Eur J Orthod. 2016;38(4):429–34.
40. Mangano F, et al. Intraoral scanners in dentistry: a review of the current literature. BMC Oral Health. 2017;17(1):149.
41. Mormann WH, et al. Chairside computer-aided direct ceramic inlays. Quintessence Int. 1989;20(5):329–39.
42. Puri S. Evolutions in CAD/CAM hardware, software, and materials. Dent Today. 2011;30(5):116–8, 120–1.
43. Ramiro GP, et al. Computer-aided design in restorative dentistry. In: Tamimi F, Hirayama H, editors. Digital restorative dentistry: a guide to materials, equipment, and clinical procedures. Cham: Springer International Publishing; 2019. p. 41–54.
44. Coachman C, Calamita M. Digital smile design: a tool for treatment planning and communication in esthetic dentistry. QDT 2012 Quintes. 2012;35:1–9.
45. Kurbad A, Kurbad S. Cerec Smile Design--a software tool for the enhancement of restorations in the esthetic zone. Int J Comput Dent. 2013;16(3):255–69.
46. Zimmermann M, Mehl A. Virtual smile design systems: a current review. Int J Comput Dent. 2015;18(4):303–17.
47. Masri R. Clinical applications of digital dental technology. Ames, IA: Wiley-Blackwell; 2015.
48. Prajapati A, et al. Dentistry goes digital: a Cad-Cam way - a review article. J Dent Med Sci. 2014;13(8):53–9.
49. Grant GT. Direct digital manufacturing; 2015. p. 41–56.
50. McLaren EA, Terry DA. CAD/CAM systems, materials, and clinical guidelines for all-ceramic crowns and fixed partial dentures. Compend Contin Educ Dent. 2002;23(7):637–41.
51. Reich S, et al. Clinical fit of all-ceramic three-unit fixed partial dentures, generated with three different CAD/CAM systems. Eur J Oral Sci. 2005;113(2):174–9.
52. Bindl A, Mormann WH. Marginal and internal fit of all-ceramic CAD/CAM crown-copings on chamfer preparations. J Oral Rehabil. 2005;32(6):441–7.
53. Stappert CF, et al. Marginal adaptation of different types of all-ceramic partial coverage restorations after exposure to an artificial mouth. Br Dent J. 2005;199(12):779–83, discussion 777.
54. Tinschert J, et al. Marginal fit of alumina-and zirconia-based fixed partial dentures produced by a CAD/CAM system. Oper Dent. 2001;26(4):367–74.
55. Fasbinder DJ, et al. A clinical evaluation of chairside lithium disilicate CAD/CAM crowns: a two-year report. J Am Dent Assoc. 2010;141(Suppl 2):10s–4s.

56. Alageel O, et al. Fabrication of dental restorations using digital technologies: techniques and materials. In: Tamimi F, Hirayama H, editors. Digital restorative dentistry: a guide to materials, equipment, and clinical procedures. Cham: Springer International Publishing; 2019. p. 55–91.
57. Fasbinder DJ. Chairside CAD/CAM: an overview of restorative material options. Compend Contin Educ Dent. 2012;33(1):50, 52–8.
58. Fasbinder DJ, Neiva GF. Surface evaluation of polishing techniques for new resilient CAD/CAM restorative materials. J Esthet Restor Dent. 2016;28(1):56–66.
59. Sailer I, et al. Five-year clinical results of zirconia frameworks for posterior fixed partial dentures. Int J Prosthodont. 2007;20(4):383–8.
60. Vult von Steyern P, Carlson P, Nilner K. All-ceramic fixed partial dentures designed according to the DC-Zirkon technique. A 2-year clinical study. J Oral Rehabil. 2005;32(3):180–7.
61. Jang GW, et al. Fracture strength and mechanism of dental ceramic crown with zirconia thickness. Proc Eng. 2011;10:1556–60.
62. Ozkurt-Kayahan Z. Monolithic zirconia: a review of the literature. Biomed Res. 2016;27(4):1427–36.
63. Mehl A, et al. In vivo tooth-color measurement with a new 3D intraoral scanning system in comparison to conventional digital and visual color determination methods. Int J Comput Dent. 2017;20(4):343–61.
64. Yilmaz B, Irmak O, Yaman BC. Outcomes of visual tooth shade selection performed by operators with different experience. J Esthet Restor Dent. 2019;31:500.
65. Liberato WF, et al. A comparison between visual, intraoral scanner, and spectrophotometer shade matching: a clinical study. J Prosthet Dent. 2019;121(2):271–5.
66. Global medical device company launches new iTero element 5D imaging system. Br Dent J. 2019;226(5):379.
67. Prudente MS, et al. Influence of scanner, powder application, and adjustments on CAD-CAM crown misfit. J Prosthet Dent. 2018;119(3):377–83.
68. Santos GC Jr, et al. Overview of CEREC CAD/CAM chairside system. Gen Dent. 2013;61(1):36–40, quiz 41.
69. Skramstad MJ. Welcome to Cerec Primescan AC. Int J Comput Dent. 2019;22(1):69–78.

Endodontic Guides and Software Planning

4

Niraj Kinariwala, Jørgen Buchgreitz, Lars Bjørndal, Bertold Molnár, and Suresh Ludhwani

4.1 Introduction

Advances in information technology, including the availability of inexpensive/ open-source software, have permitted inter-operability between 3D imaging devices, 3D virtual planning systems and 3D printers to efficiently create, manipulate and process data for the design and production of 3D printed guides.

CBCT scan converts data into DICOM file. The DICOM format facilitates the transfer of medical images and related data between computer devices built by various manufacturers and operating on different platforms.

The volumetric data (DICOM format) from CBCT scans is acquired by 3D virtual planning software to convert the data to the Standard Tessellation Language (STL) file format representing the virtual 3D surface shape. 3D imaging data from optical intra-oral/plaster model scans, existing as STL formats, are also acquired by 3D virtual planning systems. Using specialized software, the CBCT and corresponding intra-oral/plaster model STL data sets are matched to eliminate streak and void artefacts caused by metallic restorations through the precise alignment of

---

Electronic Supplementary Material The online version of this chapter (https://doi.org/10.1007/ 978-3-030-55281-7_4) contains supplementary material, which is available to authorized users.

N. Kinariwala (✉) · S. Ludhwani
Karnavati School of Dentistry, Karnavati University, Gandhinagar, Gujarat, India
e-mail: niraj@ksd.ac.in

J. Buchgreitz
Allerød, Denmark

L. Bjørndal
Section of Cariology and Endodontics, Department of Odontology, Faculty of Health and Medical Sciences, University of Copenhagen, Copenhagen, Denmark
e-mail: labj@sund.ku.dk

B. Molnár
Budapest, Hungary

© Springer Nature Switzerland AG 2021
N. Kinariwala, L. Samaranayake (eds.), *Guided Endodontics*,
https://doi.org/10.1007/978-3-030-55281-7_4

anatomical landmarks. The resultant computer-generating 3D image is then edited with computer-aided design (CAD) or implant planning software to create a blueprint of the 3D printed object. 3D printed guides or templates for endodontic purpose are called Endoguides or endodontic guides.

4.1.1 Definition

3D endodontic guide or endoguide is a template fabricated to guide drills into pre-planned positions for localization and exploration of root canal orifices or bone trephination and root end re-section. It is method of static navigation in endodontics (Fig. 4.1).

4.1.2 Synonyms

- Endodontic guide
- Endoguide
- Endodontic template
- 3D Endodontic guide/template
- Surgical guide

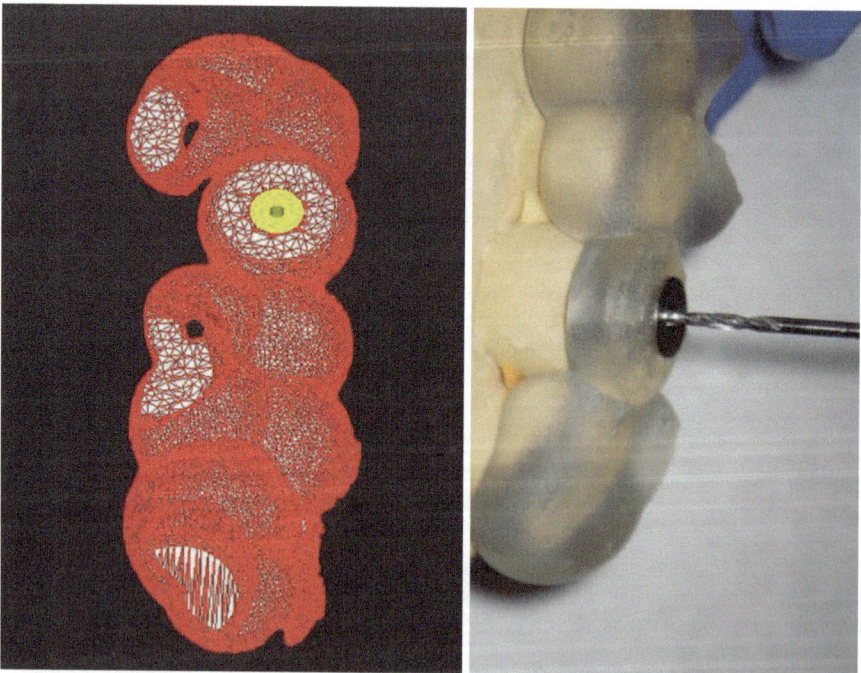

Fig. 4.1 Left: 3D Meshwork of endodontic guide on a software. Right: 3D printed endodontic guide. (Case courtesy: Dr Gergely Beyoncs, Dr Bertold)

4.2   Types of Endodontic Guides

1. Depending upon their use in endodontic treatment:
   (a) Non-surgical Guides: Used to locate calcified canals non-surgically or api-cally extended access opening cavities
   (b) Surgical Guides: Used mainly for endodontic surgeries especially for root end resection procedures
2. Depending upon their support:
   (a) Tooth supported guide: Rests over dentition of the patient. No anchor pin is required. Used mainly for non-surgical guided endodontic treatments.
   (b) Mucosa supported guide: Rests over patient's soft tissues. Fixation pins are inserted into mucosa. Not preferred for endodontic treatments.
   (c) Bone supported guide: Rests on bone surface after flap reflection. Fixation pins are inserted into bone. It can be used for surgical endodontics.
3. Classification of Surgical endodontic templates (Fig. 4.2):
   (a) Non-guiding template for soft tissue retraction
   (b) Template for cortical preparation
   (c) Template for pilot guide
   (d) Full guide for a bone trephination and root end resection

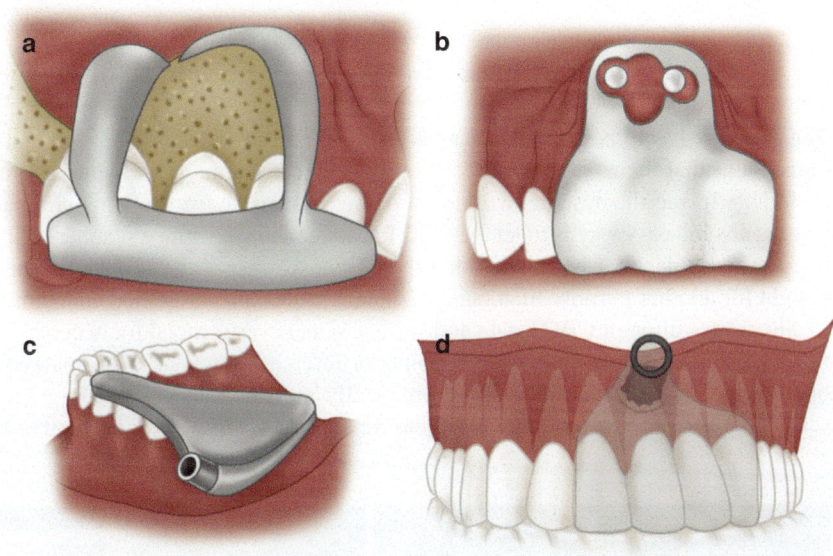

Fig. 4.2 3D printed endodontic surgical aids for different purposes. (**a**) Soft tissue retractor; (**b**) A device to orient cortical penetration; (**c**) A pilot guide; (**d**) Full guide for a bone trephine. (Image used with the permission of Springer Nature. Permission no.: 4633251128826; Drawings by Dr. Tekla Sáry; [1–4])

4.3 Steps of 3D Guide Planning and Designing

For accurate endodontic guide panning, parameters should be set for virtual panning, drills, sleeves and 3D printing. The basic steps for guided endodontics are as follows:

4.3.1 CBCT Scan of the Involved Tooth

Obtain a CBCT scan with limited field of view and high resolution. It is necessary to scan with minimal patient movement, minimal artefacts and minimal slice thickness and standard exposure parameters. It is necessary to make sure tooth has a sound and smooth tooth surface while scanning so that guide can rest on it properly.

4.3.2 The Surface Scan

It is necessary to record details of tooth surface and soft tissue surfaces. The tooth arch scanning can be done directly chairside if intra-oral scanner is available or indirectly by scanning a model made after an impression (Fig. 4.3). The scan has to cover at least one quadrant of the tooth arch to secure a stable support for the guide.

4.3.3 Merging the CBCT Scan and Surface Scan with a Software

The software has to be compatible with the CBCT scan software. Many manufactures claim that their system works as an open source without problems, but it is preferable to see the systems working together before any investments are made. The secure and easy way is to let the CBCT scanner and the surface scanner be from the same manufacturer but often either the CBCT scanner or the surface scanner is bought for another purpose than guided implant procedures or guided endodontics.

Superimposition of CBCT data and surface scan is very crucial for accuracy and fit of the guide. In this process, 3–6 points or reference landmarks are marked on both scan file and then, software automatically merges both scans. Merging the scans takes place in the software by bringing up both scans next to each other and

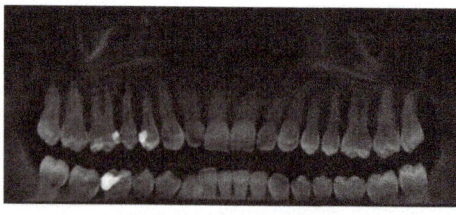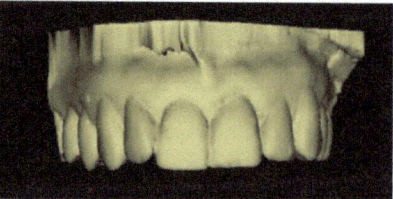

Fig. 4.3 CBCT (DICOM data) and Surface scan (STL file) of the patient

by posting markings on corresponding spots (Fig. 4.4). Evaluate superimposition of images for accurate planning (Fig. 4.5). At control of the merged image, it is checked that neither the virtual bur nor the sleeve is touching the surface scan (Fig. 4.6).

You can always crosscheck whether the data is merged properly or not in each DICOM sections. If there is any error, one can rectify it by moving the STL file in translator and rotatory movements. Once it is completed, then you can start your planning.

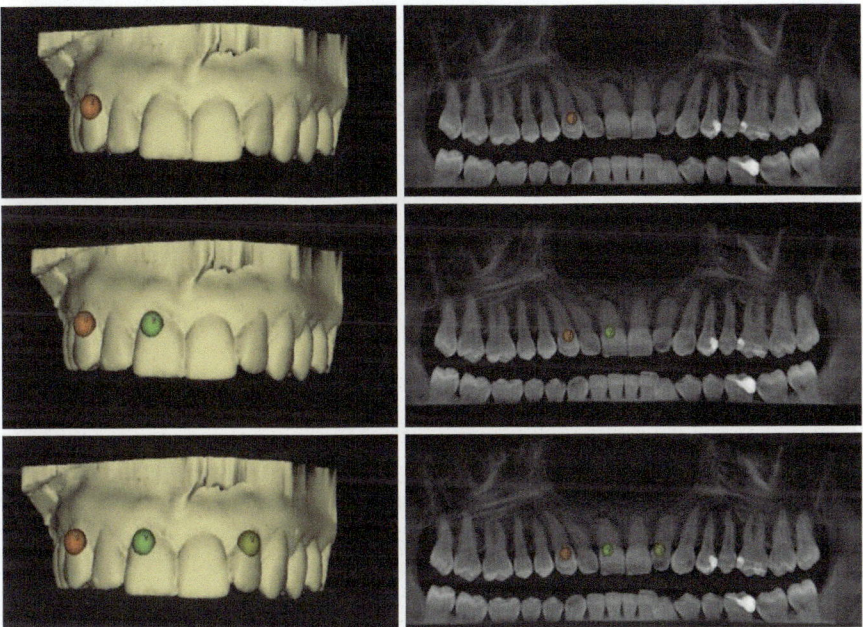

Fig. 4.4 Superimposition of CBCT data and surface scan by marking three spots on both of them

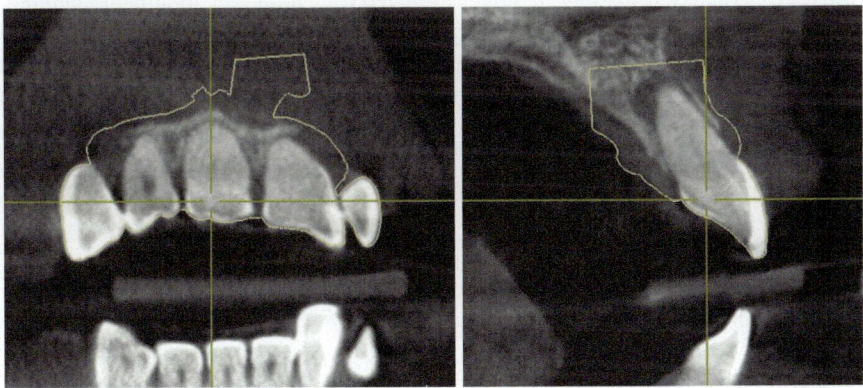

Fig. 4.5 Evaluation of data superimposition. Yellow line shows the surface scan

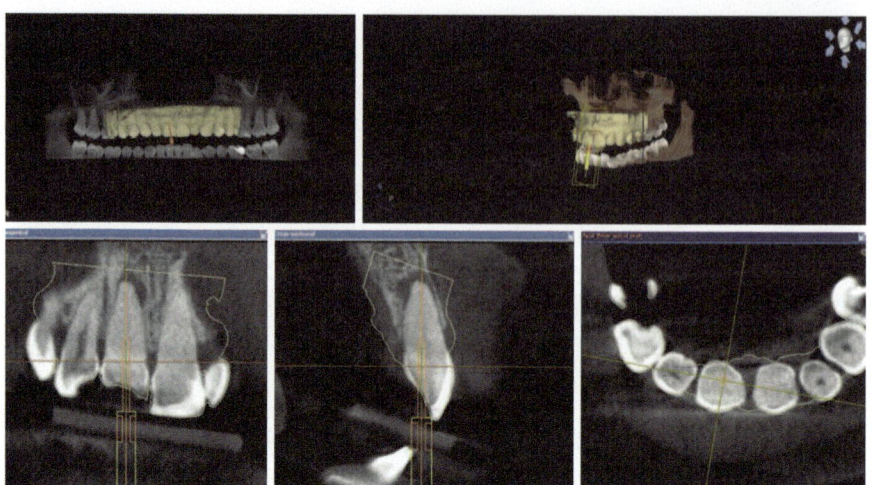

Fig. 4.6 The combined image. Surface scan is marked yellow on the panorama view and yellow line on the tangential, cross-cut and axial view

4.3.4 Designing of Endodontic Guide

4.3.4.1 Tracing the Canal

First is to locate the calcified canals on a scan. Mostly, we always can see the trace of pulp radiolucency present which helps to guide you in tracing the entire canals. It is always easy to trace and select case for guided endodontics for anterior teeth where most of the time, there is no curvature. For the canals with curvature, guided access can be provided till first curvature only. If canal is not visible even on CBCT scan, law of canal centrality should be followed while planning.

4.3.4.2 Creating Virtual Drill Path

On the CBCT scan, a virtual drill path can be planned with the help of appropriate software. As many softwares are not customized for endodontic treatment planning, implant software and virtual drills can be used. After tracing the canals, go to software implant or drill library depending upon the software and its manufacturer's instructions. Place a thin implant or drill (diameter 1.00 mm or less) mimicking as endodontic bur from the tip till the apex. Align the drill path along the path of the canal and maintain centrality within the root. Following points should be considered while planning virtual drill path for endodontic guide.

The drill path should extend from an entrance point at the incisal or occlusal surface of the tooth heading to a target point where a pulp space is assumed to exist.

Depending on the software, different procedures are possible, but the following general points have to be decided:

1. The target point
2. The angle of the drill path (deciding the entrance point) in three dimensions
3. The diameter of the drill.

The Target Point

The target point must be placed at the first visible part of the pulp canal space. If there is an apical pathosis, it can be presumed that there is a pulp canal space with remnants of necrotic infected pulp tissue, even if it not visible neither on the radiograph nor on the CBCT scan (Fig. 4.7). The reason can be diameter of the pulp canal, which is smaller than the resolution of the radiograph and the voxel size of the CBCT scan. The axial view of the CBCT can be used in these cases (Fig. 4.7b),

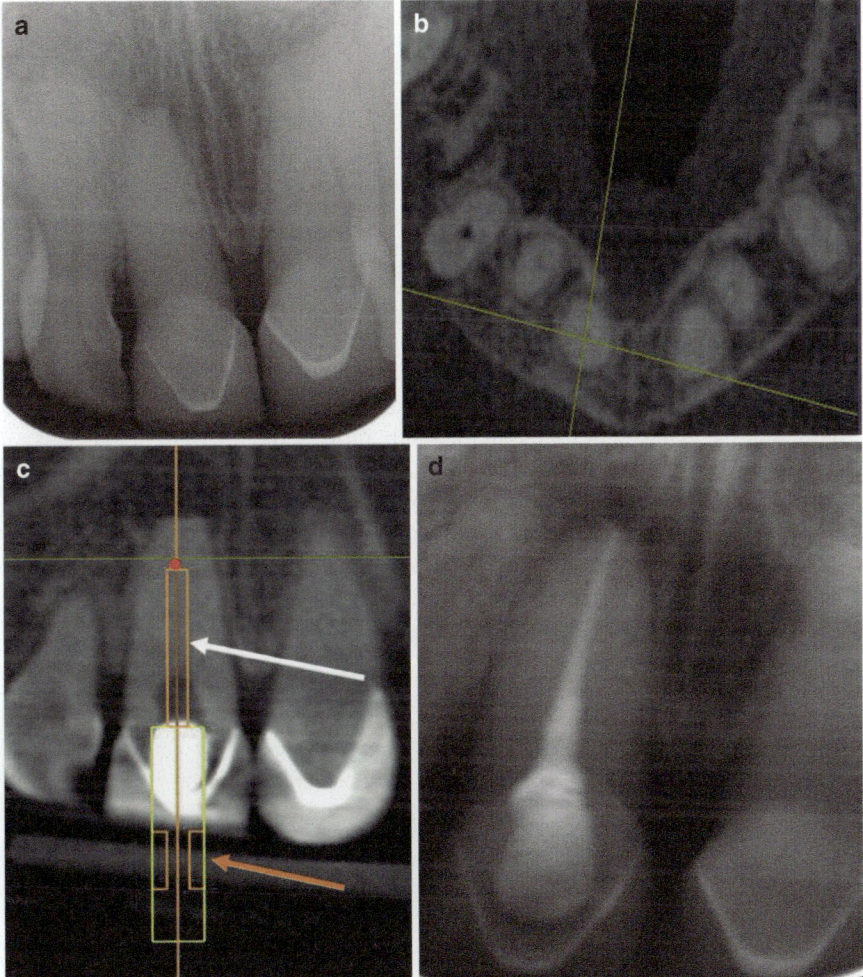

Fig. 4.7 (**a**) A radiograph of tooth no 8 with an apical pathosis. There is no visible space of the root canal neither on the radiograph nor on the CBCT. The apical pathosis is a sign of remaining pulp tissue in the pulp space. (**b**) The pulp space is located at the centre of the axial view of the root, that is the long axis of the root, even if it is neither seen at the axial view nor at the tangential view. (**c**) The virtual drill path (white arrow) reaching the target point (red dot). Yellow part is the virtual sleeve (orange arrow). (**d**) The final root canal filling

where the remnants of the root canal are in the centre of the periphery of root. This only applies to teeth with one single root canal. If the periphery of the root has concavities, reflecting the presence of separation structures, it can be presumed that the root has more than one canal.

The Angle of the Path

The ideal angle of the virtual path ensures that the drill path stays in the axis of the root from the target point to the entrance point and that the drilling thereby reaches the root canal space, short of the target point if possible (Fig. 4.7c). If the canal cannot be scouted, the drill will stay in the axis of the root and thereby lower the risk of perforations even if it turns out to be necessary to drill beyond the target point.

Often, a drill path placed in the axis of an incisor will interfere with the incisal edge and as a result, the drilling will damage the tooth needless. In these cases, the angle of the drill path can be changed by tilting the virtual drill path. But, at the same time more, caution is needed: not to drill over the target point (Figs. 4.8 and 4.9).

The Diameter of the Drill

The diameter of the drill has to be big enough to avoid bending of the drill during use. On the contrary, as the drill hole will weaken the tooth, there is an upper limit of drill size, depending on the remaining tooth substance and size of the tooth. To secure that the diameter is usable in the tooth, most of the software brands make it possible to do a rotating slice view around the axis of the virtual drill path. In this way, it is possible to assure that the drill path leaves sufficient dentin even at concavities of the root. For non-surgical endodontics treatment, recommended diameter of drill is 1.00 mm or less. Once the above parameters are determined, we can use those diameters and design the guide over tooth surface.

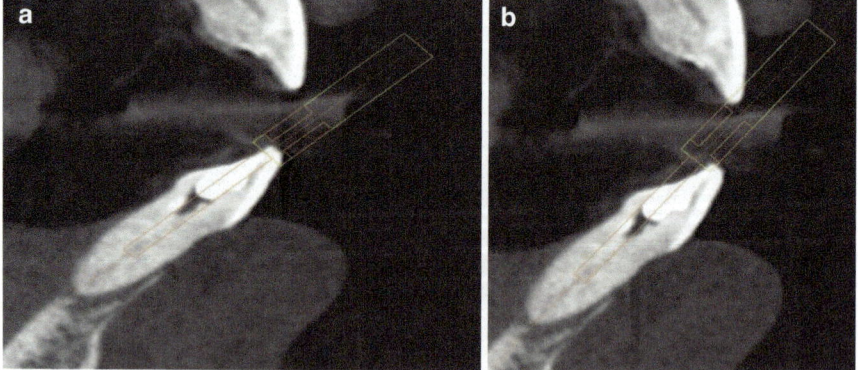

Fig. 4.8 (a) A drill path in the centre line of the tooth will involve the incisal edge. (b) The virtual drill path can be tilted to avoid the incisal edge

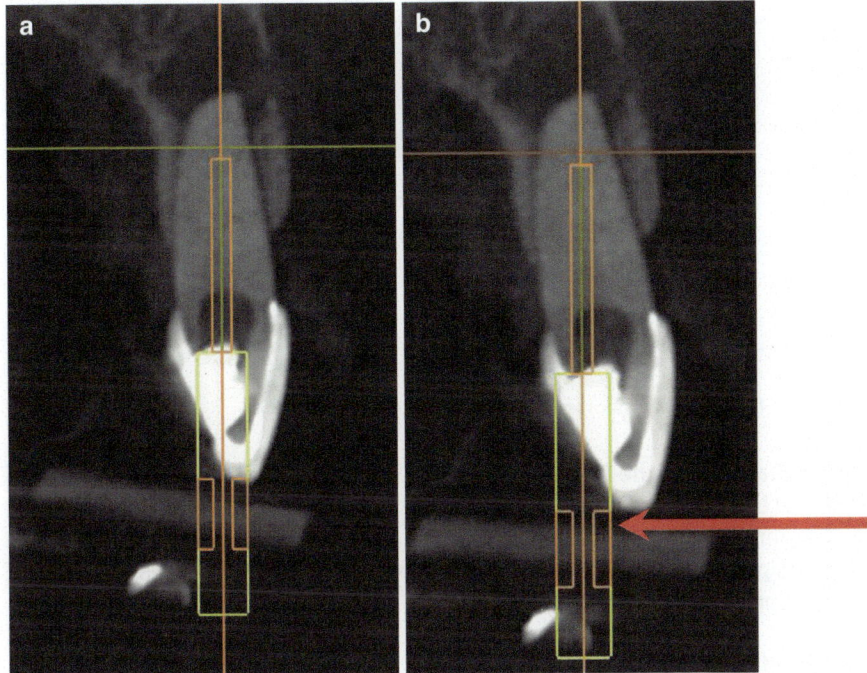

Fig. 4.9 (**a**) A drill path in the centre line of the tooth will involve the incisal edge. (**b**) The virtual drill path can be tilted to avoid the incisal edge (red arrow). Note the wrong direction of the original attempt to negotiate the root canal

4.3.4.3 Sleeve Selection
When the target, the angle and the diameter of the bur are decided, a virtual sleeve is added to the scan. For sleeve selection, there are three important parameters.

Sleeve Inert Type
There are two type of sleeve inserts (Fig. 4.10):

1. Hand-hold sleeve inserts (drill key)
2. Drill-hold sleeve inserts (guide sleeve)

Hand-hold sleeve does not provide good stability and that can lead to inaccurate drilling. Guide sleeves are recommended for endodontic treatments.

Inner Diameter of the Sleeve
Inner diameter of the sleeve corresponds to the chosen bur/drill diameter. Recommended inner diameter should be 0.1 mm larger diameter than the diameter of the bur. If virtual drill diameter is 1.0 mm, inner diameter of the metal sleeve should be 1.1 mm.

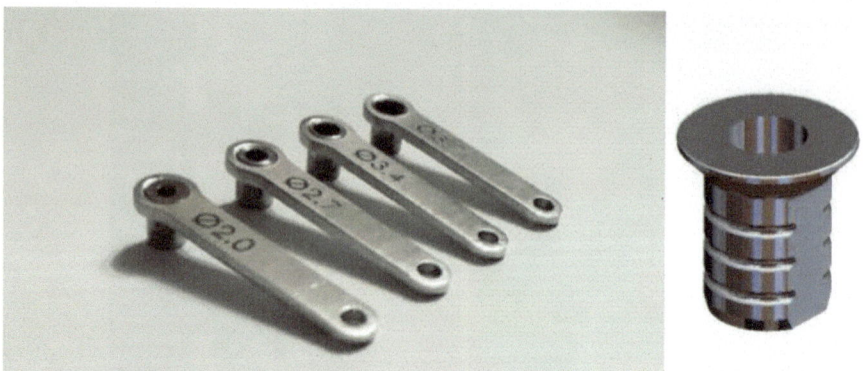

Fig. 4.10 Drill key (Left side) and guide sleeve (Right side)

Outer Diameter of the Sleeve

It should be minimum 0.1 mm larger than inner diameter for stability. It is necessary to determine the outer diameter as we need to provide that space in guide designing. It also depends upon the type of 3D printer, printer settings and resin used for guide fabrication.

Height of the Sleeve

Increase in height of the sleeve reduces apical and coronal deviation of the drill and improves angulation of the drill as well [5]. Recommended sleeve height for endodontic treatment is 5–7 mm. For posterior teeth, due to lack of inter-occlusal distance, it can be reduced.

4.3.4.4 Other Parameters To Be Considered for Endoguide Planning

Offset of the Guide

Offset can be adjusted to set the clearance between guide and the contact surface. This affects the fit of the guide. The author's experience is that 0.15 mm is ideal (Fig. 4.11). If it is less, then it is too difficult to put in or take out the guide. If offset is more than 0.15 mm, the stability of guide may be compromised.

Thickness of the Guide

Thickness of the guide affects the stability of the manufactured guide against torsion. Thickness of the guide around the sleeve is also crucial. If thickness around sleeves is less, guide may fracture or break during drilling procedure. After adjusting the wall thickness of the guide, recommended thickness of the guide is 3.5 mm. Sometimes, it needs to be changed because of the weakness of the printing material.

Coverage of the Guide

It is necessary to cover the adjacent teeth in the guide design for stability of the guide. Improper coverage can lead to unstable guide and inaccurate drilling.

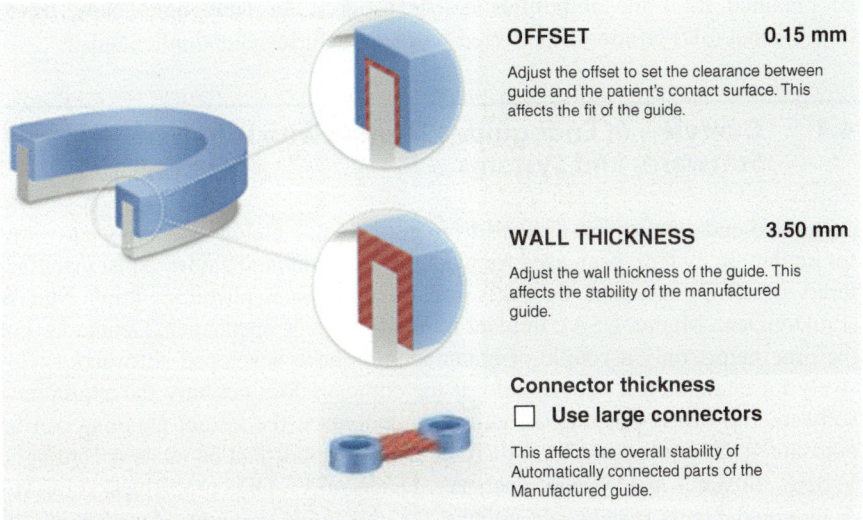

OFFSET   **0.15 mm**

Adjust the offset to set the clearance between guide and the patient's contact surface. This affects the fit of the guide.

WALL THICKNESS   **3.50 mm**

Adjust the wall thickness of the guide. This affects the stability of the manufactured guide.

Connector thickness

☐ **Use large connectors**

This affects the overall stability of Automatically connected parts of the Manufactured guide.

Fig. 4.11 Offset, wall thickness and large connectors can be set

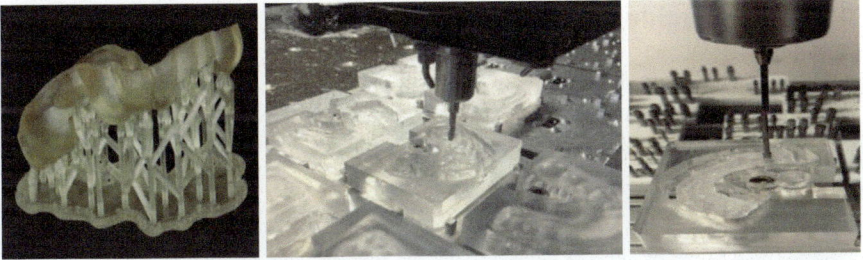

Fig. 4.12 3D printed model and CNC milling

Inspection Window

It is useful to add custom inspection window to evaluate the surface of the tooth. It helps to inspect fit of the guide. Inspection window can also be useful to dissipate heat generated from drilling. It also allows use of extra coolant from that surface, if needed. Improper and over-extended inspection window may lead to weakening of the guide.

Custom Labels

Custom labels can also be added to distinguish between different surgical guides, or to customize guided by labelling patent's name or length of the drill.

After incorporating all the parameters and designing endodontic guide, re-check the design of endodontic guide. This design is exported (as an STL file) to a print house or dental laboratory or an in-house 3D printer. Initially, CNC milling machines were used to fabricate endodontic guide (Fig. 4.12). Certificate of accuracy has to be obtained from the authorities before using it for endoguide. Now, three-dimensional (3D) printing is preferred for manufacturing endodontic guide.

4.4 Overview of Endoguide Planning with Different Softwares and Systems

As guided endodontics has evolved from guided implantology, planning softwares for implantology have been used for planning of endodontic guides. Most manufacturers of CBCT scanners deliver software for implant planning: Impla Station (ProDigiDent, Miami, USA), Implant Studio (3shape, Copenhagen, Denmark). For the time being, only a couple of manufacturers have developed softwares exclusively for endodontics: SICATEndo. If the clinician does not have the appropriate software for virtual planning of guided endodontics, the virtual planning can be outsourced. After approval from the clinician, the guide can be made accordingly. Various softwares and systems, such as coDiagnostiX®, DDS pro, Blueskybio, AIS Acteon and 2Ingis system, are popular for endoguide planning. An overview of endoguide planning with different softwares and systems has been given below.

4.4.1 Endoguide Planning with coDiagnostiX®

coDiagnostiX® is a guide designing software from Dental Wings GmbH, a Straumann group company. It was mainly developed for implant planning, but we can use it for endoguide designing as well (Fig. 4.13).

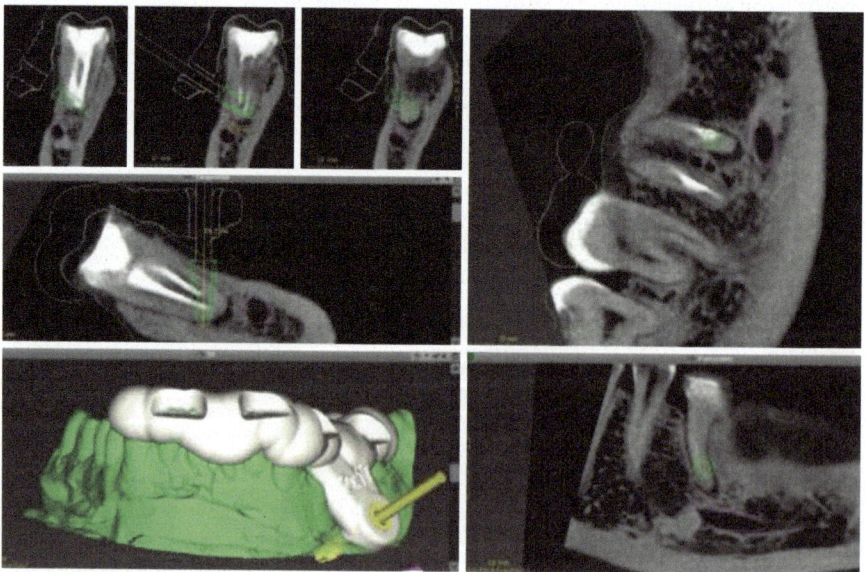

Fig. 4.13 Surgical endoguide planning with coDiagnostiX® for root end resection surgery in mesial root of lower first molar

- **Step 1: Import CBCT data**

  From options, load CBCT data (DICOM file). CBCT should not be taken in occlusion. Try to place cotton rolls or mouth pop, and take CBCT in open position with smaller field of volume (FOV) and higher resolution. It helps in easier segmentation during planning (Fig. 4.14).

- **Step 2: Selection of the arch**

  Select upper or lower arch. It is vital as the system defines all the later steps related to the chosen arch (e.g., segmentation, alignment, positioning and virtual guide) (Fig. 4.15).

- **Step 3: Segmentation**

  This step helps to clear up the 3D picture from the noise (Fig. 4.16).

- **Step 4: Alignments**

  Superimpose data in axial, sagittal and coronal views (Fig. 4.17). Not only the hard tissue but also the soft tissue can help to have accurate alignment, but the latter is only secondary.

- **Step 5: Virtual drill path planning and sleeve selection**

  Target point and virtual drill path planning has been explained detail in this chapter (Figs. 4.7, 4.8, and 4.9). Different sleeve systems can be used, or new ones can be designed (Fig. 4.18).

- **Step 6: Design Endoguide**

  Design endoguide with proper support from adjacent teeth. Offset of guide and thickness of material should be considered before printing the guide. Check alignment of the guide and re-evaluate virtual drill path and inclination. After checking all mentioned parameters, now file can be exported to laboratory or 3D printer for printing. Custom label can also be incorporated on the guide (Fig. 4.19a).

- **Step 7: Documentation**

  This step is optional. This software has option of screenshots to document minute details of planning. On completion, PDF file can be generated to document important aspects of the planning.

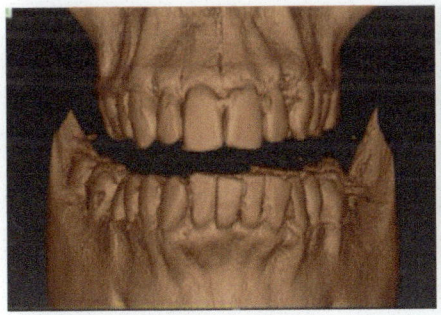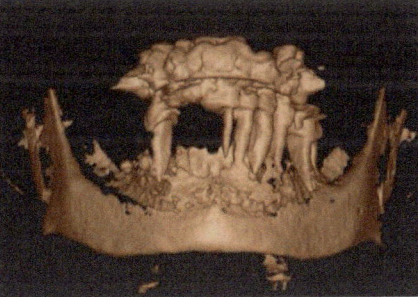

Fig. 4.14 CBCT with open and closed positions. Open position CBCT allows easy segmentation with this software

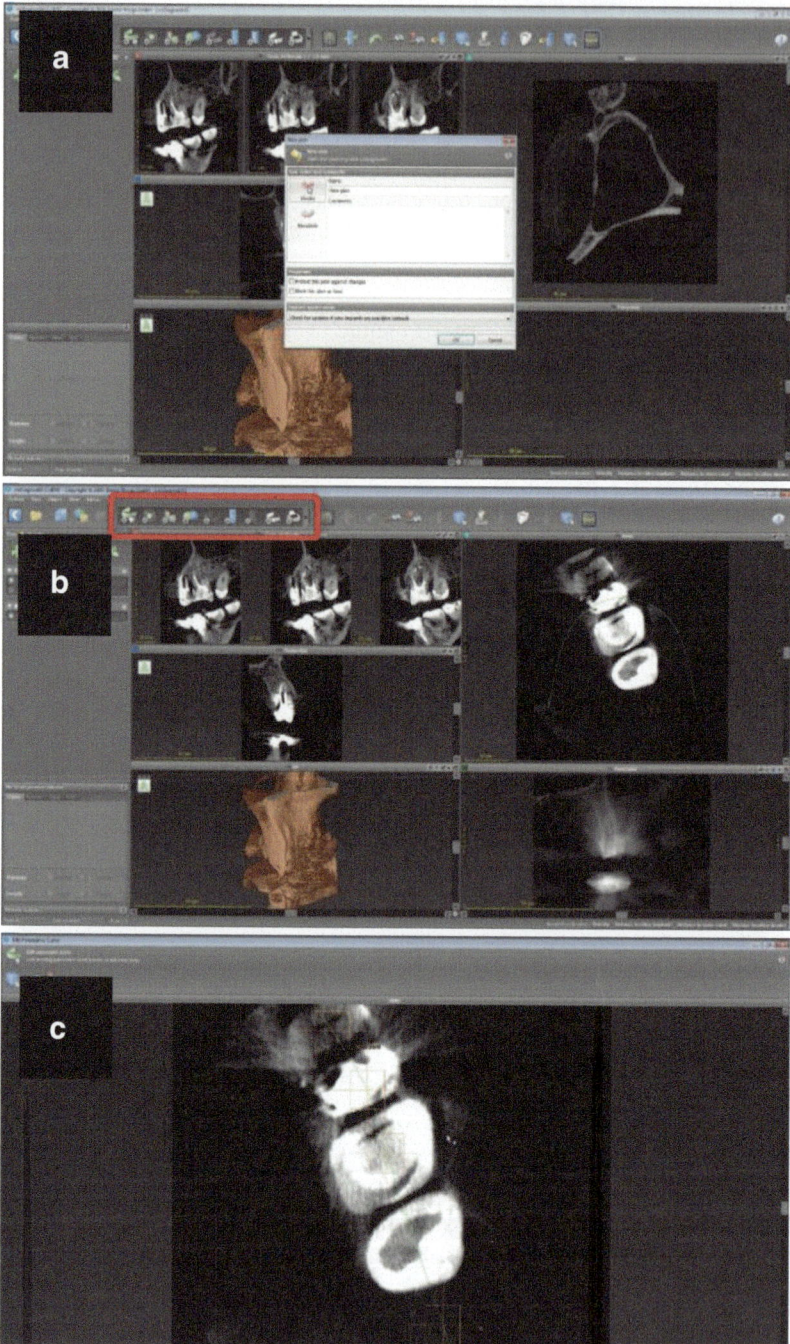

Fig. 4.15 (**a**) Selection of the arch. (**b**) Red box highlights the working line suggested by the software. It helps in step-by-step planning of the guide. (**c**) During segmentation, place the tooth of interest in the centre

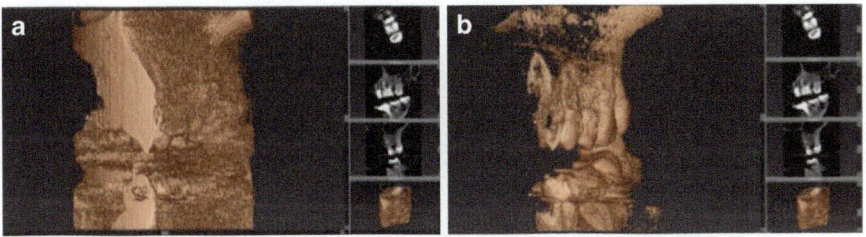

Fig. 4.16 (**a**) Noisy CBCT scan. (**b**) Noise has been cleared to evaluate intra-oral surfaces

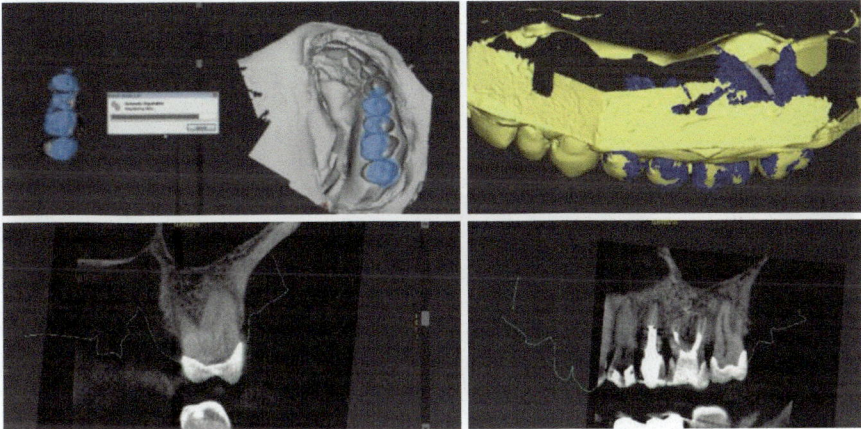

Fig. 4.17 Superimposition and alignment of surface scan and CBCT scan in axial, sagittal and coronal views. Soft tissue alignment is marked by green colour on radiographs

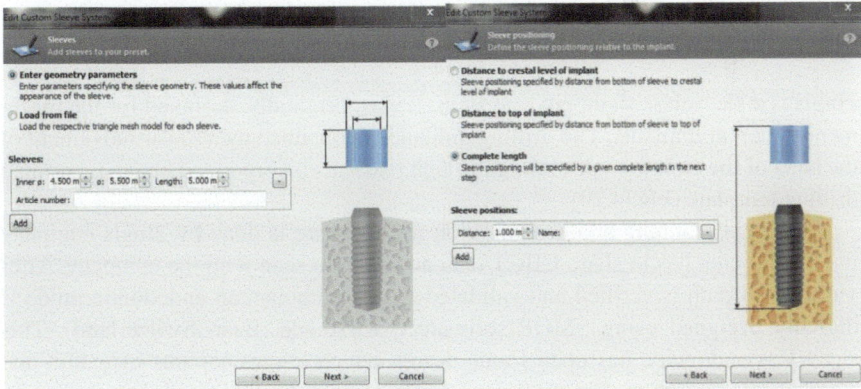

Fig. 4.18 Any parameter not listed in the database can be added to the software: inside and outside diameter or height of a sleeve. The distance of the sleeve can be given by three different aspects

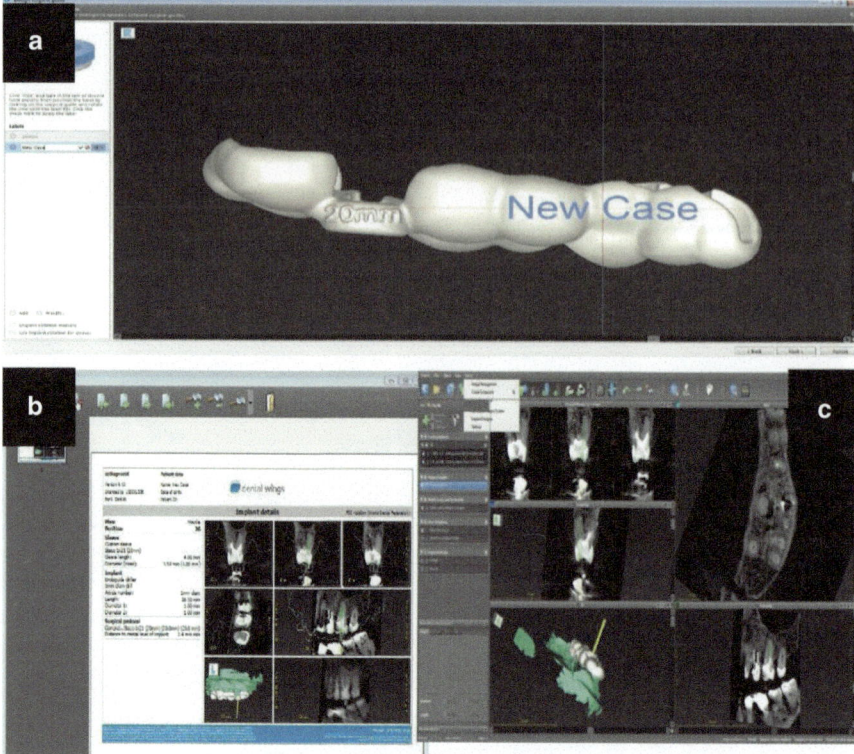

Fig. 4.19 (**a**) Custom label on the guide, (**b**) PDF file to document endoguide planning and designing, (**c**) Screenshot for documentation

4.4.2 Endoguide Planning with 2Ingis® Technology System

2Ingis is a sleeveless static guide system. It was, originally, designed for the placement of dental implants. The drilling guidance is obtained by a linear movement of the head of the contra-angle sliding through two rails incorporated in the 3D printed drilling template (Fig. 4.20).

Treatment planning and designing on the software is done by 2Ingis company itself. Clinician has to share CBCT data and surface scan with the company. After virtual drill path is verified and validated by the clinician, an endodontic guide is digitally designed using SMOP software (Swissmeda, Baar, Switzerland). This sleeveless endoguide has open frame design which allows copious irrigation and avoids heat generation (Figs. 4.21 and 4.22). Schnutenhaus S et al. has reported a mean deviation of angle of 2.85° with this system which is more precise than conventional guides with sleeves [6, 7]. Further clinical trials are required for this new promising technology.

Fig. 4.20 The 2Ingis guide designed to direct head of contra-angled handpiece for guided endodontics

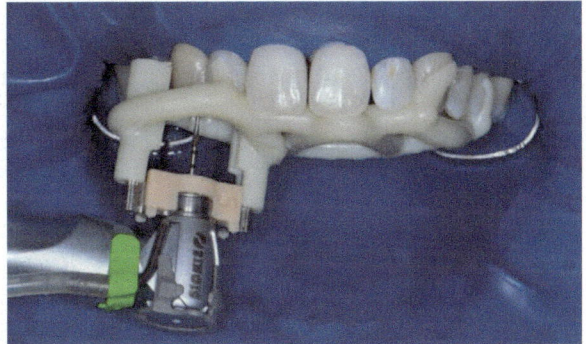

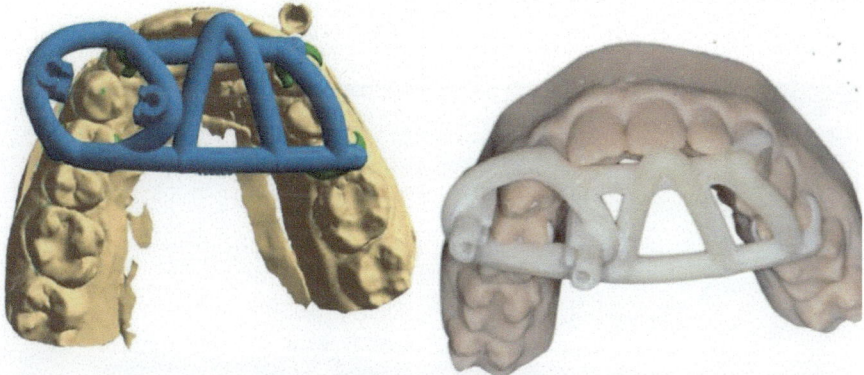

Fig. 4.21 The digital design of the 2Ingis guide and its 3D impression. The guide is digitally designed using certain teeth for support. (Courtesy: Philippe De Moyer)

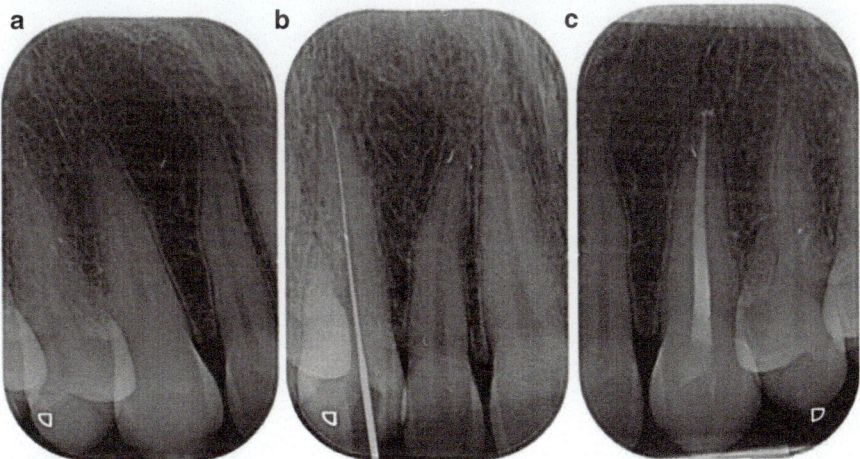

Fig. 4.22 (**a–c**) Management of calcified canal in maxillary canine. Pre-operative, patency and post-operative radiographs of the case planned and treated with 2Ingis system. (Courtesy: Antonietta Bordone, Cyril Perez)

4.4.3   Endoguide Planning with DDS Pro Software

4.4.4   Endoguide planning with Acteon® Imaging Software (AIS)

Figure 4.23 and 4.24 depicts endoguide planning and designing with DDS Pro software and Acteon® Imaging Software (AIS), respectively.

Though science of guided endodontics has evolved over the past few years, still there is limited availability of specialized software for endodontic guide designing. In the currently available software, there is limited availability of endodontic file library. Planning of endodontic guide for surgical endodontics has been explained in Chap. 8. Guided endodontics only helps in exploration of calcified canal, but one should always remember that cleaning of the root canal system is of utmost importance for success of the root canal treatment.

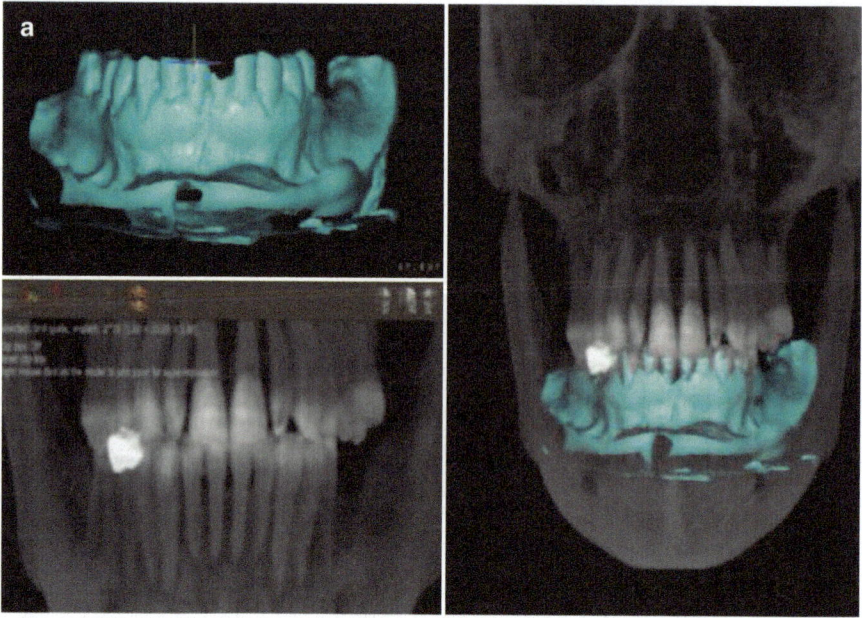

Fig. 4.23   (**a**) Superimposition of surface scans with DDS Pro software, (**b**) Target point selection for mesial root of mandibular molar, (**c**) Design of endodontic guide for mesial root canal system

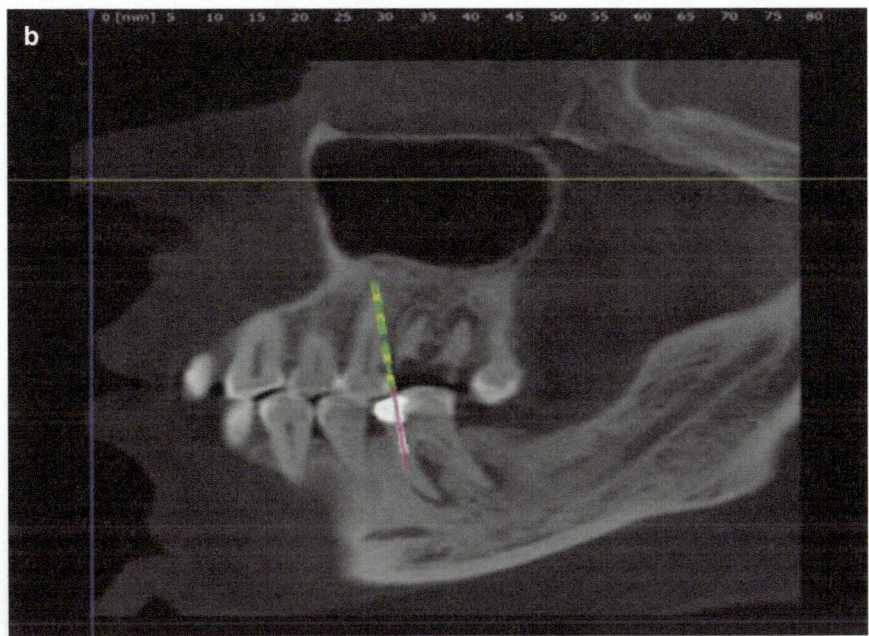

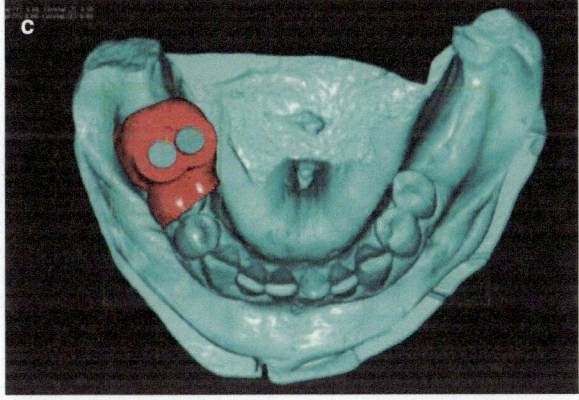

Fig. 4.23 (continued)

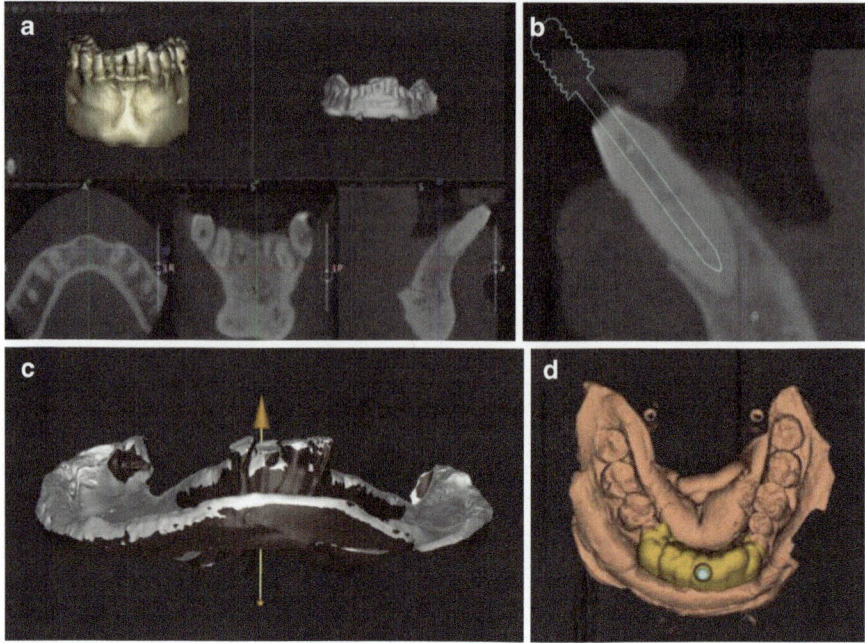

Fig. 4.24 (**a**) Superimposition of scans, (**b**) Virtual drill path for calcified canal, (**c**) Determining the placement path and undercut determination, (**d**) Designing of endoguide

References

1. Patel S, Aldowaisan A, Dawood A. A novel method for soft tissue retraction during periapical surgery using 3D technology: a case report. Int Endod J. 2017;50(8):813–22.
2. Strbac GD, Schnappauf A, Giannis K, Moritz A, Ulm C. Guided modern endodontic surgery: a novel approach for guided osteotomy and root resection. J Endod. 2017;43:496.
3. Ahn SY, Kim NH, Kim S, Karabucak B, Kim E. Computer-aided Design/Computer-aided Manufacturing-guided endodontic surgery: guided osteotomy and apex localization in a mandibular molar with a thick buccal bone plate. J Endod. 2018;44(4):665–70. https://doi.org/10.1016/j.joen.2017.12.009.
4. Giacomino CM, Ray JJ, Wealleans JA. Targeted endodontic microsurgery: a novel approach to anatomically challenging scenarios using 3-dimensional-printed guides and trephine burs-a report of 3 cases. J Endod. 2018;44:671.
5. Koop R, Vercruyssen M, Vermeulen K, Quirynen M. Tolerance within the sleeve inserts of different surgical guides for guided implant surgery. Clin Oral Implants Res. 2013;24:630–4.
6. Schnutenhaus S, von Koenigsmarck V, Blender S, Ambrosius L, Luthardt RG. Precision of sleeveless 3D drill guides for insertion of one-piece ceramic implants: a prospective clinical trial. Int J Comput Dent. 2018;21(2):97–105.
7. Schnutenhaus S, Edelmann C, Rudolph H, Dreyhaupt J, Luthardt RG. 3D accuracy of implant positions in template-guided implant placement as a function of the remaining teeth and the surgical procedure: a retrospective study. Clin Oral Investig. 2018;22(6):2363–72.

3D Printing in Endodontics

5

Gunpreet Oberoi and Hermann Agis

5.1 Introduction of 3D Printing

The embracement of 3D printing, also termed additive manufacturing, has brought an unforeseen renaissance in both treatment and diagnostic protocols in a variety of specialties in dentistry [1, 2]. Its ability to provide customization and unbeatable accuracy, while also being cost-effective, makes it a catalyst in advancing the world of medicine [3]. Its popularity is further heightened by the reproducibility of the delivered product, undemanding acquisition of skills, and unrestrained data allocation [4, 5]. Its universality is based on the fact that it interests users from every niche, from student to clinician, and even extends to the patient [6, 7]. This fact is reflected by a global increase in the procurement of 3D printers in the last decade, in both hospital and private clinical set-ups [8]. In dentistry, 3D printing has experimental, clinical, and educational applications (Fig. 5.1).

Since the advent of the use of additive manufacturing in the 1980s, dentistry, in particular endodontology, has experienced an outstanding enhancement in the advancement of workflow [9]. There has been an evolution in the technology from the development of the first 3D printing systems by Charles (Chuck) Hull in 1984 up to the cutting-edge bioprinting tools (Fig. 5.2).

To establish an additively manufactured driven workflow (Fig. 5.3), one needs access to the three basic technologies constituting the digital inventory, but without any geographical limitations:

1. 3D image acquisition with intraoral scan, computed tomography (CT) or cone beam CT (CBCT), or optical scanners such as intraoral impression scanners [11–13]

G. Oberoi (✉) · H. Agis
Department of Conservative Dentistry and Periodontology, University Clinic of Dentistry,
Medical University of Vienna, Vienna, Austria
e-mail: gunpreet.oberoi@meduniwien.ac.at; hermann.agis@meduniwien.ac.at

© Springer Nature Switzerland AG 2021
N. Kinariwala, L. Samaranayake (eds.), *Guided Endodontics*,
https://doi.org/10.1007/978-3-030-55281-7_5

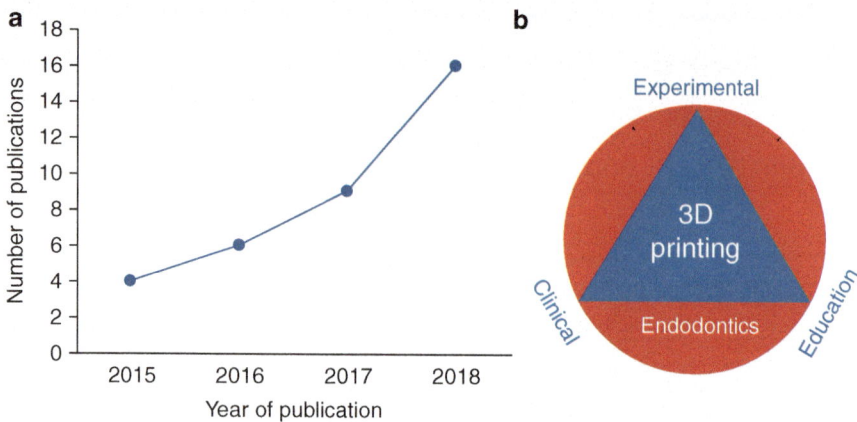

Fig. 5.1 The application of 3D printing in endodontics. The interest in the application of 3D printing in dentistry and endodontics has increased over the past years. The also becomes evident when evaluating the number of publications per year over time (**a**). The application of 3D printing in endodontics comprises the application in the clinics for the production of guides, in education for the printing of models, and for experimental purposes such as preclinical testing of 3D printed scaffolds for tissue engineering purposes (**b**). (Adopted with modifications from Oberoi et al. [2])

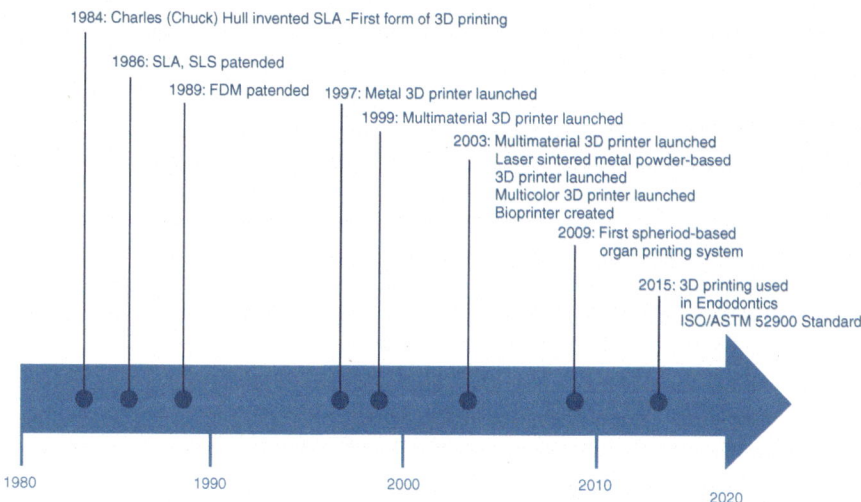

Fig. 5.2 Timeline of the evolution of 3D printing and the milestones in the application of 3D printing in endodontics

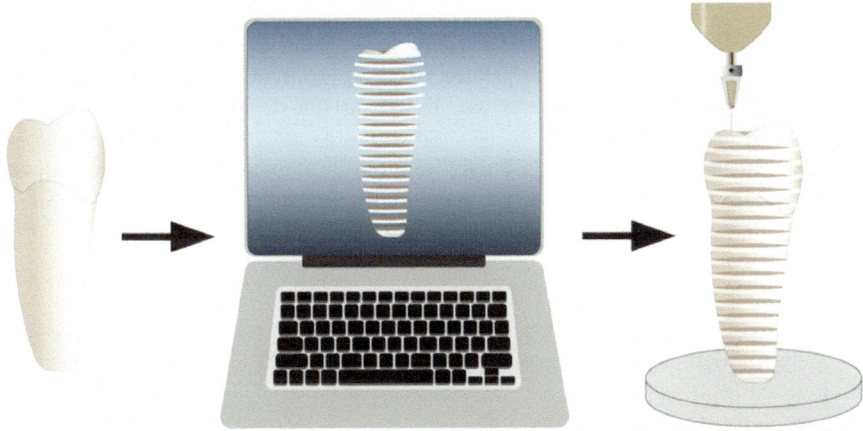

Fig. 5.3 The generic workflow of 3D printing. Based on scans by intraoral impressions or computed tomography, a digital model is designed, which is then translated into an STL file. This file is then sliced with the appropriate software and sent to the 3D printer for production. Depending on the printer-specific software, post processing may then be required. (Adopted with modifications from Ligon et al. [10])

2. A digital software for conversion of the output files the digital imaging and communications in medicine (DICOM) data of the scanners into a printable format such as the standard tessellation language (STL) files [14, 15]
3. 3D printing system

The image acquisition reverberates with 3D printing technology as the output is dependent on the quality of volumetric data obtained in the first place [9, 16]. The data source plays a crucial role from image acquisition, rendering and segmentation, designing and reconstruction, to the final printing process [17, 18]. By adjusting imaging parameters, one can optimize the desired quality of hte DICOM data for the printing process [19, 20]. There is sufficient evidence in the literature supporting high-resolution CBCT as a good imaging modality for almost all dental applications, while for research purposes, micro-CT is known to provide an in-depth image of the structure [21, 22].

The next step is the reconstruction of digital models using computer-aided software. A plethora of software programs are available, both free and licensed for image rendering, segmentation, redesigning, and conversion into an STL file [14, 15, 23]. With such software programs, it is possible to replicate the missing anatomy, redesign the data as necessary, and visualize a digital model before the printing process [24]. High-resolution micro-CT data can be remeshed and reduced to low-resolution data using these software programs, which are easier to work with, while maintaining the image quality. Certain software packages avail the clinician to perform virtual surgeries, implant placements, access cavity preparations, teeth alignment, smile designing, etc., and predict the prognosis of the treatment protocol [25–27]. Finally, the product is printed using appropriate printing materials and with the appropriate printing system, based on the desired characteristics and purpose.

With easily accessible imaging data required in almost all dental applications, additive manufacturing is gaining rapid popularity in dentistry [28–30]. 3D printers, which are now widely available, work using five basic mechanisms:

1. Fused deposition modeling (FDM)
2. Selective laser sintering (SLS)
3. Stereolithography (SLA)/direct light processing (DLP)
4. Poly-jet printing
5. Bioprinting [10, 31–36] (Fig. 5.4)

FDM printers have captured both small- and large-scale dental and medical units due to its wide availability, moderate accuracy in terms of printing resolution, technique-friendly installation, and cost-effectiveness [37]. It is capable of printing with multiple materials [38]. The filament material gets heated up and melts are heated and melted as they pass through the hot nozzle. On extrusion, it builds the object, one layer at a time. As the cost-effective option, it is recommended for anatomical model fabrication with simpler geometries [39].

In SLS and SLA, laser is the main source of light, which builds the object, layer-by-layer, from powder and liquid resin [38, 40].

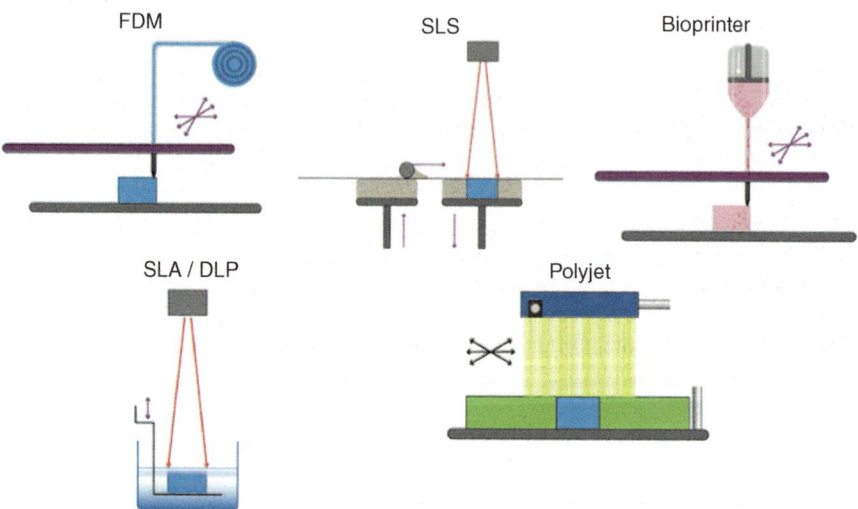

Fig. 5.4 3D printing systems. 3D printing methods applied in many fields of medicine and dentistry including fused deposition modeling (FDM), selective laser sintering (SLS), stereolithography (SLA), poly-jet, and bioprinting. (Adopted with modifications from Ligon e al. [10])

DLP uses a projector. The most advanced and robust 3D printer for polymers available today is the poly-jet printer. Here the final printed object is built from a variety of liquid polymers where the 3D model is created, one layer at a time using ultraviolet light for curing of the polymers [41]. Poly-jet printing's high cost and space requirement makes it mostly suitable for high-scale or industrial set-ups [41, 42].

Translation of tissue engineering principles into additive manufacturing, such as scaffold geometry as well as macro-, micro-, and nanolevel alterations in the design of constructed tissue, has been a huge asset for regenerative medicine [43–48]. Customization of cell-laden 3D-printed scaffolds using additive manufacturing for filling the defect leads to better vascularization and healing [46]. In this aspect, cell-ink-based bioprinters can be used with optimized printing parameters to print extra-cellular matrix for cells, providing an in-vivo-like microenvironment for growth [31, 49–56]. A multitude of materials can be bioprinted such as chitosan [57], calcium silicate complex and bioactive-agent-containing controlled-release polymeric materials [58, 59]. This technique has the future promise of saving patients from donor-site comorbidities, graft-size related issues, ethics, and accessibility of autologous grafts [60]. We will come back to the advantages and disadvantages of the specific technologies later in the chapter.

Adoption of 3D printing is not just limited to material science and prototyping, but is also used to evolve the clinical sphere of dental medicine. With neoteric innovations in technology and material science, dental surgery has met a completely new outlook. It has greatly improved the management of cases in prosthodontics, cranio-maxillo-facial surgery, orthodontics, periodontics, and, last but not the least, endodontics [22, 32, 61–64]. This development is revealed by the rapid rise in the published literature supporting the use of 3D printing in dentistry and medicine, more so in the latter. In the past decade, oral and maxillofacial surgery and prosthodontics were the cynosure of dental applications in 3D printing, but, gradually, other fields like endodontics are slowly taking leverage of this technology [1, 2, 20, 64, 65]. Inclusion of additive manufacturing into diagnostic dental and medical procedures such as 3D printed dental models based on radiographic imaging and oral scanning greatly improves the quality of data acquisition [22, 66]. This also provides an excellent tool for patient education, acquainting them with the existing problem and the proposed treatment protocol [67, 68]. The digital information acquired during diagnosis acts as a platform for virtual treatment planning, while the 3D-printed model improves the clinical and dental skills with the possibility to perform mock-procedures [1, 69, 70]. Currently, haptic simulators are gaining potential in the state-of-the-art dentistry by providing proprioception and psycho-motor skills to the clinician [1, 64]. 3D printing has the remarkable capacity to enhance oral health care in research, clinical treatment, and education of both patients and dental students. In dentistry, and specifically endodontics, compared with stereotypical treatment planning using 2D images, additive manufacturing workflow has impressively improved the understanding and interpretation of complicated anatomical structures: benefiting teaching and case management, including treatment planning and follow-up. However, owing to the relatively recent introduction of 3D printed objects and haptic simulators in endodontics, there is a paucity of published literature in this sphere. Therefore, this chapter will provide a detailed insight into the prevailing clinical, educational, and experimental aspects of additive manufacturing in endodontics (Fig. 5.1).

5.2   3D Printing Systems and Workflows

3D printing is a game-changing technique with a wide array of application [2]. Compared to traditional ways of manufacturing, including formative and subtractive manufacturing, it has several advantages, especially with regards to personalized printing. So let us evaluate the generic process of 3D printing (Fig. 5.2) [10]. First, the object is designed digitally using an appropriate software. In dentistry, several scanning systems are available including intraoral scanning and CBCT, which then require further processing to generate a digital model. This digital model is then translated into a generic file such as the STL file. Using a slicer program, the model is then sliced into layers and the parameters of the printing process are defined, as several printing systems are very specific and the control of the 3D printer is normally done with printer-specific software provided by the printer manufacturer. The object is then generated by adding layers of the printing material. Depending on the 3D printing technology and the printing material used, specific postprocessing steps are required. The first instruments became commercially available in the 1980s [10]. Over the past decades, a broad variety of technologies have been developed, which required standardized terms and nomenclature (Fig. 5.3) [10, 71]. Finally, the American Society for Testing and Materials (ASTM) International Committee F42 on Additive Manufacturing Technology defined specific terms for additive manufacturing in 2009 [10]. These terms were established in 2015 as ISO/ASTM 52900 Standard [71] (Table 5.1).

Table 5.1 Nomenclature of 3D printing technologies

Process categories according to ISO/ASTM 52900	Printing technology nomenclature
Extrusion	Fused filament fabrication (FFF), fused deposition modeling (FDM)
Vat polymerization	Stereolithography (SLA), direct light processing (DLP)
Powder bed fusion	Selective laser sintering (SLS), direct metal laser sintering (DMLS), selective laser melting (SLM), electron beam melting (EBM)
Material jetting	Material jetting (MJ), drop on demand (DOD)
Binder jetting	Binder Jetting (BJ)
Direct energy deposition	Laser engineering net shaping (LENS), Laser-based metal deposition (LBMD)
Sheet lamination	Ultrasonic additive manufacturing (UAM), laminated object manufacturing (LOM)

Adopted with modifications from [10, 71]

FDM, also known as fused filament fabrication (FFF), was one of the first 3D printing technology available for the public for a reasonable price. It is based on extrusion. Basically, a thermoplastic material such as PLA or ABS is heated and extruded through a nozzle in the print head [71]. By adjusting the nozzle diameter, print head movement speed and loading speed of the material the resolution of the printer can be optimized. FDM printers are low cost with regard to material and the printing systems. In addition, handling the system is quite easy. However, the layer-by-layer deposition results in visible lines in the object, which can only be removed by postprocessing [71]. Due to the deposition method, FDM printed objects have different physical properties depending on the orientation of the layers [71]. Therefore, printing orientation is of high relevance and needs to be adjusted to the application of the part.

SLA/DLP uses vat polymerization; in other words, it uses light to polymerize the liquid resin in a tank, thereby printing the object layer by layer [71]. Bottom-up and top-down systems are available. Some systems use a single beam, which scans the area to generate a layer, while others use light projecting systems, which polymerize the layer at once to improve the printing speed (DLP) [71]. After a layer is finished, the printing platform is moved to allow the next layer to be printed on top of the finished layer. If you compare SLA and DLP, the main difference is the source of light, which is used in the two different printing systems [71]. While SLA uses a point light beam, the DLP applies a voxel-based projector, which gives DLP a speed advantage. This is even more impressive when evaluating continuous printing systems, which do not rely on the step-by-step approach of traditional SLA systems. While FDM printers when equipped with a second print head can print more than one material per print, SLA and DLP are limited to one single material per print due to the printing technology. After printing, postprocessing is required, including washing of the printed object to remove the liquid resin and postcuring to polymerize remaining monomers and oligomers. Interestingly, this printing technology also allows for ceramic printing. Ceramic particles are mixed into a binding resin, which is then polymerized by the printing process. After cleaning, the green part is then put into a furnace and sintered to generate the final product. The chemistry of the used resins and the involved photoinitiators is reviewed by Ligon SC et al. [10] (Fig. 5.5).

Another technology is powder bed fusion, which is utilized in the SLS systems [71]. Instead of liquid resin, the SLS uses powder-based material for generating objects by fusing the powder particles by heat with different energy sources, which vary, depending on the material [71]. Typically, a laser is used, which is absorbed by the powder, thereby inducing local heating, leading to melting and solidification of the particles at the area, which is defined by the laser [10]. After this step, new powder is dispensed onto the object for the next layer [71]. Over the whole printing process, the temperature within the printing chamber is kept at a high temperature just below the melting point to limit the internal stresses and improve the printing time, and the chamber is kept under inert gas to prevent oxidation [10]. The benefits

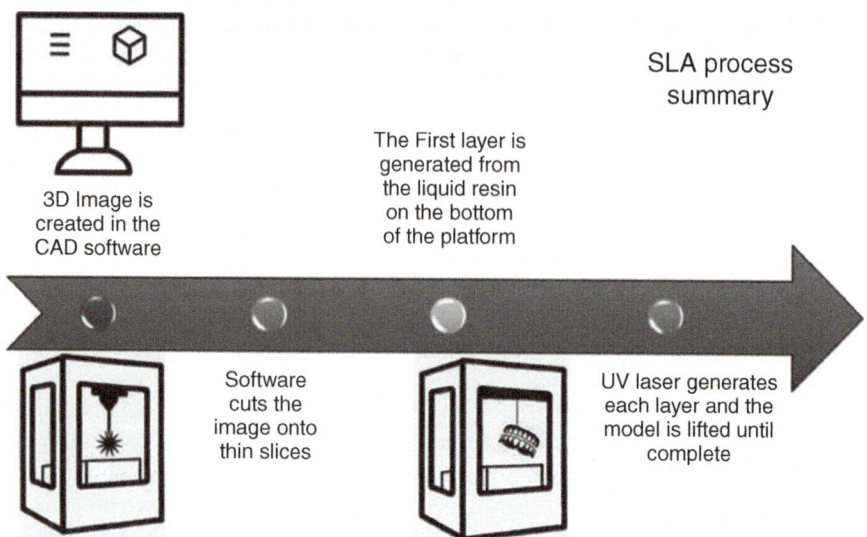

Fig. 5.5 Summary of process of 3D printing with SLA printer. (License no: 4793570032368; Courtesy: Nikoyan L et al. [72])

of this technology are the isotropy of the objects and the very high accuracy with which it prints [10]. Additionally, no support material is needed. Overall, the surface is consistent over the whole printed part. The powder materials and laser systems utilized are reviewed in [10].

The poly-jet printer builds up the object by jetting layer by layer with liquid materials, which are then polymerized by UV light. This technology allows for printing of the object with several materials with different properties. However, postprint model processing by washing and removal of solid mass support material is necessary [41]. A benefit of material jetting is that the printed object is nearly homogenous, since it is cured throughout the printing process. Due to the jetting, the surface is quite smooth, and the accuracy is the highest among all the printing systems. However, it is also one of the most expensive 3D printing technologies. As with the SLA/DLP printers, the objects are quite brittle. The chemistry of the resins used and photoinitiators is reviewed in [10].

A technology used for sand and metal printing is the binder jetting approach. Here, a binder agent is jetted onto the powder material to generate the object layer by layer [71]. This technology is used for sand and metal printing. Metal printing requires extensive postprocessing including infiltration and sintering in a furnace. In particular, shrinkage of the objects upon sintering is a big issue in this 3D printing approach. There are no residual stresses in the object as no rapid heating and cooling protocols are applied. Due to the printing technology, the surface is mainly grainy, and the objects are very fragile when taken out of the printer. The chemistry of the used materials and binders is reviewed in [10, 71].

Inspired by the idea of building a functional organ, bioprinting technologies were developed to print products that contain living cells [73, 74]. The applied technologies include cell ink-based bioprinters or spheroid/microtissue-based systems. Spheroid-/microtissue-based technologies use spheroids/microtissues as building blocks to build the construct block-by-block, similar to LEGO [75]. Spheroids are either applied by a syringe-like applicator with or without a scaffold or placed on a needle array to allow clear location of the specific spheroids. More complex approaches have been applied where honeycomb- or toroid-like shapes are used in Bio-Pick, Place, and Perfuse approaches [53]. All these approaches have to consider that spheroids and microtissues are not stable constructs, but change over time [76, 77]. Therefore, studies, which highlight the contraction dynamics of these systems, are necessary. A key issue with regard to the comparison of cell-ink- and microtissue-based approaches is the required number of cells. While in cell-ink-based approaches, the cells are suspended in the cell-ink, which serves as a scaffold, this is not the case in microtissues where the whole construct is built up by cells alone [75, 78]. Since only a limited number of stem cells can be isolated—which then require expansion with the risk of losing the required properties of the cells—it is important to have the right GMP facilities and expansion strategy available to generate enough cells for the required approach. Currently, bioprinting systems are used for experimental purposes, allowing for the generation of complex in vitro models and experimental constructs for tissue engineering approaches. The available technology and the used materials are reviewed in [36, 50, 73, 74, 79, 80].

With this technological development, 3D printing has transformed the discipline of tissue engineering and stem cell therapy. Bioprinting of tissue engineering constructs gives the flexibility to place cells into the desired functional 3D complex with exact control over the location of the cells in the construct [81]. A wide range of biomaterials. such as Chitosan [57], calcium silicate complex [58], and controlled-release polymeric materials with bioactive agents [59], can be used to generate scaffolds with a bioprinter. Also hydrogels, which can be applied as bioinks, have been developed and optimized for printing purposes [56, 78, 82]. These bioinks include fibrin-based gels, collagen-based gels as well as clay-based gels and cellulose-based gels. While the properties of kalonite seem not to be suitable for bioprinting, laponite-based gels have shown promising results [83, 84].

Using the above-mentioned technologies, 3D printing has been applied in the fabrication of human bone and skin grafts [85, 86]. With further advancements in technology, bioprinting may replace the current clinical strategies using autografts, which are associated with donor site morbidity [60].

There are challenges in the translation of 3D printing into the field of dental medicine and endodontics. These challenges include printing speed, resolution, mechanical properties, multimaterial Parts, and biocompatibility [10]. Clinical application of 3D printing in particular in dentistry requires a fast printing and post-processing to allow effective treatment in one visit. In addition, especially in guided endodontics and endodontic surgery, precision of the printing process is a key pre-requisite for success. Therefore, research and development on printing technology

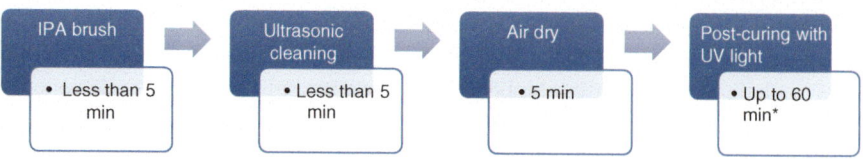

Fig. 5.6 Steps of postprocessing of 3D printed guides. It should be followed by chair-side disinfection of the guide by clinician, before clinical use. (* postcuring time may vary depending on material and manufacturer's instructions.) (Courtesy: Dr Niraj Kinariwala)

and printing material is of clinical relevance. When applying 3D printing in dental medicine, biocompatibility is a big issue, particularly since the print production process is in the hand of the hospitals, requiring distinct risk management [87].

5.2.1 Postprocessing

It is one of the most important stages of 3D printing. It can help you to get rid of both the print nuances (waviness and other defects) and the gluing traces. Another benefit of postprocessing is strengthening of a finished 3D model. Thus, postprocessing adds beauty to the finished model and additionally makes it strong.

After printing, models must be rinsed, dried, removed from support structure, and then *postcured* with curing devices containing *ultraviolet (UV) light*. Chair side disinfection of 3D printed guides should be carried out to avoid any cross-infection. After washing surgical guide, following steps can be followed (Fig. 5.6):

- Step 1: Bathe the surgical guide model in a bath of 96% isopropyl alcohol (IPA) to remove any liquid resin. Use a toothbrush to scrub the surface of the model to remove any partially cured resin. Clean with IPA for no more than 5 min.
- Step 2: Once the majority of the resin is removed, transfer the model into an ultrasonic cleaner filled with clean IPA for no more than 5 min. For this process, orient the occlusal surface of the model downward to allow resin to fall away during the agitation process. In total, the print should spend no more than 10 min in alcohol to avoid microcracks and abrasions.
- Step 3: Once cleaned, air-dry the print using compressed air. If there are any particles or residue still on the model, spray it down with more alcohol. Rinse, dry, and repeat until all uncured resin is removed.

5.3   Clinical Applications of 3D Printing in Endodontics

3D printing, with its remarkable accuracy in the production of treatment planning models and final outcomes, allows for reduction in surgical time and complications [88, 89]. Visualization and understanding of the internal root structure and tooth morphology forms the foundation of a successful endodontic treatment, and additive manufacturing has proven to be a boon in this regard [90, 91]. Geometric data from intraoral and radiographic scans used regularly for dental procedures can be harvested for multiple applications involving additive manufacturing for value-added treatment [92]. Based on this, European Society of Endodontology (ESE) stated in 2014 that CBCT should be considered in preoperative assessment and management of complex periradicular surgery. It not only overcomes the limitations of conventional 2D imaging modalities such as distortion, high noise, incomplete information, but also gives the endodontist a platform to develop numerous diagnostic and treatment planning tools, contributing toward higher prognosis in complex cases [93]. The addition of very helpful innovative patient-specific tools, such as image-based tooth and root canal models, surgical and nonsurgical guides, soft-tissue retractors, customized endodontic files, etc., to the endodontists' armamentarium, is only possible by combining 3D printing with 3D radiographic data [90].

"Guided endodontics" is defined as a novel channeled technique developed for apically extended access cavity preparation [94]. It is an adaptation of design and principles of guided implant surgeries in order to simplify complex surgical and nonsurgical endodontic procedures [3, 95]. Conventional root canal treatment offers relatively good prognosis without 3D radiographic imaging and guided endodontics, but teeth with reduced pulp spaces or obliterated canals need special modus operandi for diagnostics and treatment [96–99]. CBCT-based additively manufactured endodontic guides make the investigation of the exact anatomic coordination between each orifice and its impact on access preparation and external crown morphology easier than conventional access negotiation [100–105]. Root canals possess many anatomical variations like accessory and lateral canals, grooves, missing canals, taurodontism, C-shaped canals, bifurcations, etc. that necessitate the use of special treatment armamentarium [106–112]. These complexities are frequently neglected and procedural errors result, as these configurations are rarely detected in 2D radiographs, and, even if located by microscopes, free hand canal entrance leads to tooth structure loss [113, 114]. Navigating access opening and apicoectomy on anterior teeth is easier to navigate owing to the more accessible location and fewer canal variations. However, guided endodontic therapy optimizes the treatment procedure, providing conservative access with no tooth damage at the incisal edge in a reliable and foreseeable way, even in the presence of severe developmental anomalies or canal calcification [106, 115–118]. Use of three-dimensional imaging-based guides respects the anatomical relationship of the root apices with critical adjacent entities such as the inferior dental canal, mental foramen, and maxillary sinus [119]. In the case of surgical endodontics, presurgical 3D radiographic assessment allows groundbreaking investigation of cortical plate thickness for depth-guided drills, tooth position, and direction of root apices in the x-y-z plane, greatly improving operator skills, patient's experience, treatment time, and delivery [89, 95, 120]. Today, the dental market is flourishing with software programs specifically for planning 3D endodontic guides and drills, as well as implant planning software programs that can be applied to endodontics. These software programs, based on intraoral and radiographic scans, allow for user-friendly, structured workflow for easy identification of the shape and length of all canals and exactly determining working length, overcoming the often unreliable results from apex locators [22, 94,

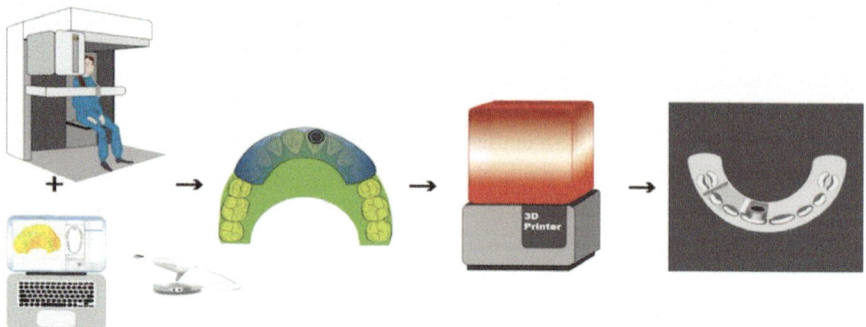

Fig. 5.7 Workflow for the generation of guides for endodontic treatment

100, 111, 115]. With the availability of cost-effective desktop 3D printers, it is possible to print customized endodontic guides, with the main objective providing navigation guidance to the operator and correct orientation to the root apex, omitting tooth structural loss and iatrogenic errors [3, 90, 114, 116]. Additively manufactured endodontic guides, similar to implant guides, consist of guide sleeves containing a customized metal tube or a 3D manufactured cylinder, providing specifically oriented access to depth-guided drills and drill keys to direct the level and angle of drills during apicoectomies (Fig. 5.7) [121–123]. Mechanical properties like structural stability of the guide, material stiffness, factors affecting design such as diameter and length of guide sleeves or drill keys, manufacturing errors, as well as operator and patient factors are known to affect their accuracy [123–125]. Miniaturization of conventional instruments allows the implementation of this technique for almost all cases of pulp canal obliteration and narrowing [96]. This technique draws a roadmap for a precise, rapid, operator-independent, yet value-based advanced endodontic treatment [65, 89]. In the case of surgical endodontics, presurgical three dimensional radiographic assessment is pre-eminent. CBCT evaluation allows thourough investigation of cortical plate thickness to determine tooth anatomy, direction of root apices and virtual drill path. This method greatly improves operator skills, patient's experience, treatment time, and delivery [85, 95, 120].

5.3.1 Guided Nonsurgical Endodontics and Retreatments

Additive manufacturing, also called rapid prototyping, coupled with a variety of CT scans such as CBCT imaging, peripheral quantitative CT imaging, and spiral CT imaging, is being increasingly promoted in the endodontic treatment of anomalous teeth [126–128]. The most common tooth anomalies occur during dental embryogenesis, root formation, or as a component of systemic syndromes, increasing the complexity of root canal treatment [129]. Some of them are root dilaceration, taurodontism, odontodysplasia, furcations, fusions, dentin dysplasia; others could be posttraumatic or senile calcifications, and pulp space obliteration [129–131]. Since tooth anatomy is the reliable blueprint for initiating a root canal treatment, endodontic management of such teeth becomes an interesting and challenging procedure partly unforeseen. Its success depends on individual clinical experience and dexterity, as well as the technical armamentarium employed. 3D printed directional guides appear to be a faithful and predictable boon for canal location during nonsurgical endodontic treatment where there are significant risks of procedural errors, like perforations and tooth structure loss [65, 90, 114, 115]. Byun et al. used an additively manufactured physical tooth model including internal root canal structures and an endodontic jig for a successful root canal treatment of a challenging tooth anomaly in the right maxillary anterior central incisor [90]. They reported that the technique of using a translucent physical model exposing the pulp chamber and root canal anatomy and an operating guide jig may be useful for better perception of the complex morphology of anomalous teeth and for carrying out the procedure with a better prognosis. In their case report, Connert et al. presented a minimally invasive treatment methodology for root canal navigation in a mandibular incisor. The tooth required advanced treatment strategies as it was diagnosed with posttraumatic severe pulp canal calcification and apical periodontitis [94, 116]. They employed a customized additively manufactured guide and drill for canal localization. In a study performed by Nayak et al., on extracted teeth, a solid tooth model (based on CBCT of extracted teeth) was sliced using a computer software program to check the deviation between the prepared root canal axis to that in simulated root canal, which was 0.07 ± 0.02 mm. The results from their study encouraged the use of 3D printing in endodontology [121]. However, it has been narrated that 3D printed endodontic depth drills are known to cause dentinal cracks in calcified root canals, which are known to cause significantly less damage as compared to postspace preparation, which weakens the tooth; moreover, they are healed by secondary dentine formation [94, 116]. The efficacy of 3D printing technology was again validated in a study carried out by Zehnder et al., on 60 extracted human teeth mounted on six maxillary jaw models. They reinforced that with guided endodontics, it was possible to negotiate all the root canals accurately up to their apical third [128]. Gok et al., contributed to the clinical success of obturating C-shaped root canals, by a study involving standardization of these canals with additively manufactured models [132]. Custom-made 3D printed guides permitted an uncomplicated and predictable canal location and management in calcified canals in a study by Meer et al. [11]. Diagnosis and management of fused mandibular second molar and premolar with concrescent supernumerary tooth using additive manufacturing of models based on CBCT were useful in promoting 3-D geometrical cognizance, enabling simulation of endodontic treatment and obtaining informed consent from the patient [113]. Yet another case report by Buchgreitz et al. imposed the importance of 3D printing in guided endodontics in the treatment of posterior teeth with pulp space obliteration and limited interocclusal distance [123]. The requirement for more interocclusal space was elucidated by converting the virtual drill path into a composite-based intracoronal guide. Data harvested from CBCT has been employed to build a 3D printed splint for salvaging a tooth diagnosed with a broken glass-fiber-reinforced composite post [133]. Position, length, and axis of the future post were virtually planned in a computer software. It was found that additive manufacturing is a feasible approach for minimally invasive endodontic revision [133].

Thus, to summarize the use of 3D printing in guided nonsurgical endodontics (Fig. 5.7), one can claim that tooth structure loss, procedural errors, and operating times are impressively reduced with a single customized drill, while the accuracy, clinical skills, and the quality of treatment is greatly increased. Certain shortcomings like elaboration of total treatment time and costs, as well as dentinal cracks arising from depth drills in calcified canals overshadow the added groundbreaking advantages.

5.3.2 Guided Surgical Endodontics and Autotransplantation

Innovations in endodontic microsurgery have steadily amassed over the past 20 years stemming from its extensive use, greater productivity, and superior outcomes [134]. It is the treatment of choice for irreversible pulpitis, pulp necrosis, and apical periodontitis in a majority of cases [135]. The unmatched results of endodontic microsurgery are enhanced by coupling it with 3D printing. As a consequence, it is possible to perform complex apicoectomy and osteotomy with augmented visualization and precision using surgical guides [89]. In large cyst-like periapical lesions, root apices are often difficult to differentiate from the adjacent bony tissues, making the level of root resection hard to determine. In nonguided periapical surgeries, navigating the root apex in a satisfactory field of view results in a large defect in the bone. Moreover, it is time consuming, depending on the operator's skills needed to transfer the 2D radiographic image perception into the clinical situation [127, 136]. 3D printed endodontic guides carry the information regarding the orientation and angle of the root apex, its arrangement in the adjacent osseous tissue, thickness of the cortical bone, and size of the periapical lesion [136]. It can reduce surgeon-dependent factors affecting the treatment prognosis, but it requires scrupulous planning and designing of the surgical guide using 3D radiographic information and computer software programs. This increases the preoperative time, but definitely reduces the chair-side time, reinforcing its usefulness [123, 137–140]. After virtual planning of the endodontic surgical guide using dedicated or implant guide-based software, it is printed using FDM, SLA, or poly-jet printer (Fig. 5.8). In the

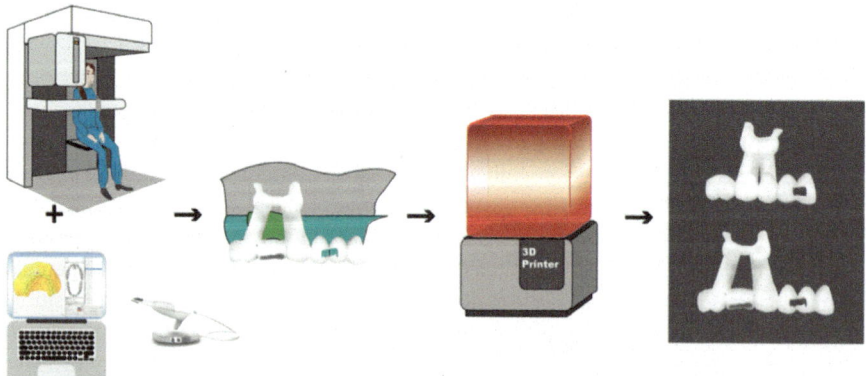

Fig. 5.8 Workflow for the generation of guides for endodontic surgery

operative field, the osteotomy site is directed by the position of the guide sleeve over the cortical plate. When using depth-calibrated drills during treatment, the position of the guide sleeve over the cortical plate helps to identify the osteotomy site. A controlled osteotomy is achieved by depth-calibrated drills analogous to the guide sleeve, which limit its field to the defined dimensions. The use of drill keys makes apicoectomy even easier by predefining the desired angle and level [89, 95, 122, 123, 128, 140].

The influence of additive manufacturing in endodontics came under light in the last decade when 3D printed endodontic surgical models were built for attaining skills and educational purposes [141].

Strbac et al. introduced this innovative surgical endodontic technique by utilizing an additively manufactured template for guided apicoectomy of an upper molar and premolar diagnosed with periapical lesions caused by extruded gutta-percha material [89]. The workflow follows a similar direction as for guided endodontics (Fig. 5.6). Here they used CBCT data and optical scanning methods for designing the guide in an adapted software originally meant for planning guided implant surgeries. Digitally planned surgical pins and piezoelectric reamers were used to accurately establish the dimensions of the osteotomy site, root resection level, and the bevel angle. The 3D printed surgical guides ultimately helped in locating the extruded part of gutta percha and its safe removal without sinus membrane perforation. Uncomplicated healing was seen during the 1-year follow-up. It strengthened the advantages of guided endodontic surgery: shortened chair side time, uncomplicated healing, and better prognosis. Later in 2018, Giacomino et al. introduced target endodontic microsurgery, using an additively manufactured surgical guide and trephine burs to accomplish a single-step apicoectomy with biopsy in complicated cases such as palatal approach to the palatal root of maxillary molar, facial approach to a fused distofacial-palatal root of a maxillary first molar, and [3] a mandibular second premolar in the vicinity of the mental foramen [140].

Later, Patel et al. developed an innovative strategy to retract soft tissue and for isolation during surgical endodontics based on the digital information harvested from CBCT and 3D printing. This tailor-made retractor improved the operative field view and manipulation of soft tissue during surgery. It highlights the fact that additive manufacturing can be garnered for multiple applications. Additive manufacturing is also gaining rapid potential in autotransplantation of heavily damaged teeth [142, 143]. It has been employed to prepare tooth sockets by using 3D printed donor tooth replicas to prevent iatrogenic damage to the actual donor teeth. This technique facilitates a straightforward and predictable results, minimizing the extra-alveolar time of the transplanted tooth. However, based on the procurement of 3D radiographic image acquisition and 3D printing armamentarium, it is less commonly employed in endodontic surgical procedures [64, 65]. Thus, it is needed to make it more cost-effective and easily accessible by the clinicians to offer their patients a state-of-the-art dental treatment.

5.4   Educational Applications of 3D Printing

Realistic models are often desired by students, clinicians, and patients for a better proprioception of the real-life situation [66, 144]. However, it has been seen that so far, dental training involved extracted teeth and simulated root canals in resin models [145–148]. Extracted teeth are associated with hygiene and ethical issues, while the latter are too idealistic and do not represent the unusual complexities regularly found in root canals [100, 102]. With the dawn of 3D printing, it is possible to print more realistic root canal simulating models with unusual anatomies that facilitate better tactile experience for the trainee [144]. There has been a rise in the replacement of typodont teeth by additively manufactured true-to-life dental models for student training protocols in various dental schools worldwide. With the advancement in material technology, it is possible to replicate both, hard and soft tissue characteristics within the same model, giving the user a better tactile sensation. The flexibility to manufacture anatomic parts such as teeth with periapical defect and cysts, in the same or magnified size, provides an unforeseen training opportunity to the student and a better understanding for the patient. The knowledge of three-dimensional spatiotemporal arrangement improves patient-clinician communication, on the one hand, and develops a superior visualization of the operative field for the clinician, on the other hand.

A lot of studies exhibit the potential for developing 3D printed biomimetic materials. Mohmmed et al. compared the physicochemical properties (zeta-potential, wettability, surface free energy) of stereolithography materials (STL) (Photopolymer, Accura) to dentine and analyzed the potential of individual material to cultivate *Enterococcus fecalis* biofilm on their surfaces [149, 150]. Both materials showed analogous physicochemical properties to dentin and substantiated their application for attachment and growth of *E. fecalis* biofilm with no statistical differences. Thus, these are a good substitute for tests requiring dentin. Research has been carried out to develop a specific ceramic shaping technique (3D printing and slip casting of a root canal mold) to reproduce canal systems with the desired shape and complexity using a microporous hydroxyapatite (HAp)-based matrix [151]. The microstructural morphology, pore size and porosity, and the Vickers microhardness of the ceramic simulators (CS) were evaluated and compared with dentin and commercial resin blocks.

It was disclosed that it is feasible to replicate the radio-opacity of a tooth and variations in root canal morphology. The endodontic treatments confirmed that the CS provided good tangible sensation during instrumentation and exhibited suitable radiological characteristics. Literature has shown that three-dimensional radiographic and optical scans can be harvested for validation of multiple instrument, technology, material, and treatment protocol efficacy [89, 92, 136, 152]. With evolution of ceramic printers and poly-jet printers, properties of dentin can be closely mimicked by 3D printing technology. This methods are being employed to fabricate 3D printed root canal models which help to investigate the cutting efficiency of latest endodontic files [22, 151, 153]. C-shaped canals come with a challenging biomechanical preparation and obturation [19, 151, 153]. To date, endodontists are endeavoring to establish standard procedures for salvaging infected teeth with such internal root anatomy. Additive manufacturing has not only proven advantageous in skill development reducing chair-side operating time, but also led to the development of the most innovative and appropriate files and obturation techniques for such cases [132, 151]. This saves iatrogenic errors like canal perforation, file breakage, and overextended obturation [153]. With the growing contest over the most apposite irrigation technique among which chemical, ultrasonic, photon-induced photo-acoustic streaming are the usually favored, realistic 3D printed models have been known to open prospects for investigation of cleaning ability [150, 154, 155]. Thus, the load on animal and human experiments is greatly reduced, decreasing the ethical issues regarding research. Researchers have used rapid prototyping for showing the stress and cleaning efficacy of files in root canal models with biofilm [23, 150, 155]. The results were analyzed with CBCT imaging and microbiological testing. These models are better as compared to extracted teeth as they are standardized and identical with respect to anatomical structure under evaluation and are accurately reproducible [121]. Extracted teeth have different dentinal and histologic characteristics based on patient age, health, and origin. 3D printed teeth model can mimick these anatomic variations and help clinicians to enhance their skills and improvise treatment protocols. Scientific reports have shown the usefulness of anatomical root canal models in determining the most suitable obturation technique for unique anatomical cases [22]. Factors affecting root fractures caused by obturation, like manual condensing force, mechanical pressure by dispensing syringe, viscosity of gutta percha, temperature, and elastic and other material properties, can be easily investigated and concluded for individual root canal structure [156]. This appears to be a boon as apical extrusion of the obturation material causes significant periapical infection, leading to endodontic treatment failure.

As compared to cone-shaped resin root canal models, 3D printed replicates of patient-specific anatomies are more representative of the real endodontic problem and prepare the dental student and clinician for challenging cases (Fig. 5.9). Thus, with tremendous potential in education and multifunctionality of models, additive manufacturing opens newer prospective in endodontics.

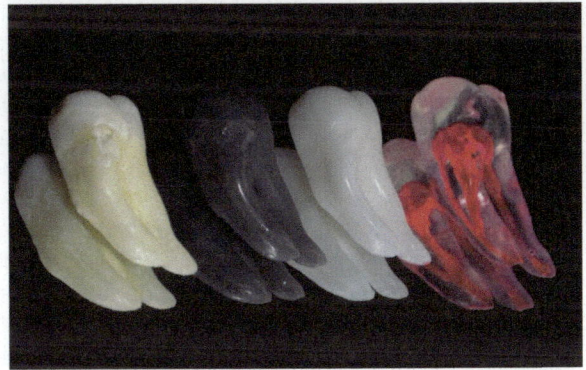

Fig. 5.9 3D printed tooth replicas for endodontic education. (Courtesy: Reymus M et al.; Adopted from 3D printed replicas for endodontic education. International Endodontic Journal, Volume: 52, Issue: 1, Pages: 123–130)

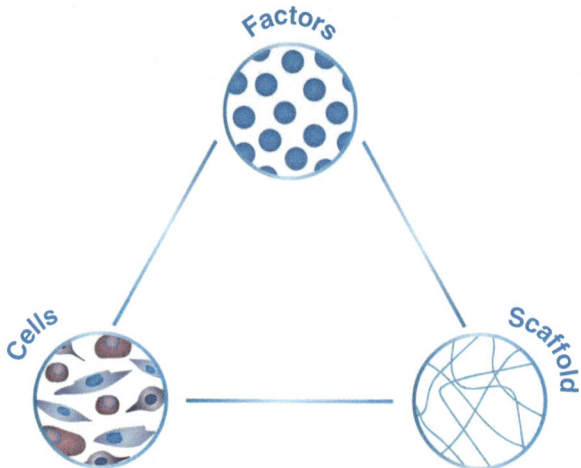

Fig. 5.10 The three pillars of tissue engineering: cells, scaffolds, and factors. (Adopted with modifications from [77])

5.5   Experimental Researches with 3D Printing Technology

3D printing has evolved tissue engineering, leading to development of bioprinters, which are further described in the Chap. 10. Tissue engineering combines the knowledge and knowhow of engineering and life sciences with the aim to restore or improve functional tissues and organs. Tissue engineering relies on three pillars, which are cells, factors, and scaffolds, which allow the generation of a vital construct for implantation (Fig. 5.10) [157].

   To ensure success, vascularization of the construct after implantation is a prerequisite. Given the current gap between repair and regeneration in endodontics, tissue engineering with the application of 3D printing can help to overcome this issue.

5.6   Future of Endodontic Renaissance

The era of digitalization in dentistry has not only transformed dental clinical practice but has also revolutionized field of dental education. More of these innovations are utilizing the technology of additive manufacturing, three-dimensional radiographic imaging, and haptic simulators [64]. Haptic simulators are commercially available computer systems that generate interactive 3D virtual simulations of teeth and skeletal tissues. They imitate complicated surgical/nonsurgical cases and offer the clinician real-time multisensory perioperative feedback [158]. The operation of haptic simulators is dependent on the digital information exchange between 3D radiography and rapidly prototyped models. A couple of studies has been presented to test the suitability of experimental haptic simulators for nonsurgical and surgical endodontic procedures [159–161]. Overall, better biomechanical preparation, shorter procedural times, conservation of tooth structure, and smaller osteotomies were shown using haptic simulators [160]. However, due to exceptionally commanding computational skills, haptic rendering of sophisticated anatomical models coupled with interactive procedures for reduction of bone is yet to be conquered [159].

Based on the advancing 3D printed materials and bioprinting technology, scientists are not far from developing a 3D printed realistic tooth bud, with automated dental embryogenesis, once in contact with the oral environment [162, 163]. Endodontics in particular can benefit from the potential of printing-customized canal obturation points and medicaments for critical cases of open apex and trauma. However, owing to initial installment costs and lack of sufficient preclinical evidence, this technology is not so popular in endodontics as compared to other dental and medical fields [65, 68, 151, 164]. Thus, it is evident that, with the integration of additive manufacturing in the endodontic training and clinical management, there is a strong prospective of establishing value-based precision dentistry.

Acknowledgment   Research of the authors on 3D printing within the M3dRES project (858060) is supported by the Austrian Research Promoting Agency (FFG). We thank Abeer El Temtamy (Columbia College of Dental Medicine) for proofreading of the chapter.

References

1. Moser N, Santander P, Quast A. From 3D imaging to 3D printing in dentistry - a practical guide. Int J Comput Dent. 2018;21(4):345–56.
2. Oberoi G, Nitsch S, Edelmayer M, Janjić K, Müller AS, Agis H. 3D printing-encompassing the facets of dentistry. Front Bioeng Biotechnol. 2018;6:172.
3. Ackerman S, Aguilera FC, Buie JM, Glickman GN, Umorin M, Wang Q, et al. Accuracy of 3-dimensional-printed endodontic surgical guide: a human cadaver study. J Endod. 2019;45(5):615–8.
4. Valdec S, Schiefersteiner M, Rücker M, Stadlinger B. Guided biopsy of osseous pathologies in the jaw bone using a 3D-printed, tooth-supported drilling template. Int J Oral Maxillofac Surg. 2019;48:1028.
5. Király L. [Three-dimensional virtual and printed models improve preoperative planning and promote patient-safety in complex congenital and pediatric cardiac surgery]. Orv Hetil 2019;160(19):747–755.
6. Aimar A, Palermo A, Innocenti B. The role of 3D printing in medical applications: a state of the art. J Healthc Eng. 2019;2019:5340616.
7. Walker M, Humphries S. 3D printing: applications in evolution and ecology. Ecol Evol. 2019;9(7):4289–301.
8. ENGINEERING.com. 2018. Was a Strong Year for the Global 3D Printer Market > ENGINEERING.com. Accessed 20 May 2019 from https://www.engineering.com/AdvancedManufacturing/ArticleID/18279/2018-Was-a-Strong-Year-for-the-Global-3D-Printer-Market.aspx
9. Dawood A, Marti Marti B, Sauret-Jackson V, Darwood A. 3D printing in dentistry. Br Dent J. 2015;219(11):521–9.
10. Ligon SC, Liska R, Stampfl J, Gurr M, Mülhaupt R. Polymers for 3D printing and customized additive manufacturing. Chem Rev. 2017;117(15):10212–90.

11. van der Meer WJ, Vissink A, Ng YL, Gulabivala K. 3D Computer aided treatment planning in endodontics. J Dent. 2016;45:67–72.
12. Anssari Moin D, Verweij JP, Waars H, van Merkesteyn R, Wismeijer D. Accuracy of computer-assisted template-guided autotransplantation of teeth with custom three-dimensional designed/printed surgical tooling: a cadaveric study. J Oral Maxillofac Surg. 2017;75(5):925.e1–7.
13. Kulczyk T, Rychlik M, Lorkiewicz-Muszyńska D, Abreu-Głowacka M, Czajka-Jakubowska A, Przystańska A. Computed tomography versus optical scanning: a comparison of different methods of 3D data acquisition for tooth replication. Biomed Res Int. 2019;2019:4985121.
14. Tardieu PB, Vrielinck L, Escolano E, Henne M, Tardieu A. Computer-assisted implant placement: scan template, simplant, surgiguide, and SAFE system. Int J Periodontics Restorative Dent. 2007;27(2):141–9.
15. Shaheen E, Sun Y, Jacobs R, Politis C. Three-dimensional printed final occlusal splint for orthognathic surgery: design and validation. Int J Oral Maxillofac Surg. 2017;46(1):67–71.
16. Filippou V, Tsoumpas C. Recent advances on the development of phantoms using 3D printing for imaging with CT, MRI, PET, SPECT, and ultrasound. Med Phys. 2018;45(9):e740.
17. Wang KC, Jones A, Kambhampati S, Gilotra MN, Liacouras PC, Stuelke S, et al. CT-based 3D printing of the glenoid prior to shoulder arthroplasty: bony morphology and model evaluation. J Digit Imaging. 2019;32:816–26.
18. Chang D, Tummala S, Sotero D, Tong E, Mustafa L, Mustafa M, et al. Three-dimensional printing for procedure rehearsal/simulation/planning in interventional radiology. Tech Vasc Interv Radiol. 2019;22(1):14–20.
19. Metzger Z, Zary R, Cohen R, Teperovich E, Paqué F. The quality of root canal preparation and root canal obturation in canals treated with rotary versus self-adjusting files: a three-dimensional micro-computed tomographic study. J Endod. 2010;36(9):1569–73.
20. Kamio T, Hayashi K, Onda T, Takaki T, Shibahara T, Yakushiji T, et al. Utilizing a low-cost desktop 3D printer to develop a "one-stop 3D printing lab" for oral and maxillofacial surgery and dentistry fields. 3D Print Med. 2018;4(1):6.
21. Nilsson J, Richards RG, Thor A, Kamer L. Virtual bite registration using intraoral digital scanning, CT and CBCT: in vitro evaluation of a new method and its implication for orthognathic surgery. J Craniomaxillofac Surg. 2016;44(9):1194–200.
22. Liang X, Liao W, Cai H, Jiang S, Chen S. 3D-printed artificial teeth: accuracy and application in root canal therapy. J Biomed Nanotechnol. 2018;14(8):1477–85.
23. Eken R, Sen OG, Eskitascioglu G, Belli S. Evaluation of the effect of rotary systems on stresses in a new testing model using a 3-dimensional printed simulated resin root with an oval-shaped canal: a finite element analysis study. J Endod. 2016;42(8):1273–8.
24. Bateman MG, Durfee WK, Iles TL, Martin CM, Liao K, Erdman AG, et al. Cardiac patient-specific three-dimensional models as surgical planning tools. Surgery. 2020;167:259.
25. van Steenberghe D, Glauser R, Blombäck U, Andersson M, Schutyser F, Pettersson A, et al. A computed tomographic scan-derived customized surgical template and fixed prosthesis for flapless surgery and immediate loading of implants in fully edentulous maxillae: a prospective multicenter study. Clin Implant Dent Relat Res. 2005;7(Suppl 1):S111–20.
26. Strbac GD, Schnappauf A, Giannis K, Bertl MH, Moritz A, Ulm C. Guided autotransplantation of teeth: a novel method using virtually planned 3-dimensional templates. J Endod. 2016;42(12):1844–50.
27. Martorelli M, Gerbino S, Giudice M, Ausiello P. A comparison between customized clear and removable orthodontic appliances manufactured using RP and CNC techniques. Dent Mater. 2013;29(2):e1–10.
28. Tunchel S, Blay A, Kolerman R, Mijiritsky E, Shibli JA. 3D printing/additive manufacturing single titanium dental implants: a prospective multicenter study with 3 years of follow-up. Int J Dent. 2016;2016:8590971.
29. Revilla León M, Klemm IM, García-Arranz J, Özcan M. 3D metal printing - additive manufacturing technologies for frameworks of implant-borne fixed dental prosthesis. Eur J Prosthodont Restor Dent. 2017;25(3):143–7.

30. Xia J, Li Y, Cai D, Shi X, Zhao S, Jiang Q, et al. Direct resin composite restoration of maxillary central incisors using a 3D-printed template: two clinical cases. BMC Oral Health. 2018;18(1):158.
31. Knowlton S, Onal S, Yu CH, Zhao JJ, Tasoglu S. Bioprinting for cancer research. Trends Biotechnol. 2015;33(9):504–13.
32. Rasperini G, Pilipchuk SP, Flanagan CL, Park CH, Pagni G, Hollister SJ, et al. 3D-printed bioresorbable scaffold for periodontal repair. J Dent Res. 2015;94(9 Suppl):153S–7S.
33. Visscher DO, Farré-Guasch E, Helder MN, Gibbs S, Forouzanfar T, van Zuijlen PP, et al. Advances in bioprinting technologies for craniofacial reconstruction. Trends Biotechnol. 2016;34(9):700–10.
34. Moroni L, Boland T, Burdick JA, De Maria C, Derby B, Forgacs G, et al. Biofabrication: a guide to technology and terminology. Trends Biotechnol. 2018;36(4):384–402.
35. Smith EE, Zhang W, Schiele NR, Khademhosseini A, Kuo CK, Yelick PC. Developing a biomimetic tooth bud model. J Tissue Eng Regen Med. 2017;11(12):3326–36.
36. Derakhshanfar S, Mbeleck R, Xu K, Zhang X, Zhong W, Xing M. 3D bioprinting for biomedical devices and tissue engineering: a review of recent trends and advances. Bioact Mater. 2018;3(2):144–56.
37. Morgan AJL, Hidalgo San Jose L, Jamieson WD, Wymant JM, Song B, Stephens P, et al. Simple and versatile 3D printed microfluidics using fused filament fabrication. PLoS One. 2016;11(4):e0152023.
38. Kalsoom U, Hasan CK, Tedone L, Desire CT, Li F, Breadmore MC, et al. A low-cost passive sampling device with integrated porous membrane produced using multi-material 3D printing. Anal Chem. 2018;90(20):12081–9.
39. Masood SH. Advances in fused deposition modeling. In: Comprehensive materials processing. Amsterdam: Elsevier; 2014. p. 69–91.
40. Mazzoli A. Selective laser sintering in biomedical engineering. Med Biol Eng Comput. 2013;51(3):245–56.
41. Ionita CN, Mokin M, Varble N, Bednarek DR, Xiang J, Snyder KV, et al. Challenges and limitations of patient-specific vascular phantom fabrication using 3D Polyjet printing. Proc SPIE. 2014;9038:90380M.
42. Ibrahim D, Broilo TL, Heitz C, de Oliveira MG, de Oliveira HW, Nobre SMW, et al. Dimensional error of selective laser sintering, three-dimensional printing and PolyJet models in the reproduction of mandibular anatomy. J Craniomaxillofac Surg. 2009;37(3):167–73.
43. Lopez CD, Witek L, Torroni A, Flores RL, Demissie DB, Young S, et al. The role of 3D printing in treating craniomaxillofacial congenital anomalies. Birth Def Res. 2018;110(13):1055–64.
44. Urkasemsin G, Ferreira JN. Unveiling stem cell heterogeneity toward the development of salivary gland regenerative strategies. Adv Exp Med Biol. 2019;1123:151–64.
45. Chen S, Shi Y, Luo Y, Ma J. Layer-by-layer coated porous 3D printed hydroxyapatite composite scaffolds for controlled drug delivery. Colloids Surf B: Biointerfaces. 2019;179:121–7.
46. Chen H, Zhang J, Li X, Liu L, Zhang X, Ren D, et al. Multi-level customized 3D printing for autogenous implants in skull tissue engineering. Biofabrication. 2019;11:045007.
47. Lipskas J, Deep K, Yao W. Robotic-assisted 3D bio-printing for repairing bone and cartilage defects through a minimally invasive approach. Sci Rep. 2019;9(1):3746.
48. Noh I, Kim N, Tran HN, Lee J, Lee C. 3D printable hyaluronic acid-based hydrogel for its potential application as a bioink in tissue engineering. Biomater Res. 2019;23:3.
49. Datta P, Ayan B, Ozbolat IT. Bioprinting for vascular and vascularized tissue biofabrication. Acta Biomater. 2017;51:1–20.
50. Huang Y, Zhang X-F, Gao G, Yonezawa T, Cui X. 3D bioprinting and the current applications in tissue engineering. Biotechnol J. 2017;12(8):1600734.
51. Wenz A, Borchers K, Tovar GEM, Kluger PJ. Bone matrix production in hydroxyapatite-modified hydrogels suitable for bone bioprinting. Biofabrication. 2017;9(4):044103.
52. Itoh Y, Sasaki JI, Hashimoto M, Katata C, Hayashi M, Imazato S. Pulp regeneration by 3-dimensional dental pulp stem cell constructs. J Dent Res. 2018;97(10):1137–43.

53. Blakely AM, Manning KL, Tripathi A, Morgan JR. Bio-pick, place, and perfuse: a new instrument for three-dimensional tissue engineering. Tissue Eng Part C Methods. 2015;21(7):737–46.
54. Nguyen D, Hägg DA, Forsman A, Ekholm J, Nimkingratana P, Brantsing C, et al. Cartilage tissue engineering by the 3D bioprinting of ips cells in a nanocellulose/alginate bioink. Sci Rep. 2017;7(1):658.
55. Thrivikraman G, Athirasala A, Twohig C, Boda SK, Bertassoni LE. Biomaterials for cranio-facial bone regeneration. Dent Clin N Am. 2017;61(4):835–56.
56. Athirasala A, Tahayeri A, Thrivikraman G, França CM, Monteiro N, Tran V, et al. A dentin-derived hydrogel bioink for 3D bioprinting of cell laden scaffolds for regenerative dentistry. Biofabrication. 2018;10(2):024101.
57. Intini C, Elviri L, Cabral J, Mros S, Bergonzi C, Bianchera A, et al. 3D-printed chitosan-based scaffolds: an in vitro study of human skin cell growth and an in-vivo wound healing evaluation in experimental diabetes in rats. Carbohydr Polym. 2018;199:593–602.
58. Chen Y-W, Shen Y-F, Ho C-C, Yu J, Wu Y-HA, Wang K, et al. Osteogenic and angiogenic potentials of the cell-laden hydrogel/mussel-inspired calcium silicate complex hierarchical porous scaffold fabricated by 3D bioprinting. Mater Sci Eng C Mater Biol Appl. 2018;91:679–87.
59. Rahman SU, Nagrath M, Ponnusamy S, Arany PR. Nanoscale and macroscale scaffolds with controlled-release polymeric systems for dental craniomaxillofacial tissue engineering. Materials (Basel). 2018;11(8):E1478.
60. Chiarello E, Cadossi M, Tedesco G, Capra P, Calamelli C, Shehu A, et al. Autograft, allograft and bone substitutes in reconstructive orthopedic surgery. Aging Clin Exp Res. 2013;25(Suppl 1):S101–3.
61. Bill JS, Reuther JF, Dittmann W, Kübler N, Meier JL, Pistner H, et al. Stereolithography in oral and maxillofacial operation planning. Int J Oral Maxillofac Surg. 1995;24(1 Pt 2):98–103.
62. Wang G, Li J, Khadka A, Hsu Y, Li W, Hu J. CAD/CAM and rapid prototyped titanium for reconstruction of ramus defect and condylar fracture caused by mandibular reduction. Oral Surg Oral Med Oral Pathol Oral Radiol. 2012;113(3):356–61.
63. Fahmy MD, Jazayeri HE, Razavi M, Masri R, Tayebi L. Three-dimensional bioprinting materials with potential application in preprosthetic surgery. J Prosthodont. 2016;25(4):310–8.
64. Shah P, Chong BS. 3D imaging, 3D printing and 3D virtual planning in endodontics. Clin Oral Investig. 2018;22(2):641–54.
65. Anderson J, Wealleans J, Ray J. Endodontic applications of 3D printing. Int Endod J. 2018;51(9):1005–18.
66. Kröger E, Dekiff M, Dirksen D. 3D printed simulation models based on real patient situations for hands-on practice. Eur J Dent Educ. 2017;21(4):e119–25.
67. Alrasheed AS, Nguyen LHP, Mongeau L, Funnell WRJ, Tewfik MA. Development and validation of a 3D-printed model of the ostiomeatal complex and frontal sinus for endoscopic sinus surgery training. Int Forum Allergy Rhinol. 2017;7(8):837–41.
68. Decurcio DA, Lim E, Chaves GS, Nagendrababu V, Estrela C, Rossi-Fedele G. Pre-clinical endodontic education outcomes between artificial versus extracted natural teeth: a systematic review. Int Endod J. 2019;52:1153.
69. Mitsouras D, Liacouras P, Imanzadeh A, Giannopoulos AA, Cai T, Kumamaru KK, et al. Medical 3D printing for the radiologist. Radiographics. 2015;35(7):1965–88.
70. Sánchez-Sánchez Á, Girón-Vallejo Ó, Ruiz-Pruneda R, Fernandez-Ibieta M, García-Calderon D, Villamil V, et al. Three-dimensional printed model and virtual reconstruction: an extra tool for pediatric solid tumors surgery. Eur J Pediatr Surg Rep. 2018;6(1):e70–6.
71. Redwood B, Schöffer F, Garret B. The 3d printing handbook: technologies, design and applications. 1st ed. Amsterdam: 3d Hubs; 2017.
72. Nikoyan L, Patel R. Intraoral scanner, three-dimensional imaging, and three-dimensional printing in the dental office. Dent Clin N Am. 2020;64(2):365–78.

73. Ozbolat IT, Moncal KK, Gudapati H. Evaluation of bioprinter technologies. Addit Manufact. 2017;13:179–200.
74. Ozbolat IT, Peng W, Ozbolat V. Application areas of 3D bioprinting. Drug Discov Today. 2016;21(8):1257–71.
75. Mironov V, Visconti RP, Kasyanov V, Forgacs G, Drake CJ, Markwald RR. Organ printing: tissue spheroids as building blocks. Biomaterials. 2009;30(12):2164–74.
76. Oberoi G, Janjić K, Müller AS, Schädl B, Andrukhov O, Moritz A, et al. Contraction dynamics of rod microtissues of gingiva-derived and periodontal ligament-derived cells. Front Physiol. 2018;9:1683.
77. Oberoi G, Janjić K, Müller AS, Schädl B, Moritz A, Agis H. Contraction dynamics of dental pulp cell rod microtissues. Clin Oral Investig. 2020;24:631.
78. Ji S, Guvendiren M. Recent advances in bioink design for 3D bioprinting of tissues and organs. Front Bioeng Biotechnol. 2017;5:23.
79. Moldovan NI. Progress in scaffold-free bioprinting for cardiovascular medicine. J Cell Mol Med. 2018;22(6):2964–9.
80. Zhang YS, Yue K, Aleman J, Moghaddam KM, Bakht SM, Yang J, et al. 3D bioprinting for tissue and organ fabrication. Ann Biomed Eng. 2017;45(1):148–63.
81. Murphy SV, Atala A. 3D bioprinting of tissues and organs. Nat Biotechnol. 2014;32(8):773–85.
82. Ahlfeld T, Cidonio G, Kilian D, Duin S, Akkineni AR, Dawson JI, et al. Development of a clay based bioink for 3D cell printing for skeletal application. Biofabrication. 2017;9(3):034103.
83. Müller AS, Gashi M, Janjić K, Edelmayer M, Moritz A, Agis H. The impact of clay-based hypoxia mimetic hydrogel on human fibroblasts of the periodontal soft tissue. J Biomater Appl. 2019;33:1277.
84. Müller AS, Artner M, Janjić K, Edelmayer M, Kurzmann C, Moritz A, et al. Synthetic clay-based hypoxia mimetic hydrogel for pulp regeneration: the impact on cell activity and release kinetics based on dental pulp-derived cells in vitro. J Endod. 2018;44(8):1263–9.
85. Almela T, Al-Sahaf S, Brook IM, Khoshroo K, Rasoulianboroujeni M, Fahimipour F, et al. 3D printed tissue engineered model for bone invasion of oral cancer. Tissue Cell. 2018;52:71–7.
86. Lee V, Singh G, Trasatti JP, Bjornsson C, Xu X, Tran TN, et al. Design and fabrication of human skin by three-dimensional bioprinting. Tissue Eng Part C Methods. 2014;20(6):473–84.
87. Kurzmann C, Janjić K, Shokoohi-Tabrizi H, Edelmayer M, Pensch M, Moritz A, et al. Evaluation of resins for stereolithographic 3D-printed surgical guides: the response of L929 cells and human gingival fibroblasts. Biomed Res Int. 2017;2017:4057612.
88. Vasak C, Watzak G, Gahleitner A, Strbac G, Schemper M, Zechner W. Computed tomography-based evaluation of template (NobelGuide™)-guided implant positions: a prospective radiological study. Clin Oral Implants Res. 2011;22(10):1157–63.
89. Strbac GD, Schnappauf A, Giannis K, Moritz A, Ulm C. Guided modern endodontic surgery: a novel approach for guided osteotomy and root resection. J Endod. 2017;43(3):496–501.
90. Byun C, Kim C, Cho S, Baek SH, Kim G, Kim SG, et al. Endodontic treatment of an anomalous anterior tooth with the aid of a 3-dimensional printed physical tooth model. J Endod. 2015;41(6):961–5.
91. Loios G, Martins RF, Ginjeira A, Dragoi MV, Buican G. Fatigue resistance of rotary endodontic files submitted to axial motion in multiplanar canals manufactured by 3D printing. Proc Eng. 2016;160:117–22.
92. Patel S, Aldowaisan A, Dawood A. A novel method for soft tissue retraction during periapical surgery using 3D technology: a case report. Int Endod J. 2017;50(8):813–22.
93. Huumonen S, Orstavik D. Radiological aspects of apical periodontitis. Endod Top. 2002;1(1):3–25.
94. Connert T, Zehnder MS, Amato M, Weiger R, Kühl S, Krastl G. Microguided Endodontics: a method to achieve minimally invasive access cavity preparation and root canal location in mandibular incisors using a novel computer-guided technique. Int Endod J. 2018;51(2):247–55.

95. Ahn S-Y, Kim N-H, Kim S, Karabucak B, Kim E. Computer-aided Design/Computer-aided Manufacturing-guided endodontic surgery: guided osteotomy and apex localization in a mandibular molar with a thick buccal bone plate. J Endod. 2018;44(4):665–70.

96. McCabe PS, Dummer PMH. Pulp canal obliteration: an endodontic diagnosis and treatment challenge. Int Endod J. 2012;45(2):177–97.

97. Hsieh C-Y, Wu Y-C, Su C-C, Chung M-P, Huang R-Y, Ting P-Y, et al. The prevalence and distribution of radiopaque, calcified pulp stones: a cone-beam computed tomography study in a northern Taiwanese population. J Dent Sci. 2018;13(2):138–44.

98. Jannati R, Afshari M, Moosazadeh M, Allahgholipour SZ, Eidy M, Hajihoseini M. Prevalence of pulp stones: a systematic review and meta-analysis. J Evid Based Med. 2019;12:133.

99. Tassoker M, Magat G, Sener S. A comparative study of cone-beam computed tomography and digital panoramic radiography for detecting pulp stones. Imaging Sci Dent. 2018;48(3):201–12.

100. Yang H, Tian C, Li G, Yang L, Han X, Wang Y. A cone-beam computed tomography study of the root canal morphology of mandibular first premolars and the location of root canal orifices and apical foramina in a Chinese subpopulation. J Endod. 2013;39(4):435–8.

101. Eaton JA, Clement DJ, Lloyd A, Marchesan MA. Micro-computed tomographic evaluation of the influence of root canal system landmarks on access outline forms and canal curvatures in mandibular molars. J Endod. 2015;41(11):1888–91.

102. Boschetti E, Silva-Sousa YTC, Mazzi-Chaves JF, Leoni GB, Versiani MA, Pécora JD, et al. Micro-CT evaluation of root and canal morphology of mandibular first premolars with radicular grooves. Braz Dent J. 2017;28(5):597–603.

103. Zhang Y, Xu H, Wang D, Gu Y, Wang J, Tu S, et al. Assessment of the second mesiobuccal root canal in maxillary first molars: a cone-beam computed tomographic study. J Endod. 2017;43(12):1990–6.

104. Rusu D, Surlin P, Stratul S-I, Boariu M, Calniceanu H, Kasaj A, et al. Changes in anatomic position of root canal orifices in pluriradicular teeth following re-location during endodontic treatment. Ann Anat. 2018;217:29–33.

105. Su C-C, Huang R-Y, Wu Y-C, Cheng W-C, Chiang H-S, Chung M-P, et al. Detection and location of second mesiobuccal canal in permanent maxillary teeth: a cone-beam computed tomography analysis in a Taiwanese population. Arch Oral Biol. 2019;98:108–14.

106. Tassoker M, Sener S. Analysis of the root canal configuration and C-shaped canal frequency of mandibular second molars: a cone beam computed tomography study. Folia Morphol (Warsz). 2018;77(4):752–7.

107. Zhang W, Tang Y, Liu C, Shen Y, Feng X, Gu Y. Root and root canal variations of the human maxillary and mandibular third molars in a Chinese population: a micro-computed tomographic study. Arch Oral Biol. 2018;95:134–40.

108. Dos Santos OR, Maria Gomes Oliveira A, Cintra Junqueira JL, Kühl Panzarella F. Association between the anatomy of the mandibular canal and facial types: a cone-beam computed tomography analysis. Int J Dent. 2018;2018:5481383.

109. Al Qahtani A, Abdulrab S, Alhadainy H. Management of a failed endodontic treatment for a maxillary second molar with two separate palatal roots. Clin Case Rep. 2018;6(9):1735–8.

110. Sathyanarayanan K, Poornima L. Endodontic management of maxillary second molar with vertucci type VI root canal morphology diagnosed using cone-beam computed tomography. Contemp Clin Dent. 2018;9(3):494–7.

111. Marceliano-Alves MF, de Lima CO, Augusto CM, Almeida Barbosa AF, Vieira Bruno AM, Rosa AM, et al. The internal root canal morphology of single-rooted mandibular canines revealed by micro-computed tomography. J Conserv Dent. 2018;21(6):588–91.

112. Saber SEDM, Ahmed MHM, Obeid M, Ahmed HMA. Root and canal morphology of maxillary premolar teeth in an Egyptian subpopulation using two classification systems: a cone beam computed tomography study. Int Endod J. 2019;52(3):267–78.

113. Kato H, Kamio T. Diagnosis and endodontic management of fused mandibular second molar and paramolar with concrescent supernumerary tooth using cone-beam CT and 3-D printing technology: a case report. Bull Tokyo Dent Coll. 2015;56(3):177–84.

114. Connert T, Krug R, Eggmann F, Emsermann I, ElAyouti A, Weiger R, et al. Guided endodontics versus conventional access cavity preparation: a comparative study on substance loss using 3-dimensional-printed teeth. J Endod. 2019;45(3):327–31.
115. Krastl G, Zehnder MS, Connert T, Weiger R, Kühl S. Guided endodontics: a novel treatment approach for teeth with pulp canal calcification and apical pathology. Dent Traumatol. 2016;32(3):240–6.
116. Connert T, Zehnder MS, Weiger R, Kühl S, Krastl G. Microguided endodontics: accuracy of a miniaturized technique for apically extended access cavity preparation in anterior teeth. J Endod. 2017;43(5):787–90.
117. Fonseca Tavares WL, Diniz Viana AC, de Carvalho MV, Feitosa Henriques LC, Ribeiro Sobrinho AP. Guided endodontic access of calcified anterior teeth. J Endod. 2018;44(7):1195–9.
118. Lara-Mendes STO, Barbosa CFM, Machado VC, Santa-Rosa CC. A new approach for minimally invasive access to severely calcified anterior teeth using the guided endodontics technique. J Endod. 2018;44(10):1578–82.
119. Mao T, Neelakantan P. Three-dimensional imaging modalities in endodontics. Imaging Sci Dent. 2014;44(3):177–83.
120. Philpott R, Gulabivala K, Leeson R, Ng YL. Prevalence, predictive factors, and clinical course of persistent pain associated with teeth displaying periapical healing following non-surgical root canal treatment: a prospective study. Int Endod J. 2018;52(4):407–15.
121. Nayak A, Jain PK, Kankar PK, Jain N. Computer-aided design-based guided endodontic: a novel approach for root canal access cavity preparation. Proc Inst Mech Eng H. 2018;232(8):787–95.
122. Fan Y, Glickman GN, Umorin M, Nair MK, Jalali P. A novel prefabricated grid for guided endodontic microsurgery. J Endod. 2019;45:206.
123. Buchgreitz J, Buchgreitz M, Bjørndal L. Guided endodontics modified for treating molars by using an intracoronal guide technique. J Endod. 2019;45(6):818–23.
124. Strbac GD, Giannis K, Unger E, Mittlböck M, Vasak C, Watzek G, et al. Drilling- and withdrawing-related thermal changes during implant site osteotomies. Clin Implant Dent Relat Res. 2015;17(1):32–43.
125. Mazzoni S, Bianchi A, Schiariti G, Badiali G, Marchetti C. Computer-aided design and computer-aided manufacturing cutting guides and customized titanium plates are useful in upper maxilla waferless repositioning. J Oral Maxillofac Surg. 2015;73(4):701–7.
126. Patel S. New dimensions in endodontic imaging: Part 2. Cone beam computed tomography. Int Endod J. 2009;42(6):463–75.
127. Patel S, Dawood A, Whaites E, Pitt FT. New dimensions in endodontic imaging: part 1. Conventional and alternative radiographic systems. Int Endod J. 2009;42(6):447–62.
128. Zehnder MS, Connert T, Weiger R, Krastl G, Kühl S. Guided endodontics: accuracy of a novel method for guided access cavity preparation and root canal location. Int Endod J. 2016;49(10):966–72.
129. Faria MIA, Borges M, Carneiro SM, Filho JMMS, et al. Endodontic treatment of dental formation anomalies. Rev Odonto Ciênc. 2011;26:88.
130. Albuquerque D, Kottoor J, Hammo M. Endodontic and clinical considerations in the management of variable anatomy in mandibular premolars: a literature review. Biomed Res Int. 2014;2014:512574.
131. Luder HU. Malformations of the tooth root in humans. Front Physiol. 2015;6:307.
132. Gok T, Capar ID, Akcay I, Keles A. Evaluation of different techniques for filling simulated c-shaped canals of 3-dimensional printed resin teeth. J Endod. 2017;43(9):1559–64.
133. Schwindling FS, Tasaka A, Hilgenfeld T, Rammelsberg P, Zenthöfer A. Three-dimensional-guided removal and preparation of dental root posts-concept and feasibility. J Prosthod Res. 2020;64:104.
134. Tsesis I, Rosen E, Schwartz-Arad D, Fuss Z. Retrospective evaluation of surgical endodontic treatment: traditional versus modern technique. J Endod. 2006;32(5):412–6.

135. Kim S, Kratchman S. Modern endodontic surgery concepts and practice: a review. J Endod. 2006;32(7):601–23.
136. Ye S, Zhao S, Wang W, Jiang Q, Yang X. A novel method for periapical microsurgery with the aid of 3D technology: a case report. BMC Oral Health. 2018;18(1):85.
137. Oh J-H. Recent advances in the reconstruction of cranio-maxillofacial defects using computer-aided design/computer-aided manufacturing. Maxillofac Plast Reconstr Surg. 2018;40(1):2.
138. Pugliese L, Marconi S, Negrello E, Mauri V, Peri A, Gallo V, et al. The clinical use of 3D printing in surgery. Updat Surg. 2018;70(3):381–8.
139. Hu YK, Xie QY, Yang C, Xu GZ. Computer-designed surgical guide template compared with free-hand operation for mesiodens extraction in premaxilla using "trapdoor" method. Medicine. 2017;96(26):e7310.
140. Giacomino CM, Ray JJ, Wealleans JA. Targeted endodontic microsurgery: a novel approach to anatomically challenging scenarios using 3-dimensional-printed guides and trephine burs-a report of 3 cases. J Endod. 2018;44(4):671–7.
141. Bahcall JK. Using 3-dimensional printing to create presurgical models for endodontic surgery. Compend Contin Educ Dent. 2014;35(8):e29–30.
142. Verweij JP, Anssari Moin D, Wismeijer D, van Merkesteyn JPR. Replacing heavily damaged teeth by third molar autotransplantation with the use of cone-beam computed tomography and rapid prototyping. J Oral Maxillofac Surg. 2017;75(9):1809–16.
143. Kim K, Choi H-S, Pang N-S. Clinical application of 3D technology for tooth autotransplantation: a case report. Aust Endod J. 2019;45:122.
144. Höhne C, Schmitter M. 3D printed teeth for the preclinical education of dental students. J Dent Educ. 2019;83:1100.
145. Arora A, Taneja S, Kumar M. Comparative evaluation of shaping ability of different rotary NiTi instruments in curved canals using CBCT. J Conserv Dent. 2014;17(1):35–9.
146. Saber SEDM, Nagy MM, Schäfer E. Comparative evaluation of the shaping ability of ProTaper Next, iRaCe and Hyflex CM rotary NiTi files in severely curved root canals. Int Endod J. 2015;48(2):131–6.
147. Pedullà E, Plotino G, Grande NM, Avarotti G, Gambarini G, Rapisarda E, et al. Shaping ability of two nickel-titanium instruments activated by continuous rotation or adaptive motion: a micro-computed tomography study. Clin Oral Investig. 2016;20(8):2227–33.
148. Alovisi M, Cemenasco A, Mancini L, Paolino D, Scotti N, Bianchi CC, et al. Micro-CT evaluation of several glide path techniques and ProTaper Next shaping outcomes in maxillary first molar curved canals. Int Endod J. 2017;50(4):387–97.
149. Mohmmed SA, Vianna ME, Hilton ST, Boniface DR, Ng Y-L, Knowles JC. Investigation to test potential stereolithography materials for development of an in vitro root canal model. Microsc Res Tech. 2017;80(2):202–10.
150. Mohmmed SA, Vianna ME, Penny MR, Hilton ST, Mordan N, Knowles JC. Confocal laser scanning, scanning electron, and transmission electron microscopy investigation of Enterococcus faecalis biofilm degradation using passive and active sodium hypochlorite irrigation within a simulated root canal model. Microbiology. 2017;6(4):e00455.
151. Robberecht L, Chai F, Dehurtevent M, Marchandise P, Bécavin T, Hornez JC, et al. A novel anatomical ceramic root canal simulator for endodontic training. Eur J Dent Educ. 2016;21:e1.
152. McMenamin PG, Quayle MR, McHenry CR, Adams JW. The production of anatomical teaching resources using three-dimensional (3D) printing technology. Anat Sci Educ. 2014;7(6):479–86.
153. Christofzik D, Bartols A, Faheem MK, Schroeter D, Groessner-Schreiber B, Doerfer CE. Shaping ability of four root canal instrumentation systems in simulated 3D-printed root canal models. PLoS One. 2018;13(8):e0201129.
154. Mohmmed SA, Vianna ME, Penny MR, Hilton ST, Mordan NJ, Knowles JC. Investigations into in situ Enterococcus faecalis biofilm removal by passive and active sodium hypochlorite irrigation delivered into the lateral canal of a simulated root canal model. Int Endod J. 2018;51(6):649–62.

155. Mohmmed SA, Vianna ME, Penny MR, Hilton ST, Mordan N, Knowles JC. A novel experimental approach to investigate the effect of different agitation methods using sodium hypochlorite as an irrigant on the rate of bacterial biofilm removal from the wall of a simulated root canal model. Dent Mater. 2016;32(10):1289–300.
156. Lertchirakarn V, Palamara JEA, Messer HH. Patterns of vertical root fracture: factors affecting stress distribution in the root canal. J Endod. 2003;29(8):523–8.
157. Janjić K, Cvikl B, Moritz A, Agis H. Dental pulp regeneration. Int J Stomatol Occlusion Med. 2016;8(1):1–9.
158. Masri R, Driscoll CF, editors. Clinical applications of digital dental technology. Chichester: John Wiley & Sons, Inc; 2015.
159. Petersik A, Pflesser B, Tiede U, Höhne KH, Heiland M, Handels H. Realistic haptic interaction for computer simulation of dental surgery. Perspective in image-guided surgery. World Scientific. 2004:261–9.
160. Suebnukarn S, Haddawy P, Rhienmora P, Gajananan K. Haptic virtual reality for skill acquisition in endodontics. J Endod. 2010;36(1):53–5.
161. Suebnukarn S, Hataidechadusadee R, Suwannasri N, Suprasert N, Rhienmora P, Haddawy P. Access cavity preparation training using haptic virtual reality and microcomputed tomography tooth models. Int Endod J. 2011;44(11):983–9.
162. Ma Y, Xie L, Yang B, Tian W. Three-dimensional printing biotechnology for the regeneration of the tooth and tooth-supporting tissues. Biotechnol Bioeng. 2019;116(2):452–68.
163. Paulsen SJ, Miller JS. Tissue vascularization through 3D printing: will technology bring us flow? Dev Dyn. 2015;244(5):629–40.
164. Reymus M, Fotiadou C, Kessler A, Heck K, Hickel R, Diegritz C. 3D printed replicas for endodontic education. Int Endod J. 2018;52(1):123–30.

Static Guided Nonsurgical Approach for Calcified Canals of Anterior Teeth

6

Jørgen Buchgreitz, Lars Bjørndal,
Antônio Paulino Ribeiro Sobrinho, Warley Luciano Tavares,
Niraj Kinariwala, and Lucas Moreira Maia

6.1   Introduction

Pulp canal obliteration (PCO) or calcified canals may present distinct diagnostic and treatment challenges [1]. In the presence of calcification, adequate access cavity preparation and identification of root canal orifice are extremely difficult. The American Association of Endodontists (AAE) Case Assessment places these cases into the high difficulty category [2]. Calcified canals pose risk of overextended access cavity preparation, incorrect alignment of the access cavity with the risk of root perforation as well as fracture of root canal instruments during canal preparation [3]. Therefore, precise and predictable preoperative planning is highly recommended, and 3D imaging may be a useful tool.

Cone-beam computed tomography (CBCT) helps the clinician to establish a proper strategy to deal with PCO with potential benefits. CBCT is a noninvasive imaging and measuring tool that can represent the tooth in all spatial planes to explore root canal anatomy [4]. Static guided endodontics can be very useful in negotiation and preparation of partly or entirely obliterated pulp chambers and canals [5, 6].

J. Buchgreitz
Allerød, Denmark

L. Bjørndal
Section of Cariology and Endodontics, Department of Odontology, Faculty of Health and Medical Sciences, University of Copenhagen, Copenhagen, Denmark

A. P. R. Sobrinho · W. L. Tavares · L. M. Maia
Department of Restorative Dentistry, Faculty of Dentistry, Universidade Federal de Minas Gerais (UFMG), Belo Horizonte, MG, Brazil

N. Kinariwala (✉)
Karnavati School of Dentistry, Karnavati University, Gandhinagar, Gujarat, India
e-mail: niraj@ksd.ac.in

© Springer Nature Switzerland AG 2021
N. Kinariwala, L. Samaranayake (eds.), *Guided Endodontics*,
https://doi.org/10.1007/978-3-030-55281-7_6

113

6.2 Review of Literature

For decades, dentists have had to locate canals, mainly, in a "tactile" manner [7]. New instruments have enhanced treatment modalities [8, 9], such as microscopy, that enrich the visibility of the pulp cavity, the microprobe DG16, and ultrasonic tips, which facilitate finding the root canal orifice with a microscope. Another diagnostic tool is cone-beam computed tomography (CBCT), which presents more accurate 3D visualization of, both, hard and soft tissues [7].

In the late 1980s and 1990s, computer-aided design/computer-aided manufacturing (CAD/CAM) and 3-dimensional (3D) printing technology were developed [10]. Since its introduction to dentistry [11], CBCT offers new possibilities in diagnosis and treatment [12]. CBCT is often used in the field of oral implantology for three-dimensional planning [13], as well as for guiding implant surgery using templates [14]. More recently, the construction of guides was introduced in endodontics for negotiating calcified root canals [5, 6]. It is vital to give the merit to Buchgreitz et al. [5], who was the first to demonstrate that guided access principles, now known as "guided endodontics," were accurate to be used in vivo. Nowadays, 3D-printing devices, based on matched 3D surface scans with CBCT data [15], can produce these templates.

Krastl et al. [16] have stated that considering the fast-paced digitization of dentistry during the last few years, it is likely that combining the information obtained from CBCTs and digital impressions shall become standard in the future. Moreover, it has been shown that when template integrates the experience of dentists and the analysis of CBCT visualization, the successful practical operation fructified [7]. Hence, a novel guided approach for the preparation of apically extended access cavities, named "guided endodontics," was introduced to overcome PCO complications [5–7]. This technique proved to be accurate, expeditious, and operator-independent in vitro settings [17, 18], as well as in vivo patients [19–24].

6.2.1 Accuracy of the Drill Path In Vitro

Based on an in vitro study [5], analyses were made to measure the accuracy of the guided concept and thereby justifying the necessary bur diameter to be used. In the particular study, the test teeth were embedded in acrylic after being supplied with a small filling in the apical part of the root. This filling performed as a target for the drill path. The drill path was placed in root dentin to mimic an obliterated root canal. Drilling was performed short of the target point with a length of the drill path extending 20 mm, simulating the length of clinically expected scenarios. Based on the diameter of the bur in use and the diameter of a radiographically barely visible root canal, an accepted distortion away from the root canal was calculated. If the size of a root canal is 0.20 mm and drill diameter is 1.2 mm (Fig. 6.15a), the highest accepted distance between the target point and the center of the drill path would be half the bur diameter and half the root canal, that is, 0.6–0.7 mm. The test was highly accurate and measured mean distance was less than 0.5 mm. In extracted single rooted teeth, accuracy of virtual drill path was evaluated and confirmed a clinically acceptable accuracy, even though a mean deviation at the tip of the bur was 0.5 mm [5].

6.2.2   Accuracy of the Clinical Drill Path in Patients

A study of guided root canal treatment, in vivo, on 50 single rooted teeth was conducted [3]. Clinical acceptable precision criteria were defined as drill path peripherally or tangentially transported. Optimal precision was defined as the drill path being centered. Optimal precision was achieved in 22 treatments, while 28 treatments showed acceptable precision. In the mandibular teeth, optimal precision was achieved in 9 out of 13 teeth, which suggests that the diameter could be reduced, for example, when treating mandibular incisors. Studies have suggested predictable clinical outcomes with use of bur or drill with diameter of 0.85 [18, 26].

6.2.3   Clinical Case Reports

Although clinical treatment trials are missing, recent clinical case reports show the successful application of this technique in endodontic practice. Table 6.1 summarizes the case reports and preclinical studies of guided endodontic access.

In ex vivo investigations of accuracy, Buchgreitz et al. [5], Zehnder et al. [6], Chong et al. [25], and Connert et al. [26] assessed stent guided access preparations by superimposing a postaccess CBCT upon preoperative designed access. Buchgreitz et al. [5] found the mean deviation of the access cavities to be lower than the 0.7-mm threshold defined by the radius of the bur plus the radius of the root

Table 6.1 Guide endodontic application

Authors	Type of study/teeth	Endodontic application
van der Meer et al. [27]	Case series/anterior teeth	Guided endodontic access
Krastl et al. [16]	Case report/anterior teeth	Guided endodontic access
Buchgreitz et al. [5]	Ex vivo	Guided endodontic access
Zehnder et al. [6]	Ex vivo	Guided endodontic access
Mena-Alvarez et al. [31]	Case report/dens evaginatus	Guided endodontic access
de Toubes et al. [28]	Case report/anterior teeth	Guided endodontic access
Shi et al. [30]	Case report/mandibular molar	Guided endodontic access
Connert et al. [26]	Ex vivo	Guided endodontic access
Lara-Mendes et al. [21]	Case report/anterior tooth	Guided endodontic access
Lara-Mendes et al. [22]	Case report/upper molar	Guided endodontic access
Connert et al. [17, 18]	Case report/mandibular incisors	Guided endodontic access
Tavares et al. [23]	Case report/anterior teeth	Guided endodontic access
Buchgreitz et al. [3]	Case series/maxillary molar	Guided endodontic access
Buchgreitz et al. [20]	Case report/maxillary molar	Guided endodontic access
Torres et al. [19]	Case report/anterior teeth	Guided endodontic access
Casadei et al. [29]	Case report/upper premolar	Guided endodontic access
Maia et al. [24]	Case report/upper molar	Guided endodontic access
Chong et al. [25]	Ex vivo	Guided endodontic access

canal. Zehnder et al. [6] and Connert et al. [26] also found small deviations from the intended access (0.12–0.34 mm at the tip of the bur) and a mean angular deviation of less than 2°. Chong et al. [25] found that conservative access cavities were achieved, and all the expected canals were successfully located in 26 teeth ($n = 29$).

van der Meer et al. [27] acquired digital impressions and CBCT scans; CAD software merged digital impression files with CBCT DICOM data to form an STL file containing boney architecture for teeth in pulp canal obliteration-affected maxillary incisors. Based on these scans, endodontic guides were created for the planned treatment through digital designing and rapid prototyping fabrication. The guides allowed for an uncomplicated and predictable canal location and management. Another report by Buchgreitz et al. [3] observed that the clinical implementation of guided root canal treatment in 50 serial cases of single-rooted teeth with pulp space obliteration was associated with a precision that, in all cases, led to the location and negotiation of the root canal and completion of the treatment.

The case reports describing the use of 3D printed guides to access obliterated maxillary and mandibular incisors [16, 18–21, 28], upper premolar [29], mandibular and maxillary molars [22, 24, 30], and type V dens evaginatus [31] support the clinical utility of the technique.

Moreover, clinicians continue to encounter difficulty in posterior molar presenting pulp canal obliteration. These conditions potentially lead to extraction of otherwise serviceable teeth. Nevertheless, premolars and molars have been efficiently treated by guide endodontics [22, 24, 29, 30]. These clinical cases show that technological evolutions should make guided endodontic procedures in posterior teeth more widespread, because their execution is relatively fast, safe, and predictable, avoiding failures in complex cases. Additionally, its success does not depend on the experience of the operator.

In complicated posterior teeth with root canal calcification, perforation, and canal deviation, guided endodontic technique has been successful [29]. Additionally, Mena-Alvarez et al. [31] described the treatment of a type V dens evaginatus by using splits as guides to perform access cavity.

The clinical reports demonstrate that 3D printed endodontic guides represent an efficient and safe means of addressing challenging endodontic scenarios. The guides enable, both, chemomechanical debridement and conservation of tooth structure. Treatment of teeth with pulp canal obliteration, malposition, or with extensive restoration may be more productive with designed targeted access guides. On the other hand, further clinical investigation in this area has to be undertaken.

6.3   Root Canal Obliteration and Clinical Challenges

Pulp canal obliteration (PCO) is characterized by the deposition of hard tissue within the root canal space [32]. It is associated with injury to the pulp and, generally, PCO has no symptoms and may be noted via tooth discoloration or routine clinical examination [33–35]. Moreover, its diagnosis can be more challenging as the response of the tooth to thermal and electric pulp tests can be diminished or even absent [36, 37].

Obliteration of the pulp space may occur as a result of the formation of tertiary dentine, due to chronic caries progression [38], or following tooth restoration [39], and after vital pulp therapy procedures [40]. Also, pulp space obliteration occurs in teeth with open apices following luxation injuries, particularly following lateral luxation, intrusion, and avulsion [41–43]. Pulp canal calcification may also arise as an adverse effect of excessive orthodontic forces, which interferes with pulpal blood supply [44, 45]. Moreover, in elderly individuals, the apposition of secondary dentine over time may lead to severe calcification of the root canal system [46, 47].

Worldwide, the number of elderly patients and their need for root canal treatment is increasing [48, 49]. Consequently, cases of calcified canals or PCO, as a result of a lifelong apposition of secondary or tertiary dentine, are increasing [47]. On the other hand, it has been shown that in young patients, 15% of traumatized permanent incisors had pulp canal obliteration [41]. In most of the cases, the PCO is related to pulp healing and does not need endodontic intervention, but, in this way, there is always a risk for the pulp to become necrotic, ranging from 1% to 27% [36, 37, 41]. The frequency of apical periodontitis has been reported to increase to approximately 10% after more than 15 years in such cases [50].

There is almost a consensus in the literature that the root canal treatment of teeth presenting with PCO is only indicated in the presence of acute symptoms or apical periodontitis [34–37, 41, 50]. Additionally, in PCO cases with severe loss of tooth structure, endodontic intervention may be indicated for postretention [51]. In these cases, even the most experienced clinicians can encounter difficulties to prepare an adequate access cavity. Additionally, it becomes hard to identify the canal orifice, which may lead to excessive loss of tooth structure, which poses risk of tooth fracture [52] and a high failure rate [53]. Root perforation and canal deviations have been reported as common complications after the treatment of PCO cases, which may result in tooth loss [54, 55].

If a seemingly obliterated tooth shows symptoms of an apical pathosis (Fig. 6.1a), it can be assumed that the pulp canal space is not hermitical closed but associated with necrotic infected remnants of the pulp tissue, indicating the need for a root canal treatment. The frequency of apical periodontitis has been reported to increase to approximately 10% after more than 15 years after the trauma [56].

Clinically, experience says that the obliterations are more pronounced in the incisal or occlusal part of the pulpal tissue. The immediate problem adhering to the superficial orifice/canal obliteration in teeth in need of a root canal treatment is to get proper access to the root canal. This can be a time-consuming and challenging task even when using an operating microscope [47]. The differences in surface hardness and color between the primary dentin and the mineralized tissue adding up in the root canal space make it possible and easier, but the result will often be overextension of the preparation with succeeding weakening of the tooth.

Usually, a root canal is only visible on two dimensional (2D) radiograph, if the diameter of the canal is more than 0.20 mm corresponding to a K-file size 20. Visibility of the root canal on 2D radiograph varies depending on the thickness of the bone and bone density of the jaws. It explains clinical ease in negotiating canals which seem calcified on 2D radiographs. Though it can be actual calcification, as well, which presents a clinical challenge for the clinician.

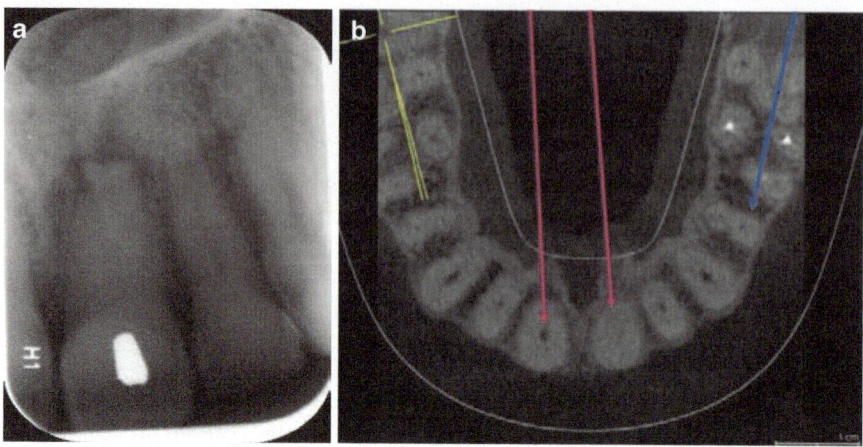

Fig. 6.1 Apical pathosis on a root without a visible root canal neither on the radiograph (**a**) nor on the CBCT (**b**). In single rooted teeth with one root canal, the canal is or was placed in the center of the axial view of the root on the CBCT scan (red arrows). If there are two canals, the cross section will have a concavity, and the canals will be placed on the bucco-lingual orientated symmetrical line of the cross section (blue arrow)

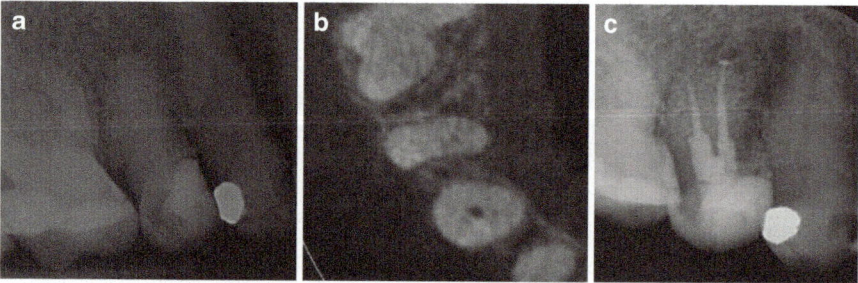

Fig. 6.2 (**a**) The surrounding structures make it difficult to localize the roots as well as the root canals. (**b**) The buccal canal is not observed at the axial view of the CBCT. (**c**) The final root canal filling

On a CBCT scan, the lowest voxel size of most manufactures is of the same order. This means that it is not always possible from a standard radiograph as well as from a CBCT scan to see the whole extent of a partly obliterated pulp space and it is not possible to assess whether a root canal is completely obliterated or not. From the axial view of the CBCT scan, it is possible to see the periphery of the root and thereby estimate the former placement of the original canal, since the canal normally is placed in the midline of the root (Fig. 6.1b). This morphological observation becomes an important landmark in the software preparation when placing a virtual drill path for guided endodontics.

As mentioned above, the surrounding bone structures may vary. On molars and premolars, it can be rather complex and sometimes, the roots are more fragile. This makes the assessment of roots and obliterations more difficult (Fig. 6.2a–c). On the

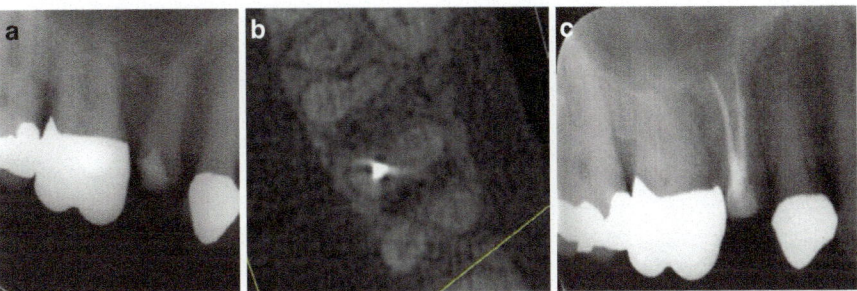

Fig. 6.3 (**a**) Calcified canal in maxillary second premolar. (**b**) The CBCT shows calcified palatal canal. (**c**) Final root canal filling

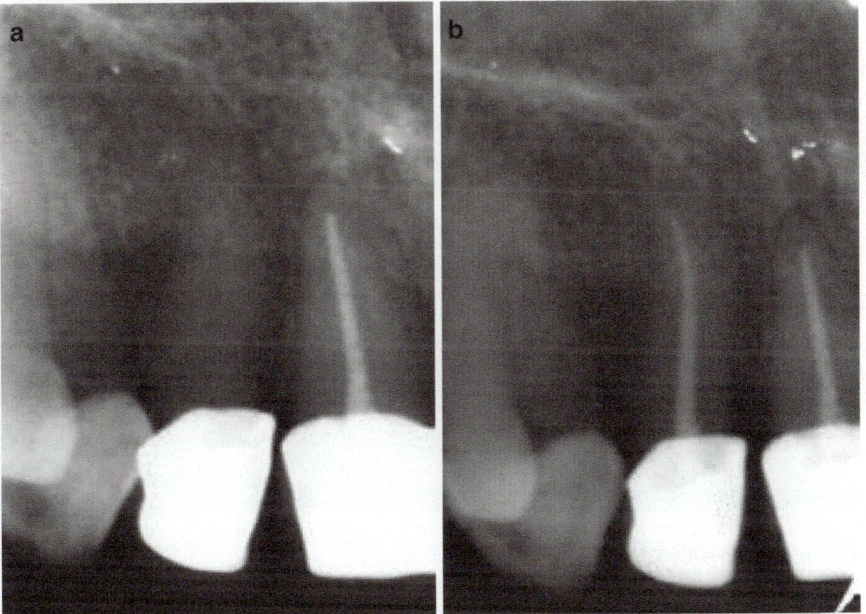

Fig. 6.4 (**a**) Superimposition of other structures may cover the apical 1/3 of the root and thereby give the impression of a root canal obliteration of the apical part. (**b**) The final root canal filling

radiographs, the roots may often cover each other (Fig. 6.3a–c). In few cases, it seems like an obliteration initiates apically, which is unusual. Actually apical canal obliteration occurs when any anatomic structures radiographically overshadow the tooth or the canal. Usually disappearance of canal reaffirms the presence of canal bifurcation or trifurcation (Fig. 6.4a, b). Splitting of canal creates the radiographic artifact of obliteration, and guided endodontics is not needed to negotiate such canals.

Sometimes, root canal is patent on two-dimensional radiograph and the conventional endodontic root canal treatment is initiated. Clinically, canal cannot be negotiated and CBCT may reveal presence of calcification in the canal. Such cases can be treated predictably with guided endodontics (Figs. 6.5a–e and 6.6).

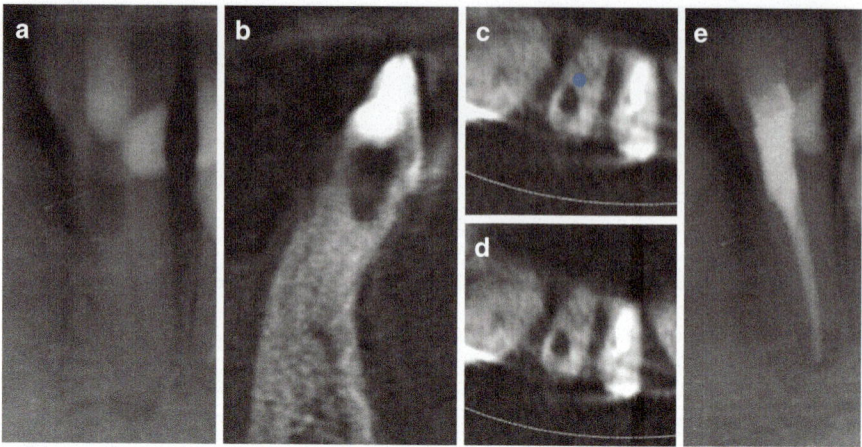

Fig. 6.5 (**a**) A lower incisal was in need of a root canal treatment, but it was not possible to localize a root canal. (**b**) The CBCT scan revealed an initial preparation off the root canal. (**c, d**) The axial view shows the direction of a new attempt. The blue dot shows the estimated position of the root canal. (**e**) The final root canal filling

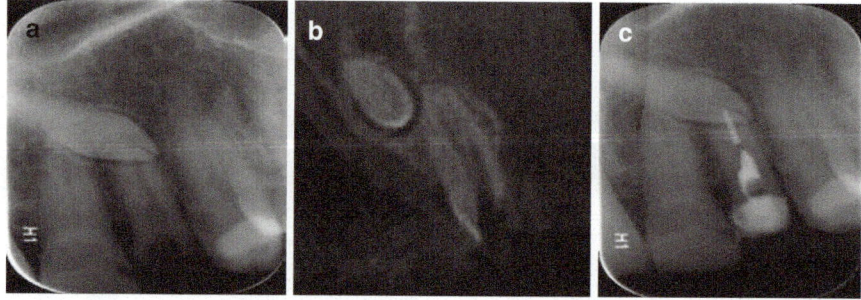

Fig. 6.6 (**a**) Maxillary lateral incisor with a seemingly apparent root canal, but, clinically, canal could not be negotiated. (**b**) The cross-sectional view of the CBCT scan revealed the position of the root canal. (**c**) Explored canal with root canal filling, postspace preparation, and temporary restoration

6.3.1   Can Obliterated Incisors Be Expected to Be Scouted?

Obliterated canals can be scouted with good technique, good armamentarium, knowledge of anatomy, and experience of the operator. With guided endodontics, the virtual drill path is extended up to first visible part of the canal from which the root canal can be scouted. The length of such an obliteration may be quite extensive and may extend up to apical third of the tooth (Figs. 6.7, 6.8, and 6.9). Smaller size stainless files should be used to scout the canal.

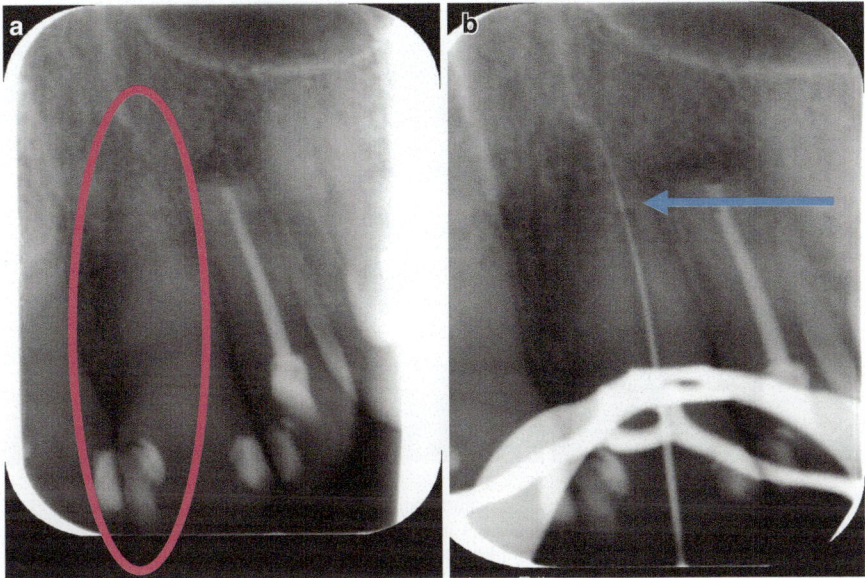

Fig. 6.7 (**a, b**) In calcified upper central incisor (#9), canal could not be scouted until 3 mm from apex (blue arrow)

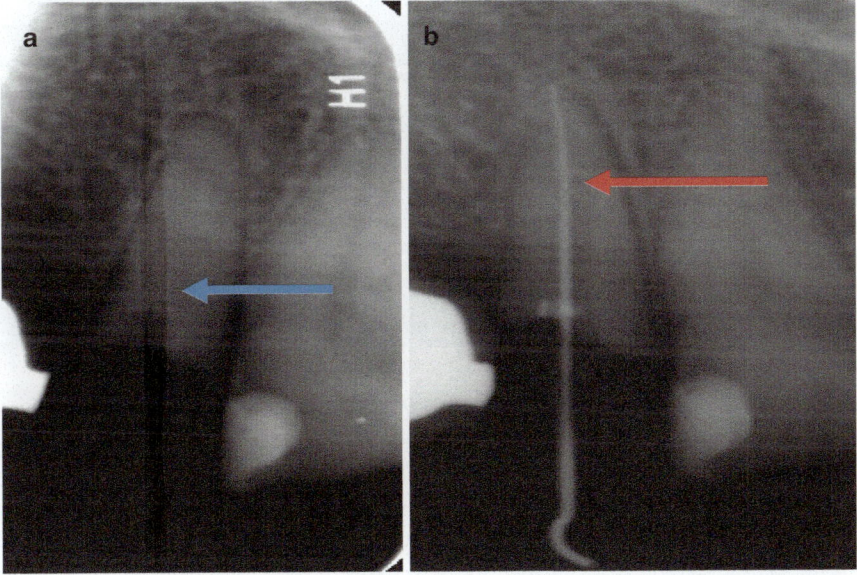

Fig. 6.8 (**a**) Extent of calcification less than 30% of root length (blue arrow). (**b**) Drill path is longer (red arrow)

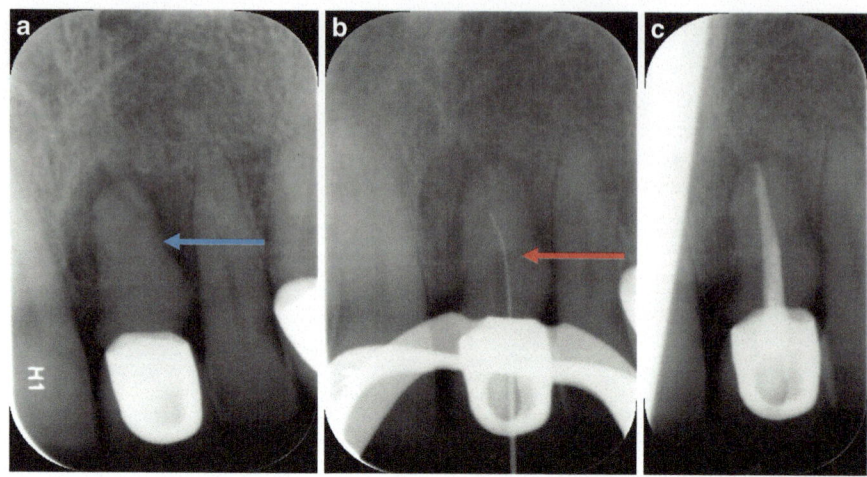

Fig. 6.9 (**a**) Calcified canal in maxillary central incisor (Extent of calcification more than 50% of the root length). (**b**) With guided endodontics, treatment was planned through existing prosthesis. Canal was scouted successfully in the middle third (Shorter drill path). (**c**) 1-year follow-up

Fig. 6.10 (**a**) A special bur produced for guided endo 1.2 mm (SICAT, Germany). (**b**) A commercially available twist bur (Busch, Germany) can be chosen and customized to fit any diameter of a guiding hole

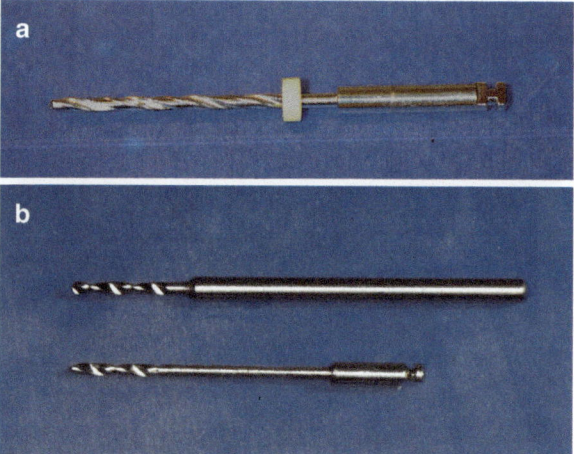

On radiographs, root canal is seen as a radiolucent line. Presence of radiopacity, in place of radiolucency of root canal, indicates presence of calcification or PCO. On conventional 2D radiograph, clinician should measure extent of obliteration from the cemento-enamel junction to the faint radiolucent line depicting canal. Notably, this visible pulp canal space is more apically placed on the CBCT, because the resolution of the 2D radiograph is lesser than the voxel size of the CBCT (Fig. 6.10). Even if extent of calcification is less than 30% of the entire root length, the drill path often extends more apically (Fig. 6.8a–c). When the extent of calcification is more than 50% of the root length, the drill path is shorter or the same in 55% of the cases (Fig. 6.9).

6.4   The Static Guiding Procedure Step by Step

Virtual planning and endodontic guide designing have been explained in Chap. 4. If the clinician does not have the appropriate software for virtual planning of guided endodontics, the virtual planning can be outsourced. Before starting clinical procedure, proper armamentarium should be selected. A practical limitation of guided endodontics is limited availability of armamentarium in the market. SICAT Endo (Dentsply Sirona Inc., Charlotte, N Carolina USA) delivers a 1.2 mm diameter drill that fits the metal sleeves of their CNC-made guides (Fig. 6.10a). Straumann Drill for Tempimplants has a diameter of 1.5 mm and a working length of 18.5 mm. The 3D printed guides can be made to fit all diameters, but still the length of the drill sets a limit of the selection. Neodent SA (Curitiba, Brazil) delivers 1.3 and 0.8 mm drills fitting the 3D printed guides. For special purposes, a commercially available twist bur can be customized (Fig. 6.10b).

Step-by-step clinical procedure is explained, below, for calcified canal in tooth number #6. First, endodontic guide is tested for stability by placing it on the tooth arch before rubber dam application (Fig. 6.11). Incorporation of inspection window or inspection holes is also helpful to evaluate fit of the guide.

The starting point of the access preparation on the tooth surface can be marked through the guiding canal by colored resin on the tip of a pin (Fig. 6.12a). After removing the guide, it is possible to make the entrance preparation with a high-speed bur and with water coolant spray (Fig. 6.12b–d). The entrance preparation should reach through the surface material whether it is enamel, dentin, ceramic, or metal. With the pin through the guide sleeve, it can be checked if the pin and later the drill can go unhindered from the surface of the tooth to the bottom of the entrance preparation.

Often, there is a previous attempt to localize the root canal and this cavity is filled with a provisional material. If the colored starting point is placed between enamel and provisional filling, it is necessary to enlarge the access cavity in order to avoid the bur from being pushed aside from the ideal direction by the harder enamel. The bur could be misled, since it needs a little push in the guiding canal to avoid heat

Fig. 6.11 Check stability of the guide on the tooth arch

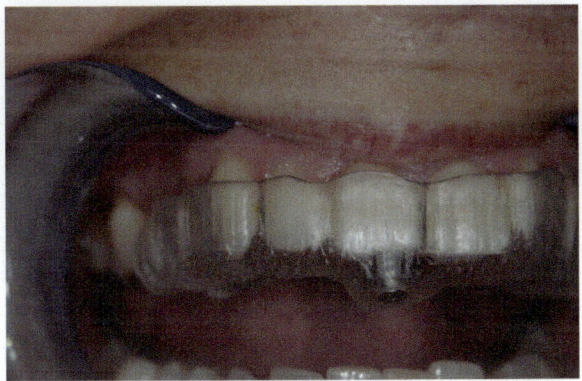

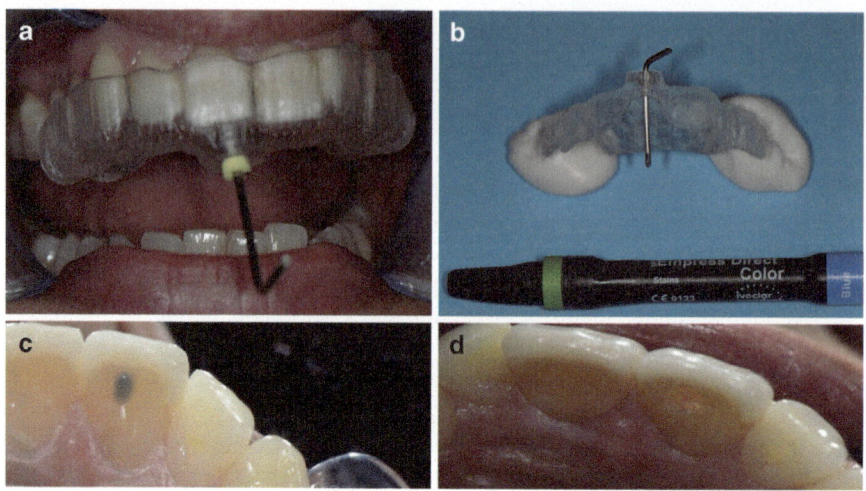

Fig. 6.12 (**a**) A marking pin with blue composite stain on the tip. (**b**) The marking pin is pressed through the guide sleeve to touch the tooth. (**c**) The blue stain marking the entrance point. (**d**) The penetration of the enamel at the entrance point

generated by the rotation. The same error may arise if the inclination of the surface is far from perpendicular to the direction of the bur. To avoid this problem of misleading a high-speed bur, a coolant spray should be used to remove the surface material at and around the starting point without the guide and before rubber dam application. Free hand drilling should be done up to dentin and base should be perpendicular to the direction of the drill path.

After adapting endodontic guide, drilling can be started directly on the dentinal surface, at low speed, without coolant spray. To avoid heat generation, drilling should be done incrementally. Initial drilling should be done short of the virtual drill path. Attempt should be made to scout the canal. If canal cannot be negotiated, further drilling should be done. After reaching the depth of virtual drill path, attempt should be made to scout the canal.

In the present case (an upper lateral incisor), the tooth was previously treated with a ceramic crown and remaining tooth structure was less. In this case, guided approach was chosen to preserve as much sound tooth structure as possible (Fig. 6.13).

6.4.1 Scouting the Root Canal

To judge depth of required drilling, before the canal can be scouted, is difficult. Based on a study of 50 single rooted teeth with seemingly obliterated pulp canal space, the relationship between the length of the obliteration and the necessary drill length was recorded [8]. In 9 out of 50 teeth, the drill path was shorter than the obliteration. Consequently, a first attempt to scout the root canal space should be

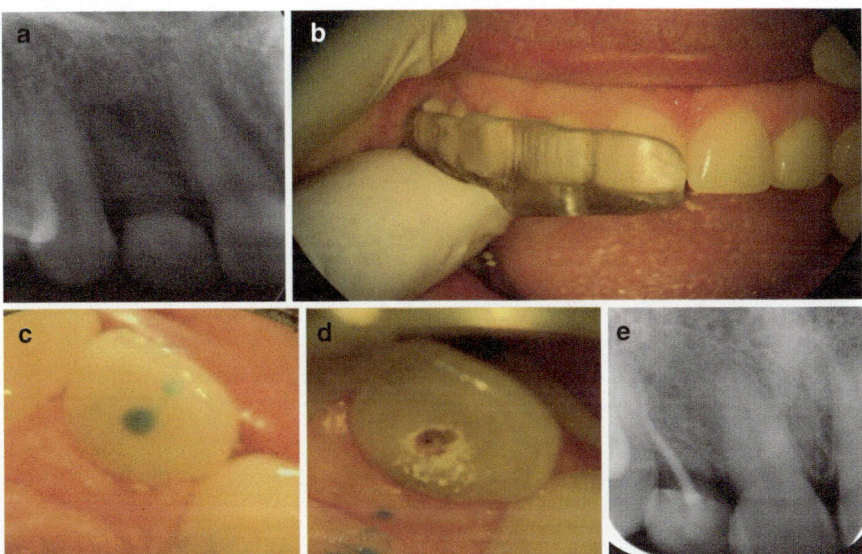

Fig. 6.13 (a) Upper right tap tooth incisor covered by a ceramic crown. (b) Checking the guide for stability. (c) Blue stain marking the entrance point. (d) The penetration of the ceramic and the enamel of the tooth. (e) The final radiograph of completed RCT

done about half the way down the planned drill path. A so-called Endo dance is very useful for scouting the canal space: Precurved K-flex file #10 is gently pushed down and up several times and use watch winding motion to scout the canal. If a canal is not found, a radiograph can be taken to ensure that the drilling is on the right track. The guided drilling continues to the level decided at the planning phase and the "Endo dance" is repeated. If canal cannot be negotiated at planned depth, drilling can be continued without the guide, since the drill path in the dentin will guide the drill. Care should be taken not to perforate the tooth, specially, at a bending of the root or at a level where the surrounding dentin is too weak.

6.4.1.1 Clinical Case Report

A female patient (25 years) was referred to the clinic to have a root canal treatment of tooth no #9 (Fig. 6.14a). The tooth was tender to percussion and the radiograph showed an apical pathosis (Fig. 6.14b). The root canal seemed partly obliterated on the radiograph but was visible in the apical half of the root. The referring dentist had failed to localize the root canal, and this treatment was finished by closing the access opening with a provisional filling (Fig. 6.14c).

Since the root canal seemed partly obliterated, it was decided to make a CBCT scan and a surface scan, to use guided approach for the case. Low noise or scattering on the CBCT was expected, since the neighboring teeth were without metal fillings or crowns. Periodontal health was good providing stability during scanning and the final drilling. The CBCT was loaded into the SICAT ENDO program. On the tangential, the cross-cut, and the axial views, only apical part of the root canal was

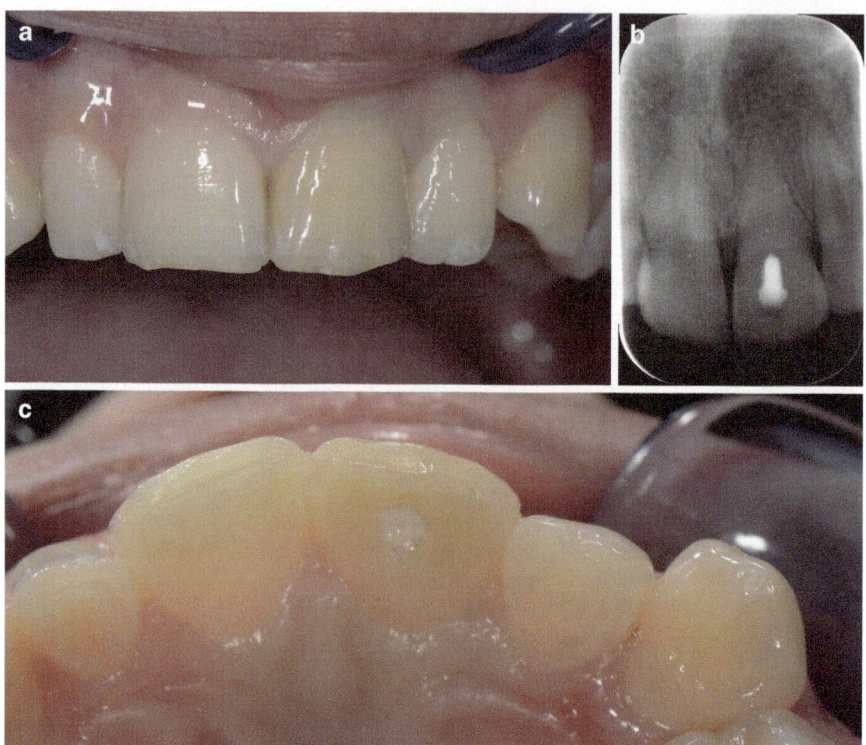

Fig. 6.14 (**a**) Discoloration of tooth no #9. (**b**) The incisal part of the root canal is seemingly obliterated. (**c**) Provisional filling following the first attempt of access opening

visible (Fig. 6.15). A virtual drill path was placed parallel to the long axis of the tooth (Fig. 6.16a), reaching the visible part of the root canal (target point) (Fig. 6.16b, c). The axial view of the CBCT is often the best view for localizing the remnants of the root canal space (Fig. 6.16d, e). To avoid interfering with the incisal edge, it was necessary to tilt the virtual drill path and thereby establish the angle of the drill path (Fig. 6.17).

6.4.2   Surface Scan in the Clinic

For this patient, a stone model from the rubber base impression was scanned and loaded into the software (Fig. 6.15). CBCT scan was merged with the surface scan, in the same way, as described earlier (Fig. 6.18). This superimposed image was re-evaluated and sent for milling to a CNC milling machine (SICAT, Bonn, Germany) to get a guide with a metal sleeve (Fig. 6.19).

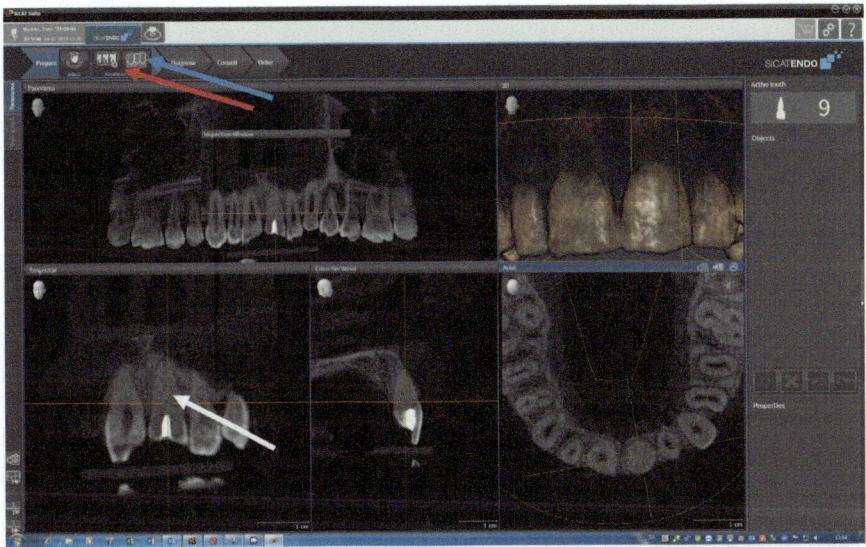

Fig. 6.15 The CBCT scan loaded into the SICATENDO program. The root canal of tooth #9 seems partly obliterated (white arrow). By clicking the box on the screen, a 2D radiograph will be superimposed on the panoramic view or the tangential view if the 2D radiograph is compatible (red arrow). By clicking the box at the blue arrow, the next screen will show the optical impression (Cerec optical impression or surface scan)

6.4.3   In the Clinic, Next Visit

The fit of the guide was checked for stability and, at the same time, a pin was placed through the sleeve. Diameter of the pin was equivalent to diameter of the virtual drill (1.2 mm). On the tip of the pin, a drop of colored composite was placed, which marked the entry point on the tooth surface (Fig. 6.20a). The preparation of the drill path was performed with the spiral drill guided through the sleeve in the guide (Fig. 6.20b). Glyde was used as a lubricant and drilling was performed at speed of 250 rpm in an endodontic hand piece. Drilling at slow speed prevents heating of both the tooth and the guide. Radiographs were taken, intermittently, to evaluate direction and depth of the drilling. Canal was scouted successfully with a hand file #10.

Rubber dam can be applied after canal negotiation or before drilling, depending on guide design and experience of the clinician. On localization of the canal, it was enlarged to the desired file size with intermittent irrigation and obturated following standard protocols of root canal treatment.

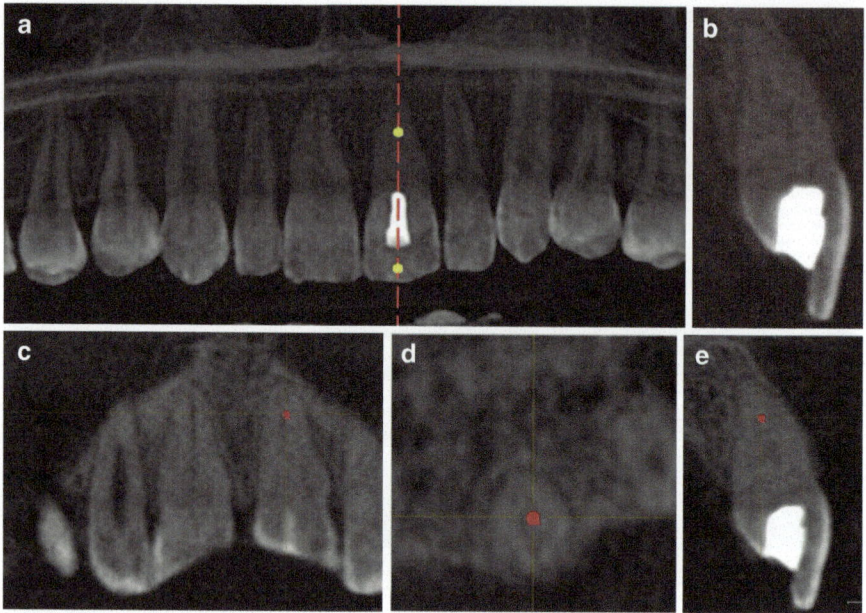

Fig. 6.16 (**a**) The panoramic view. The red dotted line represents the cut surface seen at the cross-sectional view (**b**). (**c–e**) the target (red dot) is marked by double clicking **twice** at the selected point, and can then be viewed in all three planes. The axial view (**d**) is often the most secure way to select the placement of the root canal

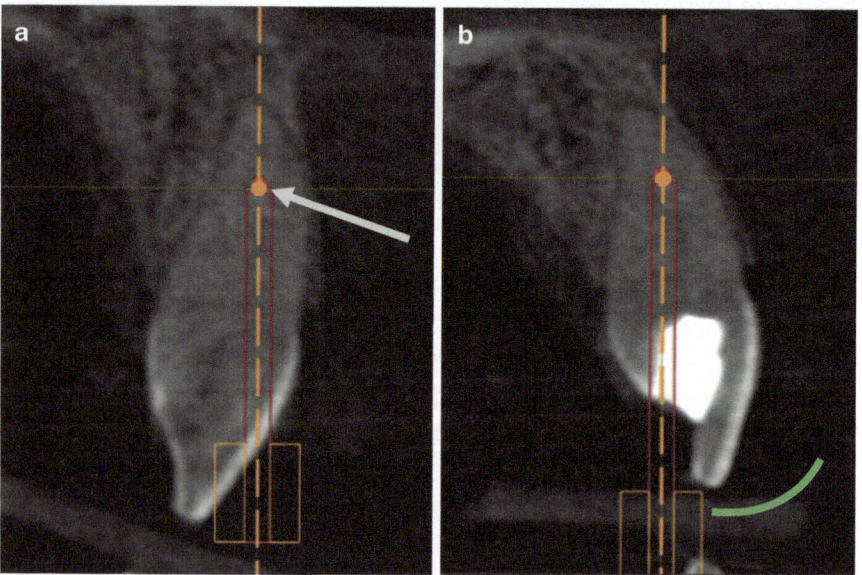

Fig. 6.17 (**a**) The drill path can be tilted around the target (white arrow) to avoid interfering with the incisal edge (green curve, **b**)

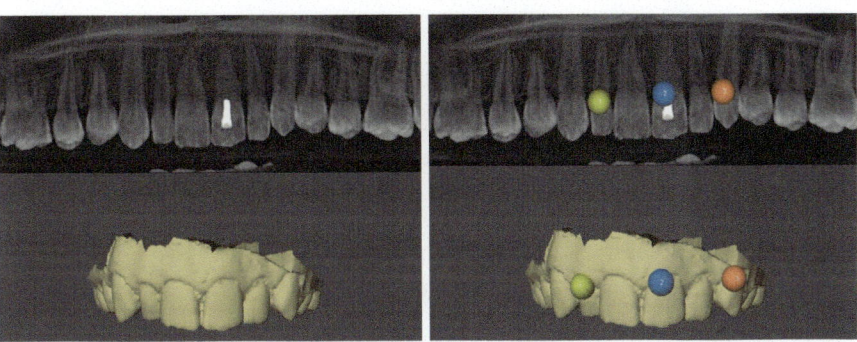

Fig. 6.18 The CBCT scan and the optical impression (left) are combined by setting markers on 3–4 corresponding teeth (right)

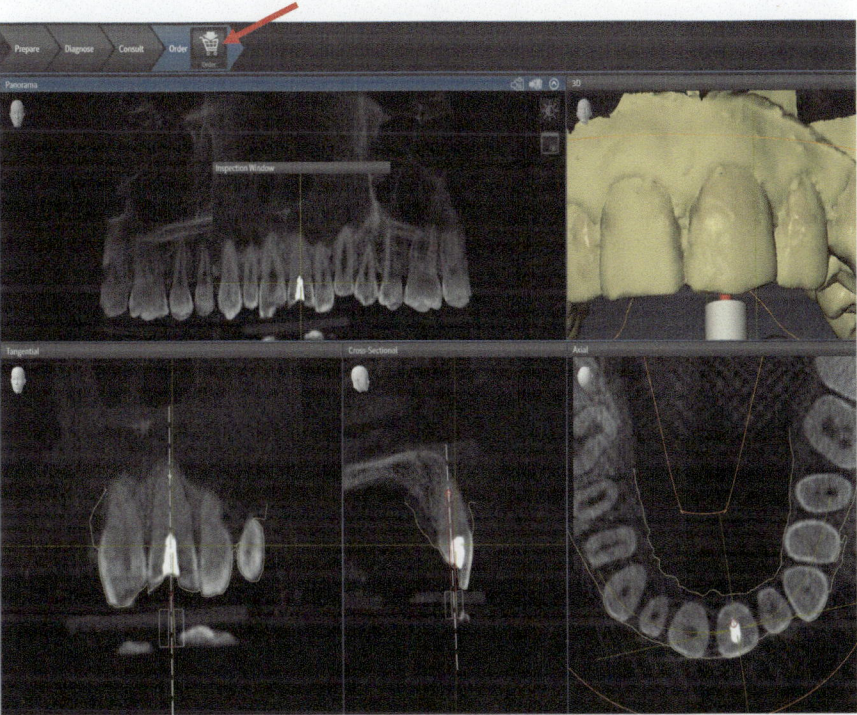

Fig. 6.19 Screenshot of the software program after planning of endodontic guide. This file can be sent to 3D printer or milling company by clicking the symbol of shopping cart (Red arrow)

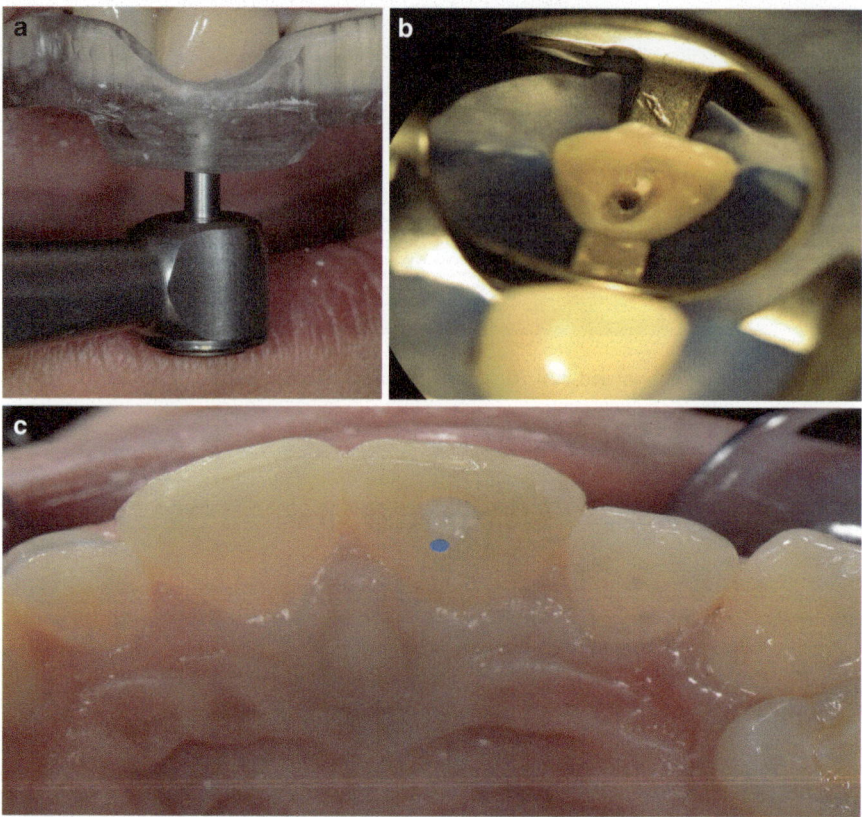

Fig. 6.20 (**a**) Marking shows point of entry for guided drilling. (**b**) The guided drilling through metal sleeve. (**c**) Canal has been negotiated successfully and shaping has been done. Note, the enamel of the access cavity was removed prior to the guided drilling and because of the selected angle, the access cavity is slightly off the first access cavity

6.5   Limitation

Every technology has its limitations. They should be considered before deciding the treatment plan. Limitations of static guidance are as follows:

1. A static guide for guided endodontics will only work for straight parts of root canals.
2. The tooth must be able to stay in a fixed position during the CBCT scanning and during the guided drilling. (Teeth with poor periodontal health should be contra-indicated to avoid errors in planning and drilling.)
3. Presence of metallic restoration or fillings of the teeth may lead to artifacts on a radiograph and may lead to inaccuracies in treatment planning.
4. Limitation of availability of armamentarium (long neck small diameter drills and sleeves).

We are looking forward to more sophisticated and customized software programs for endodontic treatments and availability of smaller long neck drills, calibrated sleeves, and precise 3D printers. "The time for the pioneers has ended. The time has come for the settlers at harvest."

References

1. McCabe PS, Dummer PMH. Pulp canal obliteration: and endodontic diagnosis and treatment challenge. Int Endod J. 2012;46:177–97.
2. American Association of Endodontists. Contemporary endodontic microsurgery: procedural advancements and treatment planning considerations. In: Endodontics. Chicago, IL: Colleagues for Excellence; 2010.
3. Buchgreitz J, Buchgreitz M, Bjørndal L. Guided root canal preparation using cone beam computed tomography and optical surface scans – an observational study of pulp space obliteration and drill path depth in 50 patients. Int Endod J. 2019;52:559–68.
4. Patel S, Durack C, Abella F, et al. Cone beam computed tomography in endodontics - a review. Int Endod J. 2015;48:3–15.
5. Buchgreitz J, Buchgreitz M, Mortensen D, et al. Guided access cavity preparation using cone-beam computed tomography and optical surface scans - an ex vivo study. Int Endod J. 2016;49:790–5.
6. Zehnder MS, Connert T, Weiger R, et al. Guided endodontics: accuracy of a novel method for guided access cavity preparation and root canal location. Int Endod J. 2016;49:966–72.
7. Shi X, Zhao S, Wang W. Novel navigation technique for the endodontic treatment of a molar with pulp canal calcification and apical pathology. Aust Endod J. 2018;44:66–70.
8. Wu D, Shi W, Wu J, et al. The clinical treatment of complicated root canal therapy with the aid of a dental operating microscope. Int Dent J. 2011;61:261–6.
9. Yang YM, Guo B, Guo LY, et al. CBCT-aided microscopic and ultrasonic treatment for upper or middle thirds calcified root canals. Biomed Res Int. 2016;2016:4793146.
10. Dawood A, Marti Marti B, Sauret-Jackson V, et al. 3D printing in dentistry. Br Dent J. 2015;219:521–9.
11. Mozzo P, Procacci C, Tacconi A, et al. A new volumetric CT machine for dental imaging based on the cone-beam technique: preliminary results. Eur Radiol. 1998;8:1558–64.
12. European Society of Endodontology. Quality guidelines for endodontic treatment: consensus report of the European Society of Endodontology. Int Endod J. 2006;39:921–30.
13. Guerrero ME, Jacobs R, Loubele M, et al. State-of-the-art on cone beam CT imaging for preoperative planning of implant placement. Clin Oral Investig. 2006;10:1–7.
14. Yatzkair G, Cheng A, Brodie S, et al. Accuracy of computer-guided implantation in a human cadaver model. Clin Oral Implants Res. 2014;26:1143–9.
15. Kühl S, Payer M, Zitzmann NU, et al. Technical accuracy of printed surgical templates for guided implant surgery with the coDiagnostiXTM software. Clin Implant Dent Res. 2015;17(Suppl 1):177–82.
16. Krastl G, Zehnder MS, Connert T, et al. Guided Endodontics: a novel treatment approach for teeth with pulp canal calcification and apical pathology. Dent Traumatol. 2016;32:240–6.
17. Connert T, Zehnder MS, Weiger R, et al. Microguided endodontics: accuracy of a miniaturized technique for apically extended access cavity preparation in anterior teeth. J Endod. 2018;43:787–90.
18. Connert T, Zehnder MS, Amato M, et al. Microguided Endodontics: a method to achieve minimally invasive access cavity preparation and root canal location in mandibular incisors using a novel computer-guided technique. Int Endod J. 2018;51:247–55.
19. Torres A, Shaheen E, Lambrechts P, et al. Microguided endodontics: a case report of a maxillary lateral incisor with pulp canal obliteration and apical periodontitis. Int Endod J. 2019;52(4):540–9.

20. Buchgreitz J, Buchgreitz M, Bjørndal L. Guided endodontics modified for treating molars by using an intracoronal guide technique. J Endod. 2019;6:818–23.
21. Lara-Mendes STO, Barbosa CFM, Machado VC, et al. A new approach for minimally invasive access to severely calcified anterior teeth using the guided endodontics technique. J Endod. 2018;44(10):1578–82.
22. Lara-Mendes STO, Barbosa CFM, Santa-Rosa CC, et al. Guided endodontic access in maxillary molars using cone-beam computed tomography and computer-aided design/computer-aided manufacturing system: a case report. J Endod. 2018;44(5):875–9.
23. Tavares WLF, Diniz Viana AC, Machado VC, et al. Guided endodontic access of calcified anterior teeth. J Endod. 2018;44(7):1195–9.
24. Maia LM, Machado VC, Alves da Silva NRF, et al. Case reports in maxillary posterior teeth by guided endodontic access. J Endod. 2019;45:214–8.
25. Chong BS, Dhesi M, Makdissi J. Computer-aided dynamic navigation: a novel method for guided endodontics. Quintessence Int. 2019;50(3):196–202.
26. Connert T, Zehnder MS, Weiger R. Microguided endodontics: accuracy of a miniaturized technique for apically extended access cavity preparation in anterior teeth. J Endod. 2017;43:787–90.
27. van der Meer WJ, Vissink A, Ng YL, et al. 3D Computer aided treatment planning in endodontics. J Dent. 2016;45:67–72.
28. de Toubes KMS, de Oliveira PAD, Machado SN. Clinical approach to pulp canal obliteration: a case series. Iran Endod J. 2017;12(4):527–33.
29. Casadei BA, Lara-Mendes STO, Barbosa CFM, et al. Access to original canal trajectory after deviation and perforation with guided endodontic assistance. Aust Endod J. 2020;46:101. https://doi.org/10.1111/aej.12360.
30. Shi X, Zhao S, Wang W, et al. Novel navigation technique for the endodontic treatment of a molar with pulp canal calcification and apical pathology. Aust Endod J. 2017;44(1):66–70.
31. Mena-Álvarez J, Rico-Romano C, Lobo-Galindo AB, et al. Endodontic treatment of dens evaginatus by performing a splint guided access cavity. J Esthet Restor Dent. 2017;29(6):396–402.
32. Langeland K, Dowden WE, Tronstad L, et al. Human pulp changes of iatrogenic origin. Oral Surg Oral Med Oral Pathol. 1971;32:943–80.
33. Holan G. Tube-like mineralization in the dental pulp of traumatized primary incisors. Endod Dent Traumatol. 1998;14(6):279–84.
34. Amir FA, Gutmann JL, Witherspoon DE. Calcific metamorphosis: a challenge in endodontic diagnosis and treatment. Quintessence Int. 2001;32(6):447–55.
35. McCabe PS, Dummer PM. Pulp canal obliteration: an endodontic diagnosis and treatment challenge. Int Endod J. 2012;45(2):177–97.
36. Oginni AO, Adekoya-Sofowora CA, Kolawole KA. Evaluation of radiographs, clinical signs and symptoms associated with pulp canal obliteration: an aid to treatment decision. Dent Traumatol. 2009;25:620–5.
37. Holcomb JB, Gregory WB Jr. Calcific metamorphosis of the pulp: its incidence and treatment. Oral Surg Oral Med Oral Pathol. 1967;24:825–30.
38. Bjørndal L, Darvann T. A light microscopic study of odontoblastic and non odontoblastic cells involved in tertiary dentinogenesis in well-defined cavitated carious lesions. Caries Res. 1999;33:50–60.
39. Fleig S, Attin T, Jungbluth H. Narrowing of the radicular pulp space in coronally restored teeth. Clin Oral Investig. 2017;21:1251–7.
40. Agamy HA, Bakry NS, Mounir MM, et al. Comparison of mineral trioxide aggregate and formocresol as pulp-capping agents in pulpotomized primary teeth. Pediatr Dent. 2004;26:302–9.
41. Andreasen FM, Zhijie Y, Thomsen BL, et al. Occurrence of pulp canal obliteration after luxation injuries in the permanent dentition. Endod Dent Traumatol. 1987;3:103–15.
42. Flores MT, Andersson L, Andreasen JO, et al. Guidelines for the management of traumatic dental injuries. I. Fractures and luxations of permanent teeth. Dent Traumatol. 2007;23:66–71.
43. Flores MT, Andersson L, Andreasen JO, et al. Guidelines for the management of traumatic dental injuries. II. Avulsion of permanent teeth. Dent Traumatol. 2007;23:130–6.

44. Delivanis HP, Sauer GJ. Incidence of canal calcification in the orthodontic patient. Am J Orthod. 1982;82:58–61.
45. Brodin P, Linge L, Aars H. Instant assessment of pulpal blood flow after orthodontic force application. J Orofac Orthop. 1996;57:306–9.
46. Johnstone M, Parashos P. Endodontics and the ageing patient. Aust Dent J. 2015;60(Suppl. 1):20–7.
47. Kiefner P, Connert T, ElAyouti A, et al. Treatment of calcified root canals in elderly people: a clinical study about the accessibility, the time needed and the outcome with a three-year followup. Gerodontology. 2017;34:164–70.
48. Allen PF, Whitworth JM. Endodontic considerations in the elderly. Gerodontology. 2004;21:185–94.
49. Wu B, Hybels C, Liang J, et al. Social stratification and tooth loss among middle-aged and older Americans from 1988 to 2004. Community Dent Oral Epidemiol. 2014;42:495–502.
50. Robertson A, Andreasen FM, Bergenholtz G, Andreasen JO, Noren JG. Incidence of pulp necrosis subsequent to pulp canal obliteration from trauma of permanent incisors. J Endod. 1996;22:557–60.
51. Naumann M, Sterzenbach G, Dietrich T, et al. Dentin-like versus rigid endodontic post: 11-year randomized controlled pilot trial on no-wall to 2-wall defects. J Endod. 2017;43:1770–5.
52. Lang H, Korkmaz Y, Schneider K, et al. Impact of endodontic treatments on the rigidity of the root. J Dent Res. 2006;85:364–8.
53. Cvek M, Granath L, Lundberg M. Failures and healing in endodontically treated non-vital anterior teeth with posttraumatically reduced pulpal lumen. Acta Odontol Scand. 1982;40:223–8.
54. Tavares WL, Lopes RC, Menezes GB, et al. Non-surgical treatment of pulp canal obliteration using contemporary endodontic techniques: case series. Dent Press Endod. 2012;2:52–8.
55. Tavares WL. Management of clinical complications following pulp canal obliteration: a report of two cases. Dent Press Endod. 2016;6:54–62.
56. Jacobsen I, Kerekes K. Long-term prognosis of traumatized permanent anterior teeth showing calcifying processes in the pulp cavity. Scand J Dent Res. 1977;85:588–98.

Static Guided Non-surgical Approach for Posterior Teeth

7

Gergely Benyőcs and Niraj Kinariwala

Static guided endodontics has been successfully used for anterior teeth. However, with caution, this method can also be applied to premolar and molar teeth if the inter-occlusal distance is optimum to accommodate endodontic guide, bur (drill) and handpiece. For guided treatment of posterior teeth, good armamentarium and adequate inter-occlusal distance are the key to success.

7.1 Considerations for Guided Approach for Posterior Teeth

7.1.1 Indications

- *Calcified canals*:
    Calcified canals predispose many clinical challenges for the operator. Guided approach will reduce risk of endodontic mishaps in calcified canals (Fig. 7.1).
- *Minimal invasive endodontic approach*:
    Minimally invasive endodontics (MIE) is a concept to preserve the healthy coronal, cervical and radicular tooth structure during the endodontic treatment. Guided endodontics can help in preserving pericervical dentin (PCD) and perform access opening according to canal projection. Figure 7.2 depicts a case of minimal invasive endodontic approach for upper second molar.

Electronic Supplementary Material The online version of this chapter (https://doi.org/10.1007/978-3-030-55281-7_7) contains supplementary material, which is available to authorized users.

G. Benyőcs
Budapest, Hungary

N. Kinariwala (✉)
Karnavati School of Dentistry, Karnavati University, Gandhinagar, Gujarat, India
e-mail: niraj@ksd.ac.in

Fig. 7.1 Calcification in distobuccal root of maxillary first molar

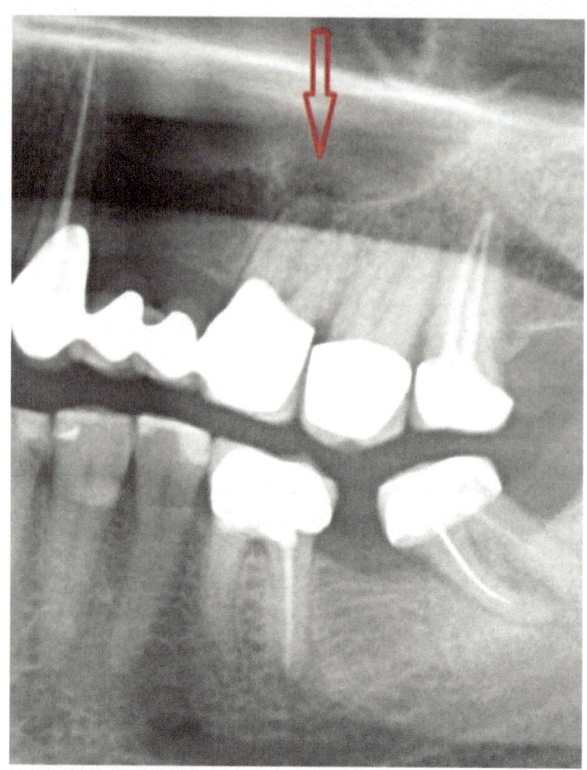

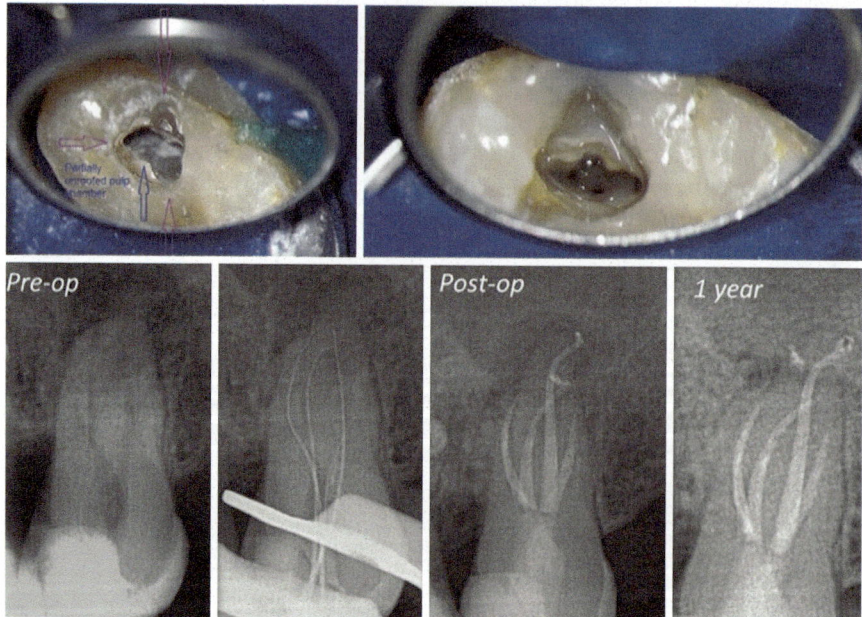

Fig. 7.2 Case of minimal invasive approach for maxillary second molar

- *Selective root re-treatments*:

    Root canal re-treatment is traditionally considered an "all or none" treatment approach. It is typically recommended that all restorative and obturation materials should be removed from all roots regardless of the presence or absence of periapical pathosis. In contrast, surgical endodontics is not viewed as an "all or none" treatment approach. Traditionally, only the diseased root(s) is addressed via root-end resection and root-end filling. The use of cone-beam computed tomographic imaging allows for a more accurate evaluation of the periapical status of individual roots associated with multi-rooted teeth. This information has introduced a novel and conservative treatment alternative for previously endodontically treated teeth with multiple roots presenting with post-treatment disease. This new approach is termed "selective root re-treatment." Advanced imaging allows the clinician to make predictable treatment decisions with respect to the presence or absence of periapical pathosis of individual roots as opposed to making assumptions about the tooth as a whole. Selective root re-treatment combines the approach of non-surgical retreatment with the selectivity of surgical root resection. In this manner, re-treatment could be limited to a single root or roots clearly showing periapical pathosis while leaving the root(s) with no visible or perceived pathosis untouched [1].

The decision to selectively treat and/or re-treat one or more diseased roots must also be based on a thorough oral examination and the clinical interpretation of tooth structure after access. Restorations with inadequate marginal integrity and/or restoration treatment planned for full replacement may not be candidates for selective root re-treatment procedure. Additionally, teeth undergoing a selective root re-treatment procedure found to have recurrent caries and/or visible leakage on access should have all restorative materials removed. Presuming that the existing restoration is of sound marginal integrity and showing no signs of recurrent caries, smaller precision slot accesses can be designed to minimize damage to the restoration and maximize its current structural integrity (Fig. 7.3).

If guided selective re-treatment has to be performed through existing restorations, metallic restorations should be removed or replaced prior to the treatment planning. Metal and zirconia restorations may create artefacts on CBCT, and they could be the potential source of inaccuracy. However, with superimposition of the scan data and experience, such inaccuracies can be minimised.[1]

7.1.2   Evaluation of Inter-occlusal Distance

To place a guide and endodontic drills in posterior teeth, adequate mouth opening is a necessity (Fig. 7.4). To use more than 10 mm long burs over the guide ring position, inter-occlusal space must be pre-evaluated. Try to place a drill intra-orally, before planning this treatment option (Video 1).

For limited inter-occlusal space, operator can use the following options:

- Use of short drills: Limited availability of such burs and drills, limit use of guided endodontic approach in posterior teeth.
- Plan angulated access for the drill, depending on canal projection (Fig. 7.5).

---

[1] Metals fused to ceramic crowns, metal posts and zirconia restorations are difficult to drill through the sleeve. It may result in over-heating or damage to existing restoration.

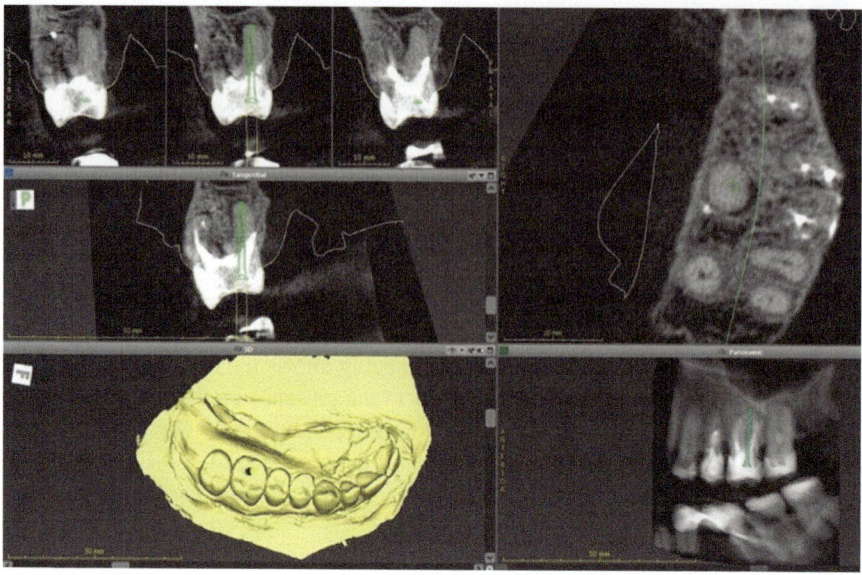

Fig. 7.3 Selective root canal retreatment of maxillary right second molar for palatal canal. CBCT reveals calcification in palatal root. After merging CBCT scan with intra-oral impression, planning was carried out on a software

Fig. 7.4 Endodontic guide and drill try-in for posterior teeth. Inter-occlusal distance should be adequate for this approach. Design of guide has been modified by incorporation of inspection window

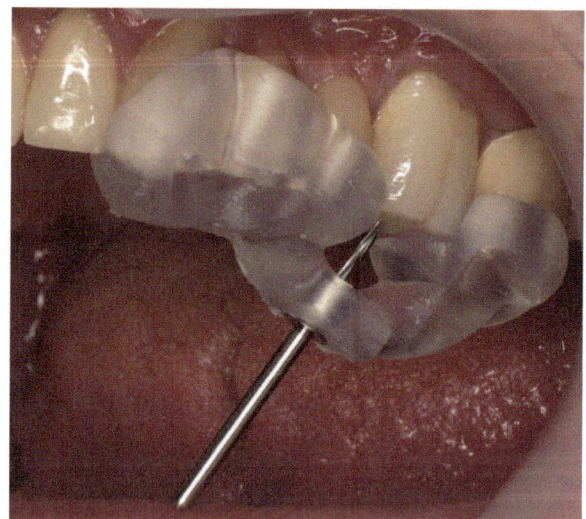

7.1.2.1 How to Evaluate Accessibility with Mock Guide and Drills?

Test inter-occlusal distance with silicon impression material by placing it on the region to be treated (Video 1). The dimensions of silicon block should be similar to the planned guides. Hold it in the mouth, and mimic drills movements. Take it out and place it along with drills, few times, to confirm accessibility. This preliminary test is important before planning guided treatment for posterior teeth.

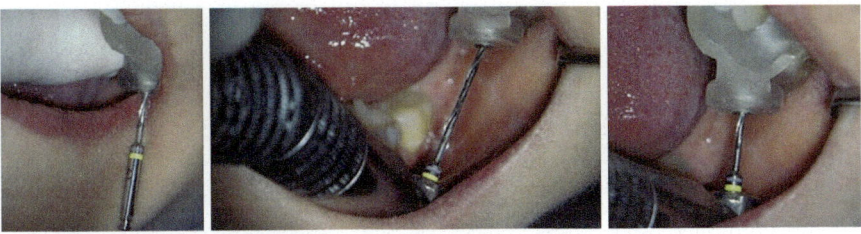

Fig. 7.5 Angulated approach for posterior guided endodontic treatments

Fig. 7.6 ATEC drill and sleeve, exclusively manufactured for non-surgical endodontic treatments. (Courtesy: Steco system-technik)

ATEC Drill 1.0 mm / Endoseal

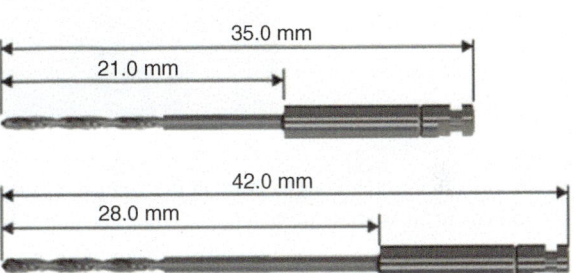

StecoGuide Endo-sleeve for ATEC Drill

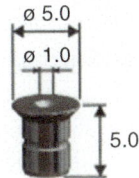

7.1.3 Burs and Sleeves Used for Static 3D Guided Approach for Posterior Teeth

Any drill with diameter ranging from 0.75 to 1.2 mm can be used for drilling. Special endo-guide burs with sleeves for guided endodontics are available in the market, manufactured by Steco (Fig. 7.6). Recommended sleeve height for posterior teeth is 5–6 mm. Few manufacturers 3D print sleeve from plastic or resin along with the guide (Fig. 7.7). This concept is interesting, but requires more studies and research to prove its accuracy.

7.1.4 How to Reduce Over-heating During Guided Treatment?

• Try to avoid using high-speed drills. After every 1 mm, stop drilling further to allow cooling.

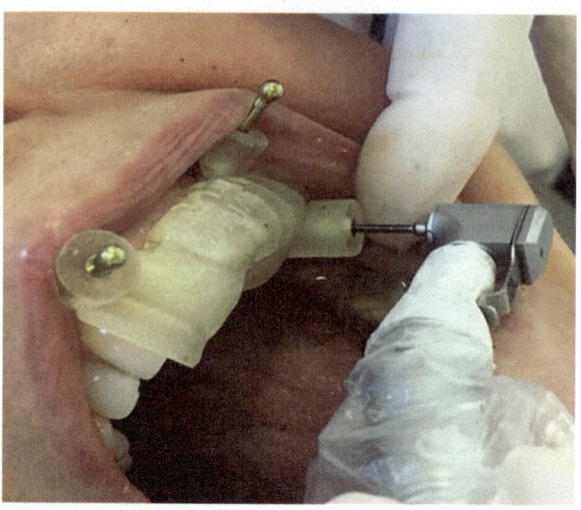

Fig. 7.7 3D printed sleeve from plastic or resin along with the guide

- Modify the guide design: Plan an inspection window around the tooth on buccal and occlusal surface to secure external cooling while drilling (Fig. 7.4). It also allows use of extra coolant while drilling (Video 2).

7.1.5 Is It Possible To Treat Premolar or Molar with a Single Endodontic Guide?

For multi-rooted teeth, usually one guide is not enough as we have to plan and design drill guide for each root canal. For example, for calcified mesiobuccal and palatal canals of maxillary first molar, usually we need two different endodontic guides. This drawback, certainly, increases the cost of the treatment (Fig. 7.13).

7.1.6 Can We Change the Drill Path During Static Guided Treatment?

Static drill guides do not allow any changes in treatment plan. To overcome this limitation, dynamic navigation in endodontics can be used.

7.2 Step-by-Step Clinical Procedure

1. Check stability of the guide on the cast and intra-orally.
2. Evaluate the dimensional accuracy of the guide bur (concentricity and run out), as increased run-out may lead to gross apical inaccuracy while drilling.
3. With the help of the guide, mark the entry point of the access through the sleeve with small bur on the enamel or on the restoration.

4. Remove the enamel or existing restoration free hand, without a guide. (To avoid over-heating, high-speed burs should not be used with the metallic sleeve.)
5. After removing enamel, place the guide. Secure it with fingers or fixation screw.
6. Insert the guide bur in the sleeve drill and drill, cautiously, into the dentine. With this approach, we can achieve directed dentin conservation.
7. To avoid over-heating, drill in short and intermittent periods. Use copious amount of water coolant. Clean the bur (drill) properly after each stroke.
8. Start drilling with a short bur. After reaching the coronal third of the root, use long bur to reach the target point. With this method, improper angulation and wobbling of the long bur can be avoided.
9. After reaching the pre-planned depth, scout the canal. If canal cannot be negotiated, try to drill further into the canal. Once canal has been negotiated, carry out biomechanical preparation.

7.2.1 Case Report 1

A 61-year-old woman reported with pain in the upper left molar region. The second and third left molars showed signs of apical periodontitis confirmed by the cone-beam computed tomographic (CBCT) scans brought to us by the patient at the initial appointment (Fig. 7.8). Conventional endodontic treatment was discontinued given the difficulty in locating the root canals. Intra-oral scanning and the CBCT scans were used to plan the access to the calcified canals by means of implant

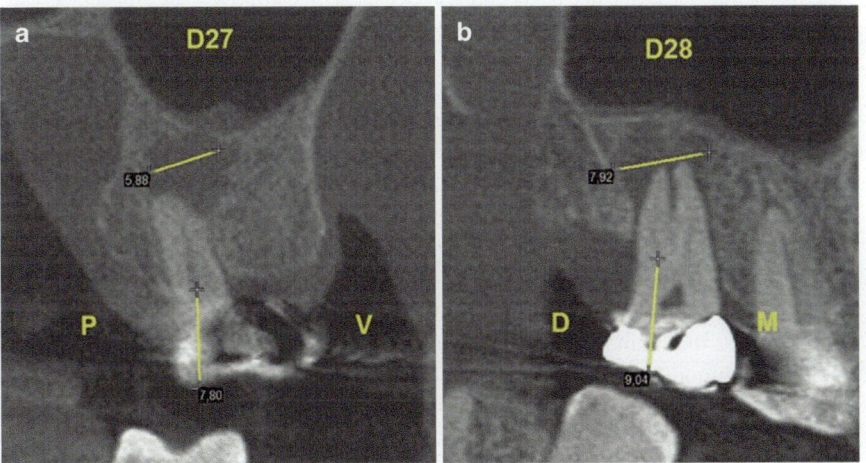

Fig. 7.8 (a) A cross-sectional cut representing the palatal root of the maxillary second molar, indicating a distance of approximately 7.80 mm from the occlusal surface to the visible light of the canal and a diameter of the lesion of 5.88 mm. (b) A cross-sectional cut representing the distobuccal root of the maxillary third molar, indicating a distance of approximately 9.04 mm from the occlusal surface to the visible light of the canal and a diameter of the lesion of 7.92 mm. (License no: 4787080843270; [2])

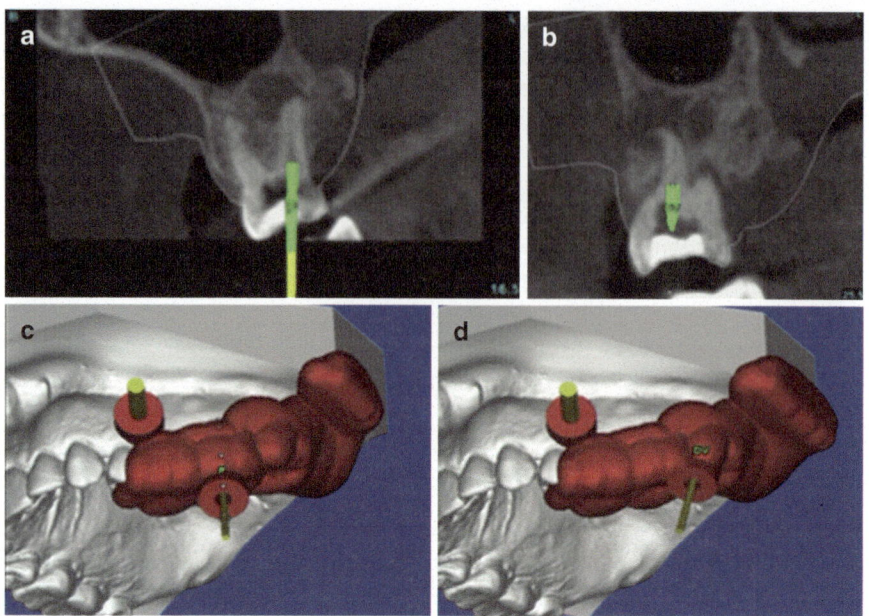

Fig. 7.9 (**a, b**) A virtual drill was designed by applying the implant designer tool of the SimPlant software and virtually superimposed on the root canal of the maxillary left second and third molar. The axis of the drill was angled in such a way that the tip of the extended drill would reach the tomographically visible lumen of the root canal. (**c, d**) After planning the position of the drill, two virtual templates were designed by applying the template designer tool of the SimPlant software. Two sleeves were integrated into both of the printed templates: one to guide the drill during cavity preparation and the other to ensure correct fixation in the patient. (License no: 4787080843270; [2])

planning software (Fig. 7.9). Guides were fabricated through rapid prototyping and allowed for the correct orientation of a cylindrical drill used to provide access through the calcifications. Second to that, the root canals were prepared with reciprocating endodontic instruments and rested for 2 weeks with intra-canal medication. Subsequently, canals were packed with gutta-percha cones using the hydraulic compression technique. Permanent restorations of the access cavities were performed. By comparing the tomographic images, the authors observed a drastic reduction of the periapical lesions as well as the absence of pain symptoms after 3 months. This condition was maintained at the 1-year follow-up (Fig. 7.10). Thus, the guided endodontic technique, in molars, can be regarded as an excellent option for the location of calcified root canals, avoiding failures in complex cases [2].

7.2.2   Case Report 2

A 56-year-old woman reported with pain in the lower left molar region. The lower left third molar showed signs of apical periodontitis confirmed by the radiographs (Fig. 7.11). Treatment planning and superimposition of surface scans was carried

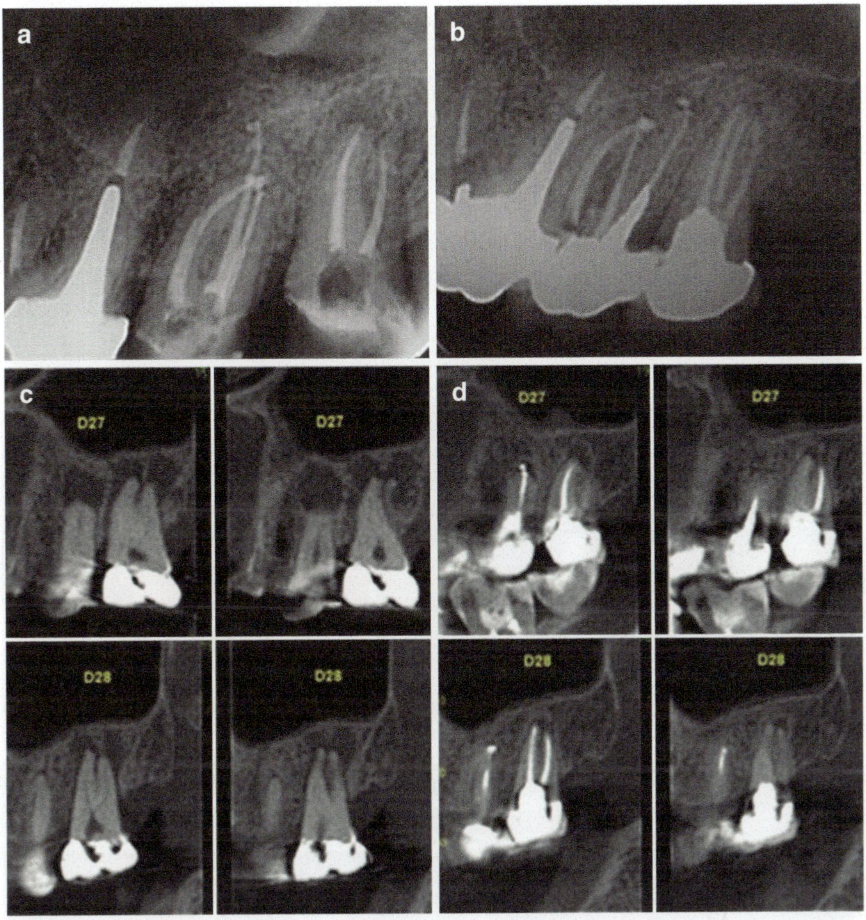

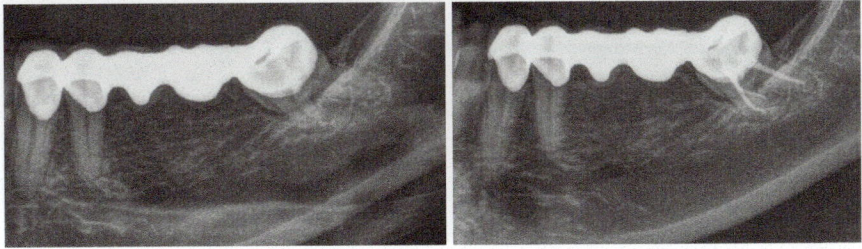

Fig. 7.10 Case follow-up. (**a**) Radiographic image at 3 months after treatment. (**b**) Radiographic control 1 year after the procedure. (**c**) Tomographic image before endodontic treatment of teeth 27 and 28. (**d**) Tomographic image of teeth 27 and 28 1 year after endodontic treatment. (License no: 4787080843270; [2])

Fig. 7.11 Pre-operative and 2 years follow-up radiograph of lower left third molar

out on a software. After segmentation and alignment, virtual bur was placed to the target points. For mesial and distal canals, two drill paths were planned (Fig. 7.12). For mesial root, target point was measured between mesiobuccal (MB) and mesio-lingual (ML) root canal orifices. Planning was carried out through zirconia crown, as per patient's preference, to preserve existing restorations. Guides were printed, and their stability was evaluated on the cast and intra-orally (Fig. 7.13). Dimensional accuracy of the drills was checked in the sleeve. Guided access opening was carried out with guide and ultrasonic tips were used to modify access to avoid file distortion and separation. The dentine bridge was preserved between mesial and distal root canal systems. This type of access is also known as "Truss Access." Follow-up was carried out after a month and after 2 years (Fig. 7.14).

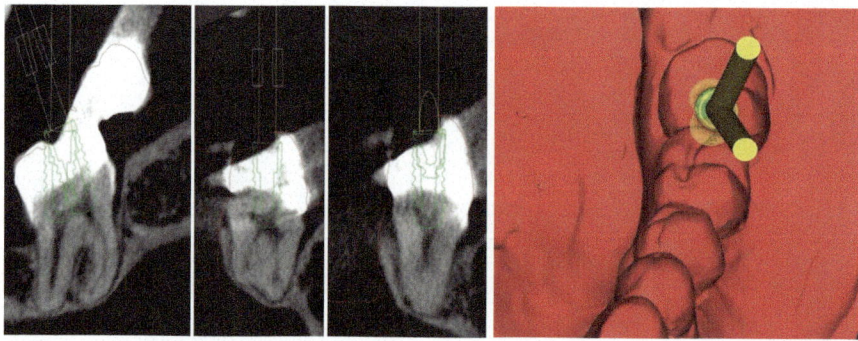

Fig. 7.12 Two separate virtual drill paths were planned for mesial and distal root canal systems

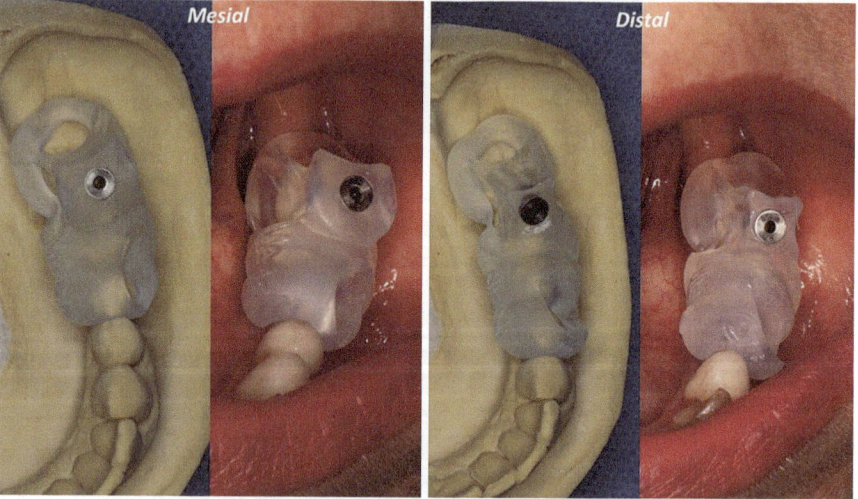

Fig. 7.13 Guide stability was checked on the cast as well as intra-orally

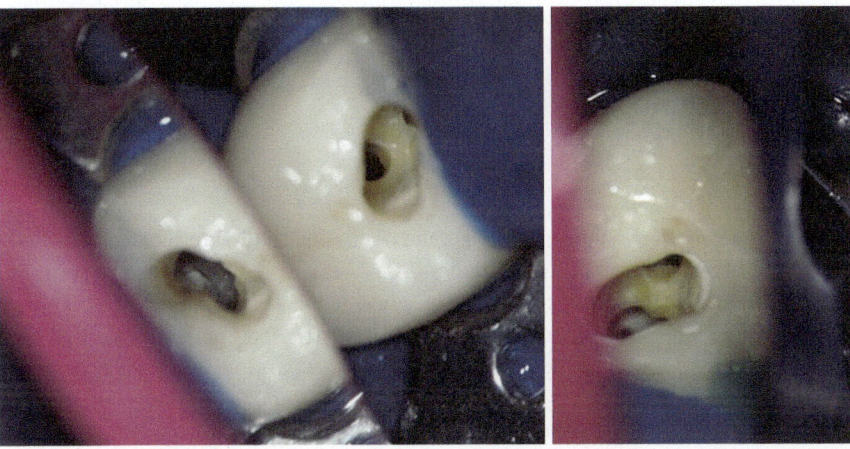

Fig. 7.14 Preservation of dentin bridge between mesial and distal root canal systems. (Truss Access)

7.3 Intra-coronal Guide Technique

Molars are the most frequent tooth that are in need of RCT. In cases of canal obliteration, they can be treated using a guided endodontic concept. If the inter-occlusal distance is reduced, the concept can be changed by using an intra-coronal guide technique developed by Jørgen Buchgreitz et al. [3].

7.3.1 Steps of Intra-coronal Guide Technique

1. Perform access opening and complete biomechanical preparation of accessible canals.
2. Block the accessible canals with calcium hydroxide or with the final root filling material.
3. Cone-beam computed tomographic scan and surface scan of the quadrant.
4. Design the guide path on the cone-beam computed tomographic scan.
5. Merge the scans and produce the guide by 3-dimensional printing or 3-dimensional milling.
6. Control the fit of the guide and the possibility of the pin to go unimpeded through the sleeve and reach the floor of the access cavity.
7. Moisten the surface of the access cavity and fill the access cavity with light-curing composite material.
8. Place the guide on the teeth and press the pin through the sleeve in the guide as well as through the composite to the floor of the access cavity.
9. Light-cure through the guide.

10. Remove the guide and the pin. Scout the canal through the guide path in the composite.
11. Remove the light-cured composite. Complete the root canal treatment.

7.3.2 Case Report

A 52-year-old patient referred, because the dentist had failed to localize the disto-buccal root canal of a maxillary molar (#3) associated with apical pathosis. After re-opening and rubber dam placement, a glide path was established for both the palatal first mesiobuccal root canal and the second mesiobuccal using a size 10 hand file and coronal flaring. Further instrumentation to the working length was achieved by reciprocating file size 25. All three canals were temporarily filled with calcium hydroxide. For the distobuccal root canal, guided endodontics was chosen in order to avoid further impairment of the tooth, because negotiation of the canal failed even with the use of the operating microscope. Following the merged data obtained from the cone-beam computed tomographic and surface scans, a translucent SICAT Optiguide (SICAT, Bonn, Germany) was constructed containing a sleeve represent-ing the proper direction of a drill path in order to reach the distobuccal root canal (Fig. 7.15). The access cavity was temporarily filled with a composite material made for light-curing. Before light curing, the Optiguide was replaced on the teeth, and a steel pin was pressed through the sleeve and the composite whereby the proper drill path direction was transferred into the composite (Fig. 7.16). After polymeriza-tion and removal of the Optiguide and pin from the composite base sleeve, the guided drilling could be performed. This case report is the first on guided access preparation in a molar with pulp canal obliteration and limited inter-occlusal space.

7.4   Potential Mishaps

7.4.1   Unstable Guide

Unstable endodontic guide may lead to complications such as over-extended cavity preparation or perforation of the tooth. Instability of endodontic guide can be attrib-uted to multiple reasons:

- Faulty impression or faulty scanning
- Improper planning of the guide, for example over-sized offset: Offset is the space which is planned between the guide surface and the tooth which can be adjusted in the planning software. Based on our experience, 0.15 mm offset is ideal for posterior teeth. Guide can be stabilized by hands on both sides, or incorporating surgical pins during planning or using chair-side composite.

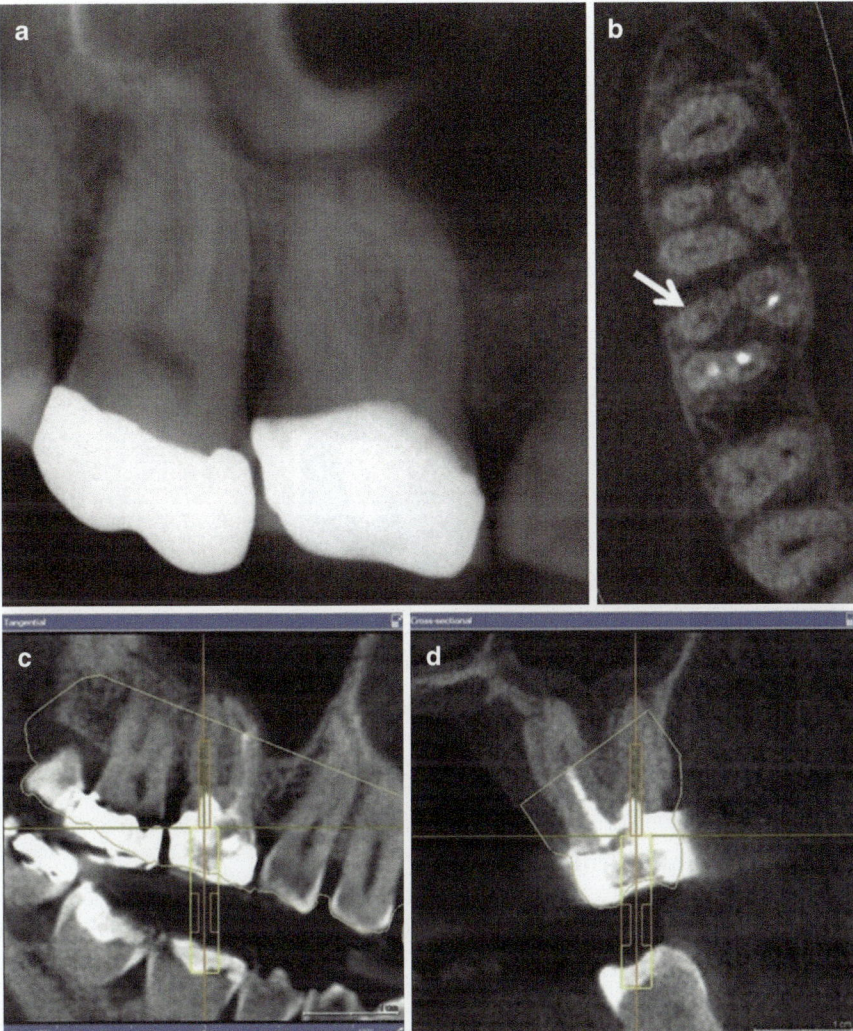

Fig. 7.15 (**a**) Radiographic presentation of tooth #3 in need of root canal treatment because of a broadened periodontal ligament and soreness to percussion. The distal root canal is seemingly obliterated. (**b**) The axial view of the CBCT image exposes the region. The distobuccal canal is marked beyond the curvature, making further instrumentation possible (arrow in **b**); the three other root canals show radiopacity reflecting the in-between calcium hydroxide. (**c**) Tangential and (**d**) cross-sectioned CBCT images show that the virtual drill path (orange outlines in **c** and **d**) is placed on the images as well as the CEREC surface scan (yellow outlines in **c** and **d**) and merged with the CBCT image by the help of special software. (License no: 4786900066761; [3])

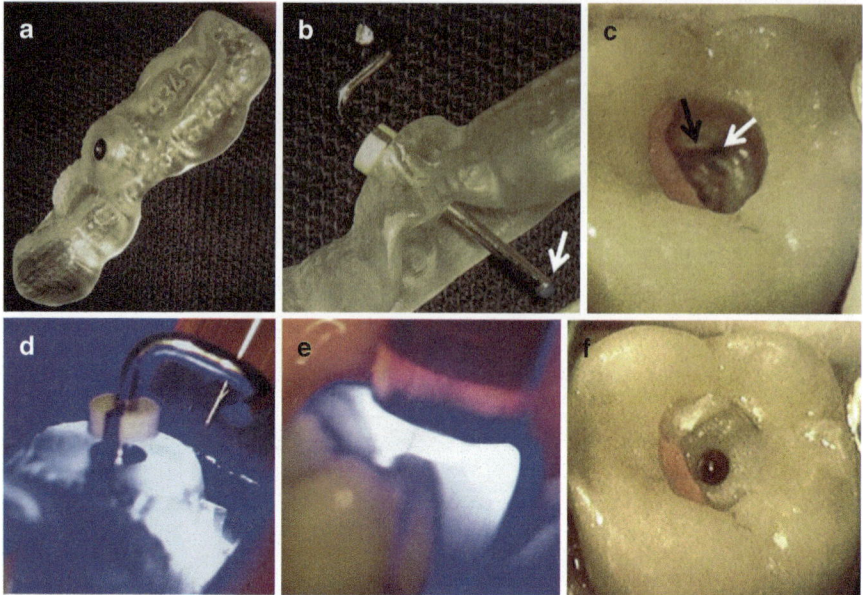

Fig. 7.16 (**a**) A view of the Optiguide with the metal sleeve. (**b**) The guide with the guide pin in the sleeve and with blue stain at the tip (arrow). (**c**) Tooth #3 with the blue mark visible (white arrow) showing that the pin could reach the floor of the access cavity but also defining the entrance of the distobuccal root canal. The original attempt to scout the canal is visible (black arrow). (**d, e**) Because of the Optiguide, the illumination was performed without a rubber dam. (**f**) A view of the access preparation filled with cured composite (the intra-coronal guide). The canal made by the guide pin is seen in the composite. (License no: 4786900066761; [3])

7.4.2 Inaccurate Drilling

Unnecessary removal of healthy tooth structure or perforation occurs due to inaccurate drilling. Following variables lead to inaccurate drilling:

- Artefacts on CBCT
- Unstable guide
- Dimensionally inaccurate bur and/or sleeve
- Faulty planning on the software

Already accessed tooth can be difficult (Fig. 7.17). The access created, before guided approach, could slide the drill into different directions. To avoid this, create a small ditch or plateau at the bottom of the original access. Intra-coronal guide technique is also helpful to treat such cases.

For implant placement, different drills and guide supports are required. In guided endodontics, we usually use tooth-supported guides and single or two drills. So, the accuracy of static guided endodontics is far better than guided implant placement in

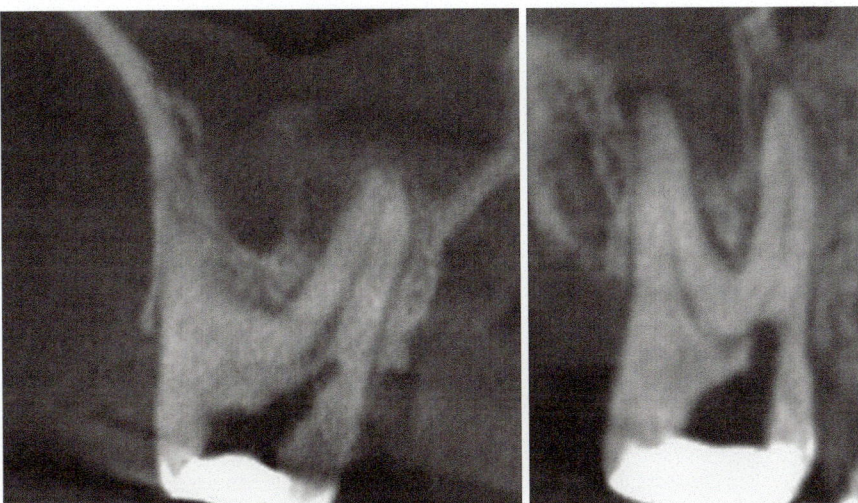

Fig. 7.17 Inaccurate drilling with guided approach

the literature [4]. With advent of shorter and smaller drills and advances in dynamic guidance technology, application of navigation for posterior teeth will get more acceptance.

References

1. Nudera WJ. Selective root retreatment: a novel approach. J Endod. 2015;41(8):1382–8.
2. Lara-Mendes STO, et al. Guided endodontic access in maxillary molars using cone-beam computed tomography and computer-aided design/computer-aided manufacturing system: a case report. J Endod. 2018;44:875–9.
3. Jørgen Buchgreitz DM. Guided endodontics modified for treating molars by using an intracoronal guide technique. J Endod. 2019;45:818–23.
4. Tahmaseb A, et al. Computer technology applications in surgical implant dentistry: a systematic review. Int J Oral Maxillofac Implants. 2014;29:24–42.

Static Guided Approach in Surgical Endodontics

8

Mark Adam Antal

Surgical endodontics has gone through spectacular development in the last decades. Earlier research indicated moderate success rates, as low as 30–40% [1]. The first step toward a more successful treatment was the evolution of concept of retrograde filling in the early 1990s [2]. However, success rates are still quite variable, ranging from 19% [3] to 96% [4].

Studies with higher success rates (more than 90%) have consistently used high-power magnification, dental operating microscope [5–7]. Microscopic root-end surgery also allowed to perform a 90° root-end resection, perpendicular to the root axis, instead of the conventional 45° bevel. Bevel of root-end resection is an important parameter in success of endodontic surgery. Success rate of surgery can increase from approximately 60–70% to 90–94%, when the cut is performed at 90° instead of 45° [8]. Length of root-end resection is also a significant factor. It has been suggested that the removal of a 3 mm of root end ensures the elimination of the ramifications and lateral canals in over 90% of the cases [9, 10].

Even with use of retrograde filling and dental operating microscope in the surgery, the operator often finds it difficult to consistently reach the documented success rates. Operator experience and anatomical variability can influence the outcome of the surgery, but it must be admitted that the osteotomy itself, especially in cases with intact cortical bone, is a challenging operation. Site and size of osteotomy with precise angulation are difficult to reach, if no aids are used. Precise root-end resection of apical 3 mm of the apex is not easy either. Furthermore, the diameter of the osteotomy should optimally be kept as small as 3–4 mm to avoid excessive postoperative pain and prolonged healing [11–13]. Accordingly, several improvements have been proposed to enhance the success of such interventions [11, 14].

M. A. Antal (✉)
Department of Operative and Esthetic Dentistry, Faculty of Dentistry, University of Szeged, Szeged, Hungary
e-mail: antal.mark@szte.hu

© Springer Nature Switzerland AG 2021
N. Kinariwala, L. Samaranayake (eds.), *Guided Endodontics*,
https://doi.org/10.1007/978-3-030-55281-7_8

The use of CBCT in endodontics was recommended in 2014 by the European Society of Endodontology [15]. This was an important departure from the panoramic/periapical era, but it solved only part of the problem. Having a CBCT image will help the operator to get a better idea of what to expect during the operation but will have to depend on knowledge and experience of operator, nevertheless. This leaves plenty of room for error, which motivates search for new aids and approaches. The first such attempt was reported by Pinsky and colleagues, who examined the use of CAD/CAM surgical templates for endodontic indications in vitro. A scan guide was fabricated for a dry human mandible with a full set of teeth. The guide was extended apically in a way that it covered the planned surgical locations (Fig. 8.1). Five operators performed freehand and guided drilling so that the accuracy of the two approaches could be compared. All apices were involved. In the guided group, the mean distance from the apex (error) was 0.79 mm, while in the

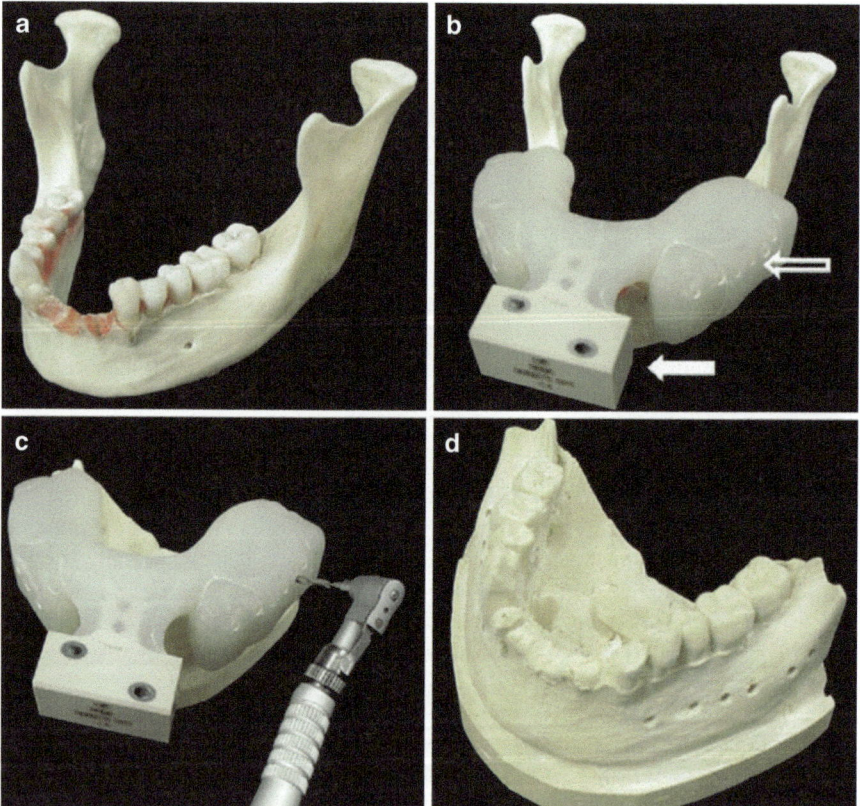

Fig. 8.1 (**a–d**) The pilot study by Pinksy et al., testing the accuracy of freehand versus guided drilling on a stone model. ([16], Image used with the permission of Elsevier. Permission no.: 4620730221742)

freehand group, it was 2.27 mm. It is noteworthy that in the freehand group, the operators missed the apex by >2 mm in 80% of the attempts and by >3 mm in 30% of the attempts [16]. The study was the first to demonstrate that the guided approach does improve accuracy. This has been recently affirmed by Hawkins et al., who have proven in a surgical simulation scenario, that targeted endodontic microsurgery provided more efficient completion of osteotomy and resection, with a more appropriate root-end resection volume and bevel angle than conventional endodontic microsurgery [17].

The interest in surgical guides for endodontic surgery has been renewed in recent years, possibly because stereolithographic manufacturing has become widely and much more readily available than it used to be. Liu et al. applied additive manufacturing to fabricate surgical guides to help osteotomy and apex location. They found that the operation time was dramatically reduced [18]. In a case report, Patel and colleagues used a 3D printed custom soft tissue retractor (without guide function) for periapical surgery (Fig. 8.2.) [19]. In another case report, Strbac and colleagues used a stereolithographically fabricated surgical template for osteotomy and root resection [20]. This template helped the operator to locate the root apices during surgery, though it did not guide the drill itself (Fig. 8.3). Ye et al. operated a left maxillary lateral incisor and canine with a 3D printed template to help the localization of the apices and to target the osteotomy by defining the entry point on the cortical bone (Fig. 8.4).

The first truly guided case of endodontic surgery was reported by Giacomino et al. [21] in 2018. The authors used a 3D printed guide for combined osteotomy and root-end resection with a round bone trephine. They concluded that the guide was useful for the control of the depth and angulation of the osteotomy. Ahn and colleagues used a surgical template to localize the apices of a mandibular molar covered by thick buccal bone plate (Fig. 8.5) [22]. Interestingly, the authors used the template according to what implantology would call the pilot protocol. That is, only the initial osteotomy was performed through the template, the rest of the procedure was done without it.

Fig. 8.2 Patel's 3D printed model to retract the soft tissue during surgery. ([19], Drawing by Dr. Tekla Sáry)

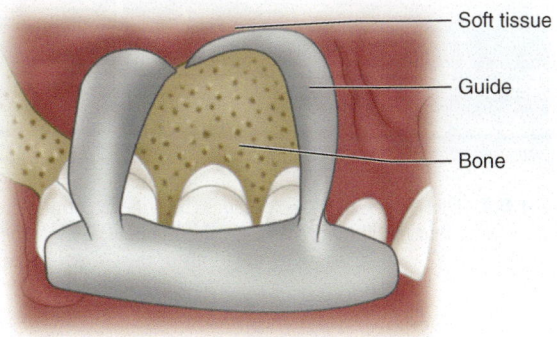

Soft tissue

Guide

Bone

Fig. 8.3 The 3D printed model by Strbac et al. for apex localization. Markings helped the operator to identify the apices of the molar tooth. ([20], Image used with the permission of Elsevier. Permission no.: 4620721384330)

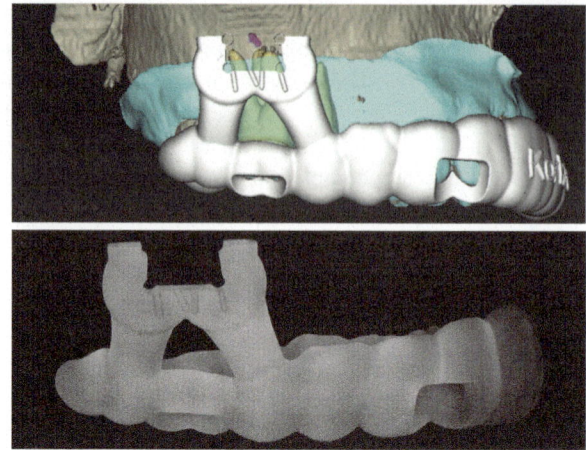

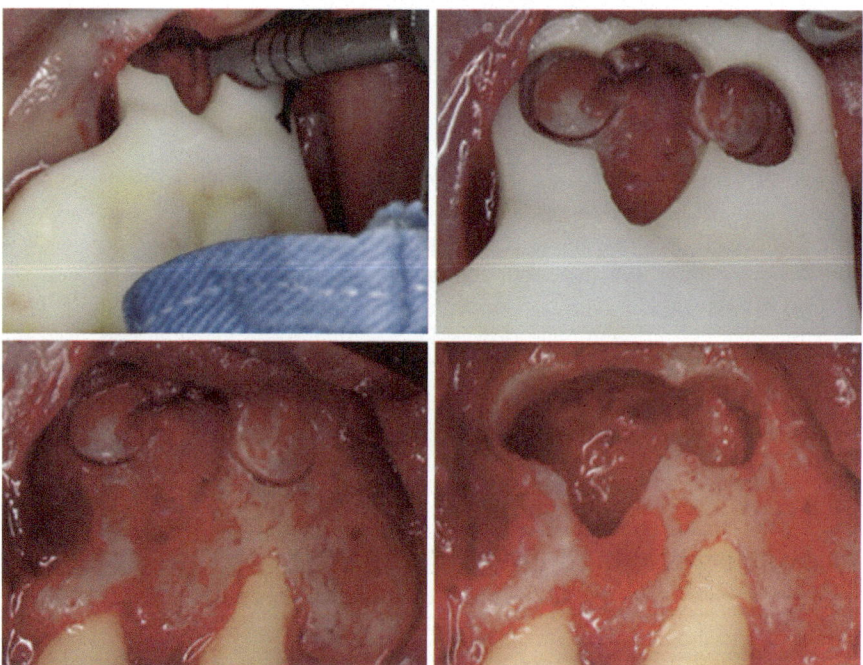

Fig. 8.4 The aid designed by Ye et al. to help the penetration of the cortical bone with the trephine [11]. Note that the aid did not guide the trephine, only helped to determine where to penetrate. (Image bye Ye et al., used under the terms of the Creative Commons BY)

Fig. 8.5 Pilot guide by Ahn et al. [22]. (Image used with the permission of Elsevier. Permission no.: 4620740751372)

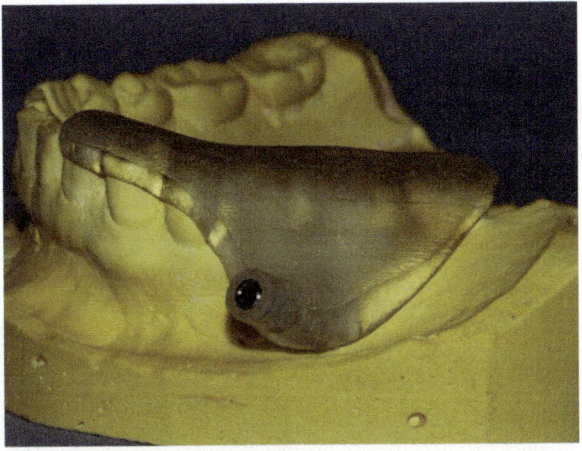

Guided approach for surgical endodontics is as safe as freehand surgery, but it allows better localization. Interestingly, with this method, it is possible to resect the root end, simultaneously, along with the bone.

8.1 Preparations for Surgical Template Production: Approaches to Imaging

CBCT is a cornerstone of 3D surgical template printing. Digital guide production workflows rely on CBCT images, which should have higher resolution. The resolution of CBCT depends on voxel size, which is influenced by the CBCT machine and the applied field of view (FOV). The smaller the FOV, the better the resolution. However, a small FOV means that only a limited portion of patient anatomy will be scanned, which can make image registration difficult. Image registration is the superimposition of the CBCT image of a dental impression or a dental scan on the anatomical image. Even more importantly, the resulting surgical template may have poor retention, which is not safe for surgery. This conflict between resolution and registration/retention can be resolved by gaining experience with the specific CBCT device and template fabrication system.

The other major problem related to this initial phase is anatomical. In contrast to guides, used in orthograde endodontics or implantology, in surgical endodontics, the access needs to be in the apical area, which should be perpendicular to the root axis. To reach this end, the apical area needs to be registered as accurately as possible, either with an oral scanner or with regular dental impression. In few cases, this can be really challenging. Distal locations, long roots, narrow vestibulum, or

Fig. 8.6 A shared anatomical difficulty of most guided endodontic cases is the undercut at the vestibular area. (Image used with the permission of Springer Nature. Permission no.: 4638290411498)

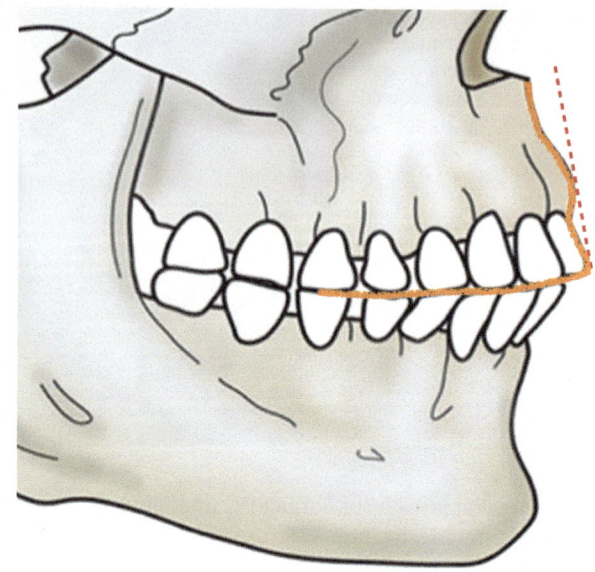

even limited mouth opening can cause difficulties in accurate registration of apical area (Fig. 8.6). For this reason, different methods should be used for different cases. CBCT image and surface scan of the arch are prerequisite for guided endodontics, as described in Chap. 4. For surgical endodontics, following methods can be employed for template planning and designing:

1. Dual CBCT with impression (one image of the patient with a markered impression[1] in the mouth, and one of the markered impression itself)
2. Dual CBCT with radiological template (one image of the patient with a markered radiological template, and one of the markered template itself)
3. Dual CBCT with custom tray and impression (one image of the patient with a markered impression in the mouth, and one of the markered impression itself)
4. Simple CBCT with impression (one CBCT image of the patient, one of the impression, separately)
5. Simple CBCT with stone model scan (one CBCT image of the patient, one extra-oral scan of the stone model)
6. Simple CBCT with intraoral scan (one CBCT image of the patient, one intra-oral scan)
7. Simple CBCT with scanned impression (one CBCT image of the patient, and one extraoral scan of the impression)

As no comparative research is available regarding the accuracy of these methods at the moment, the choice is up to the dentist. Whichever of these methods seems to

---

[1] i.e., an impression in a tray with radiopaque markers

fit the actual case the best should be applied, considering the advantages and disadvantages, as discussed below.

8.1.1 Dual CBCT with Impression

One CBCT image of the arch is taken with a markered impression in the mouth, and one CBCT scan of the markered impression itself (separately). This is one of the first methods that were introduced to prepare the production of implant guides. The basis of this method is CBCT image of the patient with the dental impression resting on the dentition (or the alveolar ridge). This tray has radiopaque markers, and rubber base impression material is used (Fig. 8.7). Prefabricated impression trays are, usually, not high enough to cover the vestibular area, so it may need customization. The easiest way to extend vestibular depth is to use Kerr Impression Compound (KerrHawe, Switzerland) (Fig. 8.7). The difficulty of this method is that the impression needs to be placed back into the oral cavity of the patient, at the precise position, for CBCT imaging. This is often not possible because the interdental spaces are filled with the impression material. Therefore, it is advisable to cut all the undercuts and interdental area of such an impression before sending the

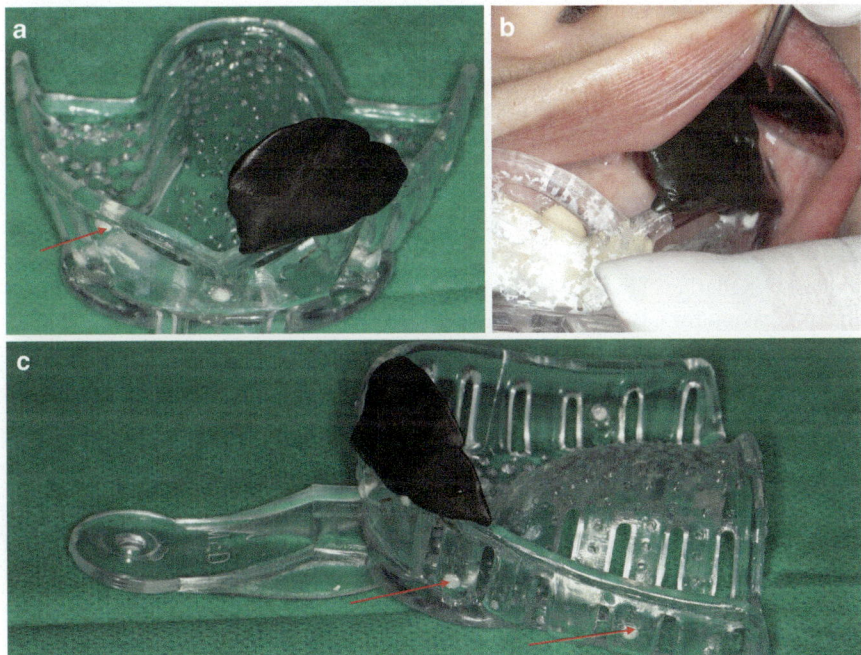

Fig. 8.7 (**a–c**) Preparations on a premarked plastic tray. The arrows point at the radiopaque markers on the trays. Extension over the target area was done with Kerr Impression Compund (KerrHawe, Switzerland)

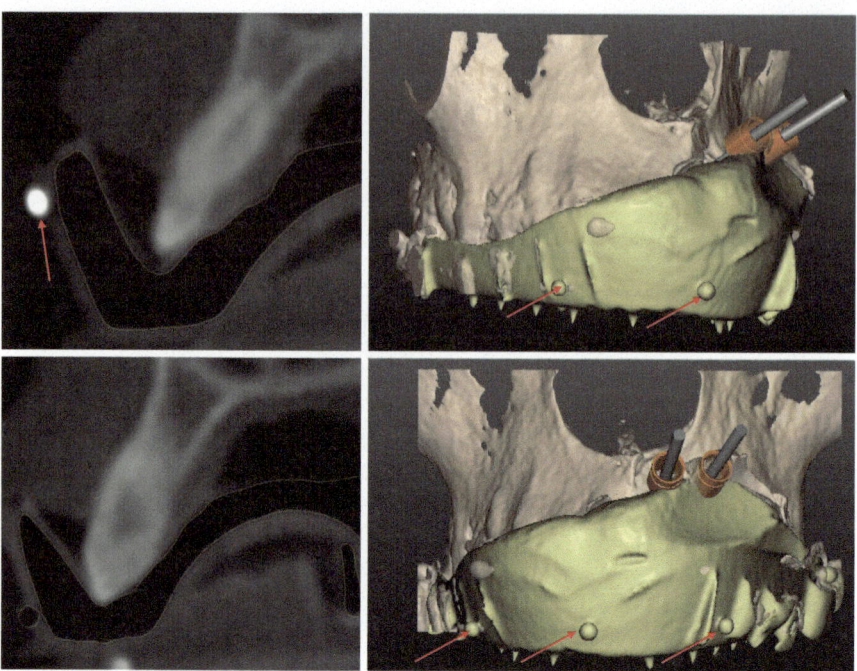

Fig. 8.8 Digital image of an impression tray in a software (SMART Guide, DicomLAB Dental, Szeged, Hungary). The arrows point at the radiopaque markers

patient for imaging. If dentist is not present when the CBCT imaging takes place, often, patient is taught how to reinsert the impression. It is easier for the patient to find the right position if the impression is taken in occlusion (i.e., the patient bites on the impression tray with the antagonists). Impression trays with radiopaque markers are either prefabricated or custom-made. If markers are custom-made, use at least 6–8 markers (Fig. 8.8). The major drawback of the method is reinsertion of the impression for CBCT, which may lead to inaccuracies and errors in guide planning and fabrication (Fig. 8.9).

8.1.2 Dual CBCT with Radiological Template

This is a very similar method to that, and it is used especially for completely edentulous cases in implant dentistry. One CBCT scan of the arch is taken along with template, placed intraorally. Second CBCT of template should be obtained separately. This template should contain radiopaque radiographic markers. After an initial impression of the patient, either in alginate or silicone, a stone model is fabricated. If needed, the tray may be extended as described before. In order to achieve maximum coverage of the surgical area, it is also possible to modify the stone model and make a deeper vestibular area (Fig. 8.10). Note that this requires extreme care, as if the end result is too deep, it will be impossible to place the

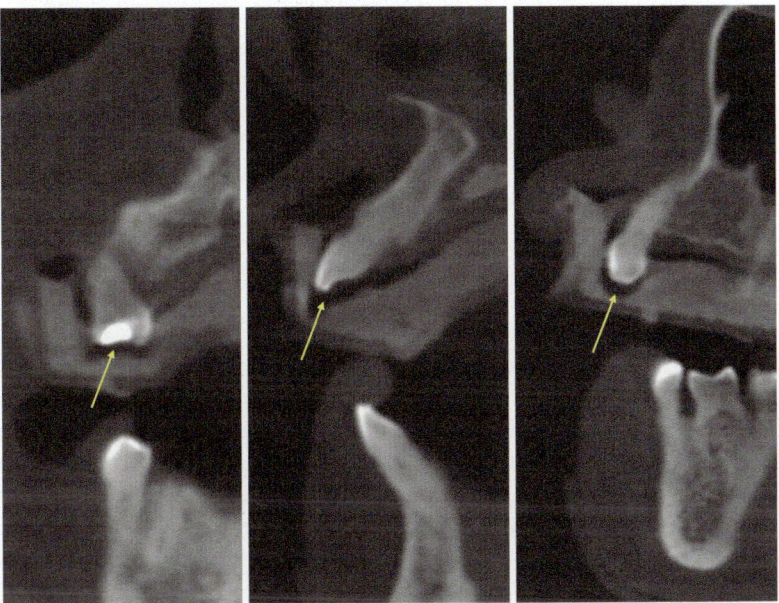

Fig. 8.9 Poor impression fit during imaging (three different cases). The arrows point at the space between the teeth and the impression. (These images could not be used for image registration)

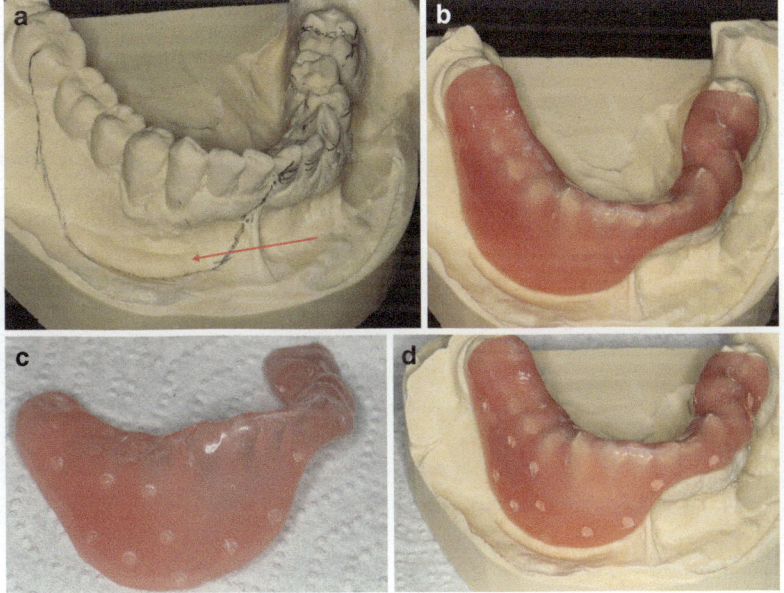

Fig. 8.10 Radiological template for endodontic surgery. (**a**) Stone model with the outline of the planned extension of the template (in pencil). Note the secondary vestibular extension performed in the lab (arrow). (**b**) Template fabricated in the dental lab. (**c**) Holes for the gutta-percha markers. (**d**) Gutta-percha markers in the template

surgical guide (it will be too narrow). The dental technician should be instructed to fabricate template with precise thickness and extension of the borders. In patients with braces or metallic restorations, it is difficult to determine the border between upper and lower teeth on the CBCT image. Use of first two methods can help in planning of such cases. The markers for the radiological template may be fabricated from gutta-percha or any sort of acrylic material (like acrylic resin).

8.1.3   Dual CBCT with Custom Tray and Impression

One CBCT image is obtained with a markered custom tray in the mouth. Second CBCT image of the markered custom tray, itself, is obtained. This method is a mixture of the both methods discussed prior methods. The initial impression is taken in alginate or silicone. A stone model is then fabricated, as this allows the modification of the margins in the vestibular area to provide optimal access to the operation site. With the help of this stone model, a custom tray is prepared, which is extended over the vestibular area at the target tooth. This custom tray is markered with gutta-percha, and a silicone impression is taken with it (Fig. 8.11). Undercuts and excessive interdental material need to be eliminated. All steps can be accomplished in the dental office,

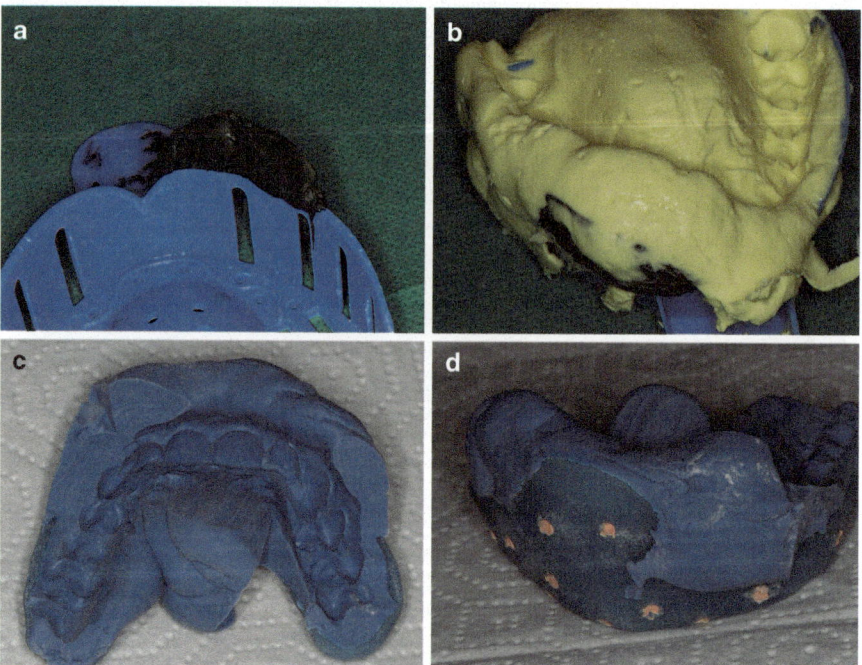

Fig. 8.11 Preparing the markered individual tray. (**a**) Custom tray extended with impression compound. (**b**) Alginate impression. (**c**) Individual tray with impression material. Note that the undercuts have been cut away. (**d**) Markers on the outer surface of the individual tray

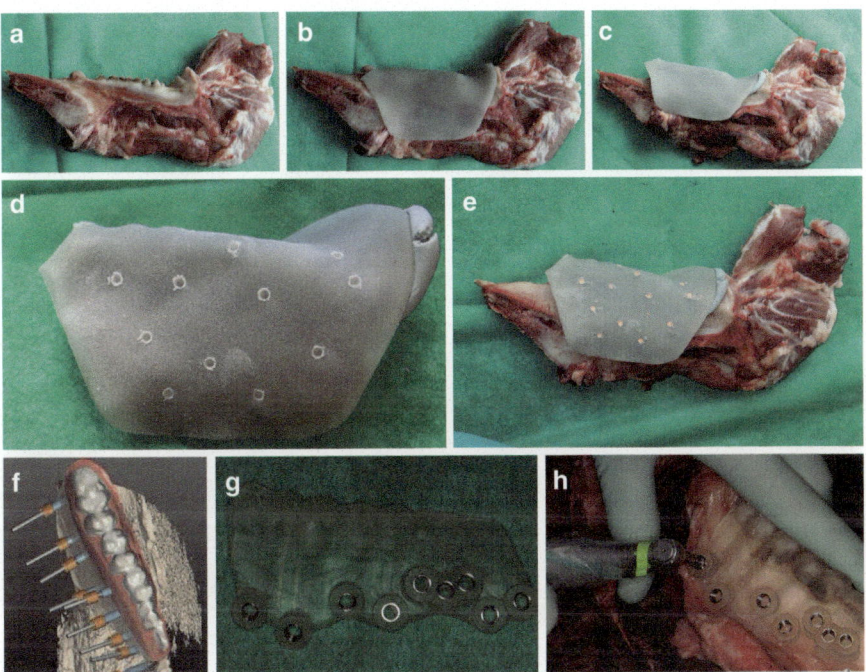

Fig. 8.12 The steps of the process steps in an in vitro experiment. (**a–e**). Preparation of the markered individual tray; (**f**) The 3D plan; (**g**) The guide; (**h**) Surgery

so it is not necessary to involve the dental technician. In our experience, though, this method is not really practical for everyday use, while it has proven to be really useful for in vitro studies (Fig. 8.12). If the CBCT device is in the same dental office, the patient can be scanned with the impression.

8.1.4   Simple CBCT with Impression

CBCT scan of the patient is obtained. Intraoral impression is also taken. This is a very simple method, as it only takes a silicone impression in any custom-made plastic impression tray. The only difficulty is that it requires at least eight or more teeth without metallic restoration (sound or restored with composite) so that image registration can be accurate. Metallic restorations or bridges, multiple crowns, or amalgam restorations cause too much noise in the CBCT image, which prevents anatomical landmarks from being used for registration. If necessary, the tray may be extended, as described earlier. Another option is to retract soft tissues of lips or the buccal area with a dental mirror. This could also help to model the whole target area of the vestibule, but as this part would not have any rigid support, it might get damaged during manipulation (transport, scanning, etc.). This can lead to a suboptimal fit of the surgical guide, especially at the operation site (Fig. 8.13).

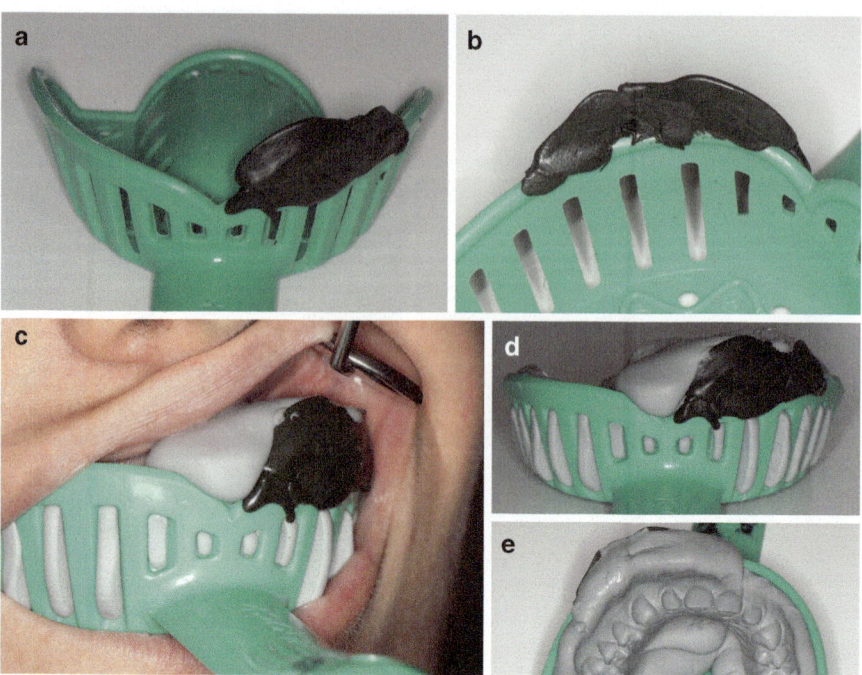

Fig. 8.13 Custom plastic tray extended with impression compound. (**a**, **b**). The tray with the extension; (**c**) Taking the impression. Note that the target area is entirely covered. (**d**, **e**) The impression with the extended vestibular part

8.1.5   Simple CBCT with Stone Model Scan

CBCT image of the patient is obtained. Extraoral scan of the stone model of the patient's dentition is taken. Reliable stone model and precision of the scanner are key factors to have good results. The same difficulties might arise as with the radiological template, as the stone model's precision relies on the initial impression (alginate or silicone) and the inclusion of the target area can be challenging. However, as mentioned earlier, it is also possible to modify the stone model (Fig. 8.14). Too few metal-free teeth can cause further difficulties, as metal artifacts can render image registration extremely difficult or even impossible.

8.1.6   Simple CBCT with Scanned Impression

CBCT image of the arch is taken and the patient's silicone impression is scanned, extraorally. It is recommended that only silicone be used for these impressions, as alginate does not always work seamlessly with scanners. The method is basically the same as the previous one, without the stone model fabrication. The advantage is that the procedure is shorter and simpler, the disadvantage is that the

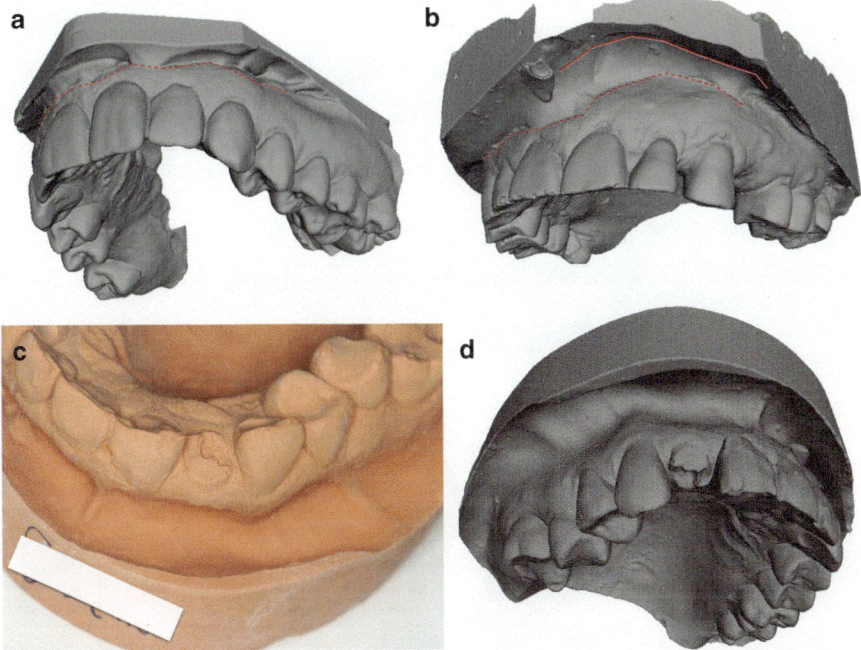

Fig. 8.14 Scanned stone models. (**a**) Scan of an unmodified stone model. Note that the vestibular area is only modeled up to the attached gingiva; (**b**) A stone model fabricated for the preparation of endodontic surgery. The dashed line shows the margin of the attached gingiva, the continuous line connects the deepest points of the modelled vestibular area. (**c, d**). The stone and scanned versions of the same model, both with deep vestibulum

post-hoc correction of the vestibular depth is not possible with this method. Tray extension and soft tissue retraction will help here as well. It must be kept in mind that the borders of the resulting impression will define the borders of the surgical guide.

8.1.7 Simple CBCT with Intraoral Scan

CBCT image of the arch is obtained. With use of the intraoral scanner, surface scan is registered. Operator has direct control over scanning procedure. It can be especially difficult, though, to scan areas covered by movable soft tissue. Small movements, swallowing of the patient, breathing, or just small stops during the scanning can cause the scanner to lose track. The scanner builds the 3D image as scanner is moved along the various intraoral surfaces. Movement disrupts the continuity of scanning, and, in some instances, the whole process needs to be started over again. A possible method to overcome this difficulty is to start scanning from the attached gingiva and move on toward the movable vestibular parts, but the procedure may be challenging to record the depth of vestibule (Fig. 8.15).

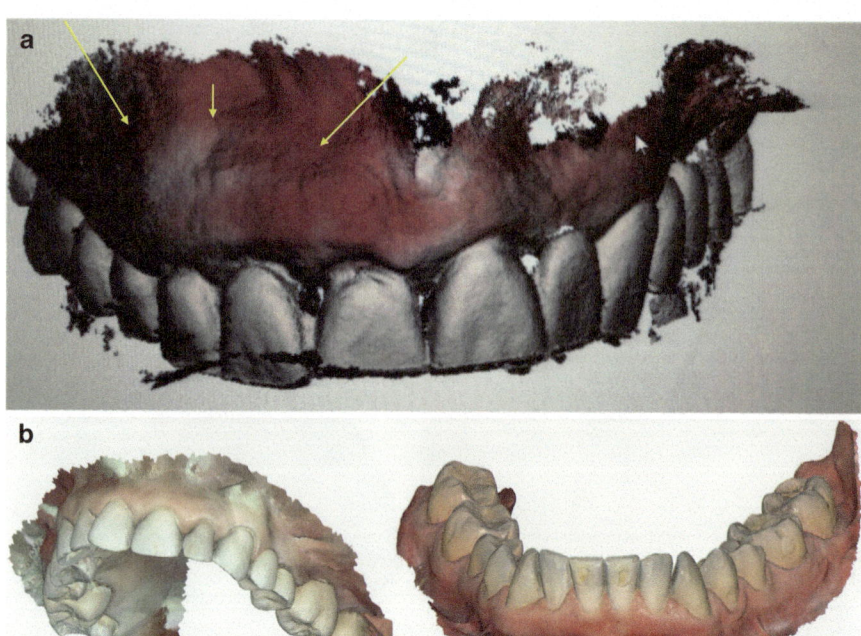

Fig. 8.15 Intraoral scanner images. (**a**) The arrows point at the deepest vestibular points in a relaxed (nonretracted) position on picture. (Adva Intraoral Scanner, GC, Tokyo, Japan) With the retraction of the soft tissues, the scan is eligible for guided endodontic surgery. (**b**) Scans, where the retraction of the soft-tissues is not sufficient for guided endodontic surgery. (Dios Intraoral Scanner, DentalDirekt, Spenge, Germany; Images with the courtesy of Dr. Örs Bajusz)

8.2   Image Registration

This is a critical step of the preparatory phase. Image registration is a term used in information technology. In this phase, data of CBCT scan and surface scan are superimposed. It must be kept in mind that not every guide manufacturing system is able to handle any kind of input, so it is recommended to gather information on this before opting for any of the methods. For instance, we had a CBCT and impression scan case where registration process was flawless, but the software was not able to extract information from the resulting model for printing. After careful examination, it was concluded that the software required counterclockwise-rotating mesh as an input. Even if such a problem is easily corrected with any 3D manipulating software, such manipulations always mean extra hassle and unwanted errors. The key is to carefully study the guide production system and understand its workflow. Workflow for different softwares has been described in Chap. 4.

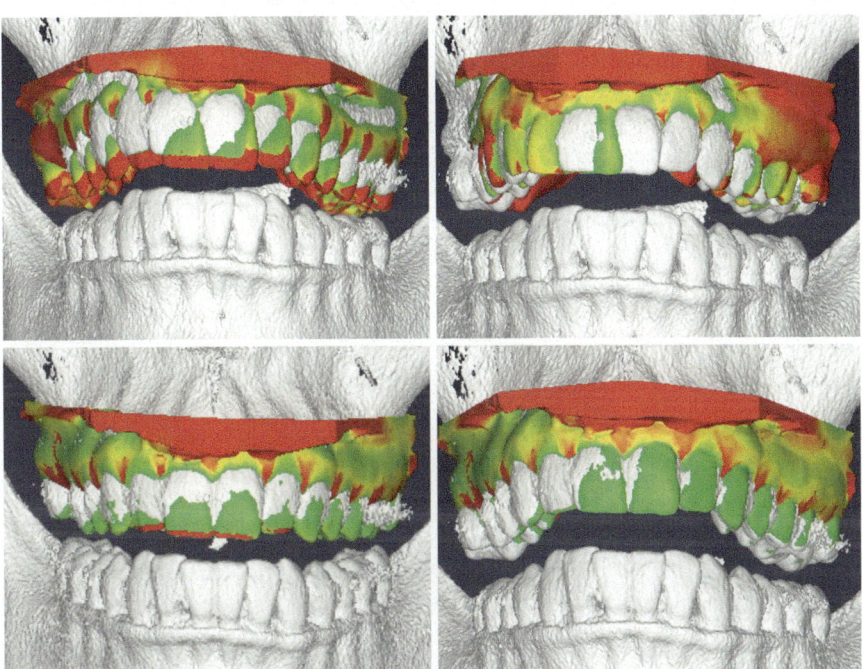

Fig. 8.16 The process of registration. The different colors indicate different degrees of match between the two models DICOM and STL. (Dentiq Guide, 3DII, Seoul, Korea)

Who should do the registration? There are softwares that require the user to manually complete image registration. It can be time-consuming, especially in the beginning, when the user lacks experience with the given software. But even with experience, image registration is best done by individual with a sound knowledge of digital image processing. There may be dentists with such knowledge, but it is safe to assume that they do not represent the majority. Some softwares offer automatic registration with minimal user involvement. Either the operator must mark three identical anatomical reference points in both of the images to be merged or move the two three-dimensional models until they almost completely overlap. To help with this procedure, such softwares use color-coding to indicate the degree of overlap (Fig. 8.16). This is a safer way for those having little knowledge of/interest in digital image processing, but it still takes extra time that the dentist could use for actual dental work. Therefore, such systems are not really practical for everyday use. To solve this problem, some companies began to offer registration as part of the guide manufacturing process. This is of considerable help and it makes guided surgery easy to use in daily practice. Such an extra service comes at a higher price. Unfortunately, such companies produce only implant guides at the moment, but the idea is readily applicable to endodontic guide production. Superimposition of CBCT scan and surface scan with different softwares have been explained in detail in Chap. 4.

8.3 3D Printed Static Aids: Applications for Endodontic Surgery

3D-printed static aids have been used for various purposes in endodontic surgery. Based on the literature, such aids may be classified as follows (Fig. 8.17):

1. Nonguiding 3D printed template to help access
2. 3D printed template for cortical preparation
3. Pilot guide
4. Full guide for a bone trephine

Below we give a brief summary of these applications.

8.3.1 Nonguiding 3D Printed Template to Help Access

These templates are designed to define the surgical area. They retract soft tissues to ensure access to the surgical site. Such surgical aids do not localize the root apex, neither do they guide a drill nor bone trephine. These aids are (or more precisely were at some point) sort of crudely localizing tissue retractors. We mention this

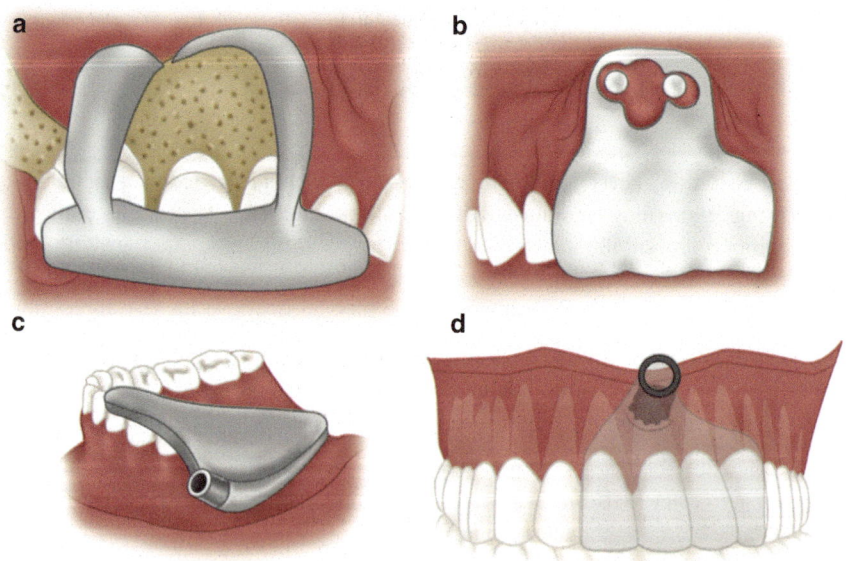

Fig. 8.17 3D printed endodontic surgical aids for different purposes. (**a**) Soft tissue retractor [19]; (**b**) A device to orient cortical penetration [20]; (**c**) A pilot guide [22]; (**d**) Full guide for a bone trephine. (Image used with the permission of Springer Nature. Permission no.: 4633251128826; [21]; Drawings by Dr. Tekla Sáry)

application here, as this was one of the attempts to use 3D printed aids in endodontic surgery [19], but with the development of the field, it had become obsolete before it could get acceptance.

8.3.2   3D Printed Template for Cortical Preparation

This guide helps to define the exact site where the cortical bone should be penetrated for root-end resection. After placing the template, a short drill or cortical trephine is applied through it to mark the cortical bone (see Figs. 8.3 and 8.4) [20, 23]. This template helps to define osteotomy site over the root apex, but they do not help the operator to find the right angulation or length of root end resection. However, such guide can be used for repeated reorientation throughout the surgery.

With this method, only initial guidance is achieved. Main drawback of this method is lack of navigation below the cortical bone. This approach cannot guarantee that the drilling will actually reach the apex, even if it was started in the right direction.

8.3.3   Pilot Guide

This surgical guide is widely used in implant surgery, which is also applicable in endodontic surgery. Here a guiding template is used for drilling with a small diameter drill (the "pilot" drill). Initial drilling is performed with this drill through the template and the resulting bony cavity provides guidance to subsequent drills (applied without the template). Pinsky et al. [16] followed this protocol in their in vitro study, and concluded that such guides could enable precise targeting of the apex. The results of Ahn and colleagues corroborate this [22]. Pilot guides are easy to get hold of, as most implant surgical guide systems have their pilot option. The only difference in an endodontic case is that the planning happens perpendicular to the axis of the tooth. Alternatively, the pin drill can be used for this purpose. Once the pilot drilling is ready, further drills are applied to extend the osteotomy, until the diameter allows the removal of the apex. Pinsky et al. [16] have shown that with this method, clinicians can reach safely within 1 mm of the root apex. Further extension is necessary until a micromirror can be introduced for orientation. Careful planning and evaluation of preoperative CBCT are the key to success as any error in planning can result in unintended damage to anatomical structures. Therefore, we recommend that when a pilot guide is used, planning should be done with a 2 mm safety margin (Fig. 8.18).

8.3.4   Full Guide for a Bone Trephine

To ensure precise osteotomy and apex removal, fully guided endodontic surgery should be planned. This approach is novel, so extensive literature on this approach

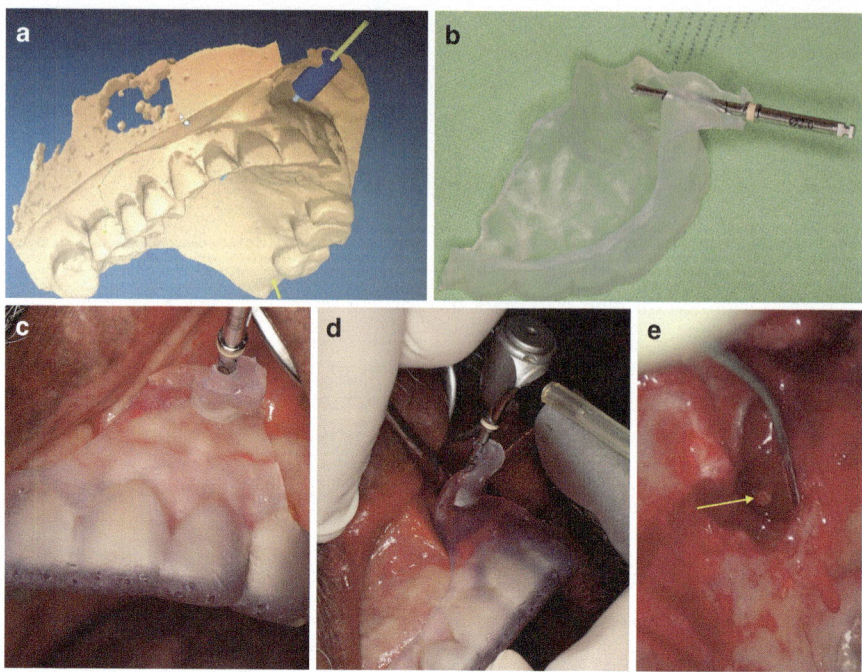

Fig. 8.18 A pilot guide. (**a**) the 3D plan in a software (Dentiq Guide, 3DII, Seoul, Korea); (**b**) The surgical template with a 2.0 mm diameter pilot drill; (**c**) The drill and the guide in situ (for cortical marking); (**d**) Drilling after flap elevation; (**e**). The apex identified in a micromirror under magnification (OPMI Pico, Zeiss, Germany). The arrow points at the gutta-percha

is not available yet. Giacomino et al. successfully used a round trephine through a 3D printed surgical guide to perform both the osteotomy and the root-end removal in the same session [21].

As for the fabrication, any of the imaging methods described above can be used, and a planning software that allows the use of drilling sleeves is required. It is important that the diameter of the drilling sleeve should correspond to the external diameter of the trephine to be used to ensure stability. Poor fit leads to poor results. Always check the actual external diameter of the trephine (e.g., with calipers), as the value shown on the trephine can be inaccurate. Care must be taken, though, that the fit is not so tight as to cause friction between the trephine and the sleeve, as this can lead to heat generation and, also, hinder the rotation of the instrument. As guiding sleeves are manufactured for the purposes of dental implantology, in our practice, we use custom-made metal sleeves whose internal diameter is greater by 0.04 mm than the external diameter of the trephine. This difference allows tension-free rotation (Fig. 8.19). Recently, the first article has been published with preliminary results about the precision of such interventions. The median angular deviation of the trephination in the

Fig. 8.19 A default sleeve of the SMART Guide system (dicomLAB Dental, Szeged, Hungary; right) and a custom-made sleeve for endodontic surgery with a bone trephine. Note that the custom-made sleeve is higher to provide additional stability to the trephine

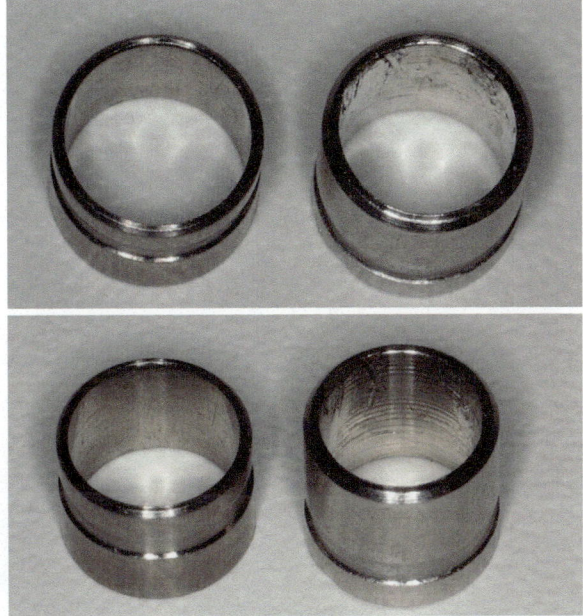

study was 3.95° (95% CI: 2.1–5.9), which makes the process comparable to the angular deviation of guided implant surgery [24].

The trephine itself may be any sort of hollow trephine in a surgical contra-angle. Sterile irrigation must always be used, and rotational speed must be kept low, not exceeding 800 RPM.

Most bone trephines have a working part that is wider than the rest of their body, as shown in Figs. 8.20 and 8.21. This raises the question if the sleeve should be planned to fit the working part or the rest of the body. If the sleeve is planned for the body of the trephine, it will necessitate that the trephine be inserted into the sleeve in a retrograde manner, which is possible only if there is enough space between the bone and the rim of the sleeve facing the bone. This is not only difficult, but also not safe.

Further drawbacks include

1. The possibility of overpenetration (regular bone trephines do not have a stop, see Fig. 8.22)
2. Difficulties with planning (until recently, no software offered the option to plan endodontic cases, so the user had to put up with generic cylindrical implant models of the same diameter as the trephine to be used, see Fig. 8.23)

These drawbacks have been addressed by developing a bone trephine for endodontic surgical purposes and integrating it into an existing planning software, as described below.

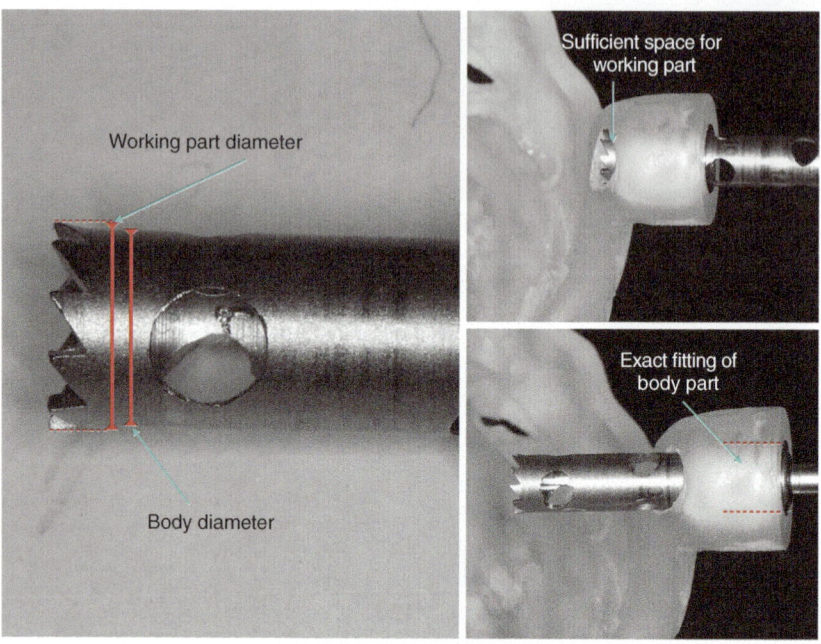

Fig. 8.20 Left: The difference between the diameter of the working part and the body of a regular bone trephine. Right: Because of the diameter difference, reverse insertion is necessary

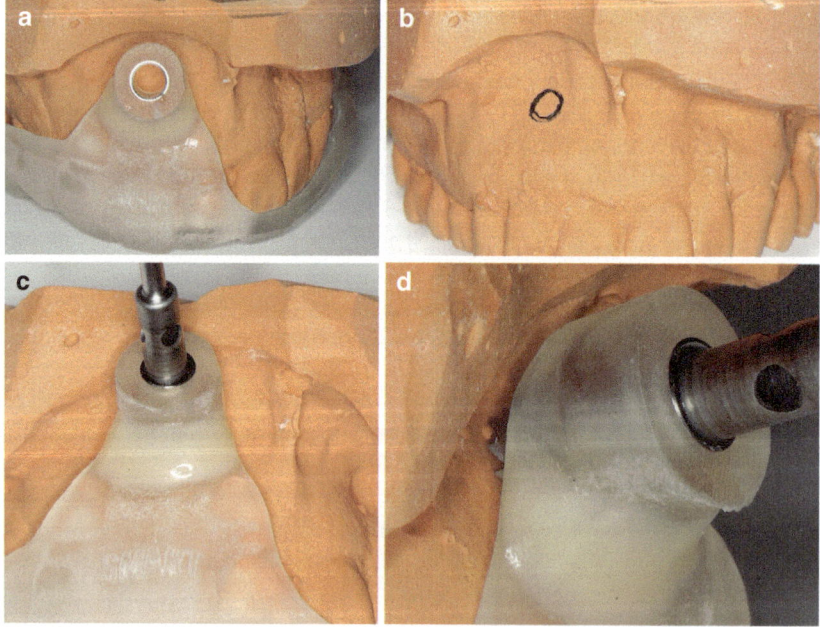

Fig. 8.21 (**a–d**) Check of fit on a stone model. Note that in this case, a bigger sleeve was applied to allow the direct insertion of the trephine (with its wider working part forward)

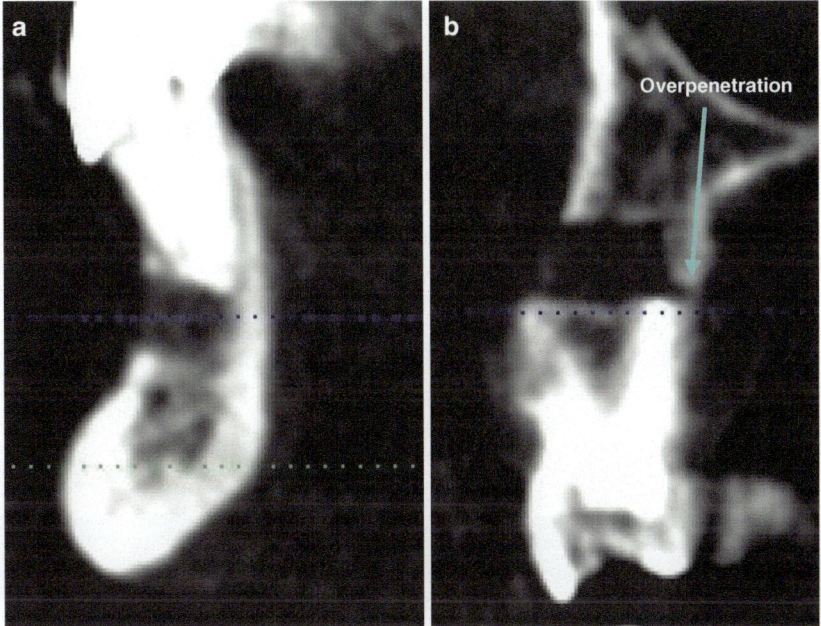

Fig. 8.22 Control CBCT images. (**a**). Penetration as planned (**b**) Overpenetration (the palatal cortical is almost perforated)

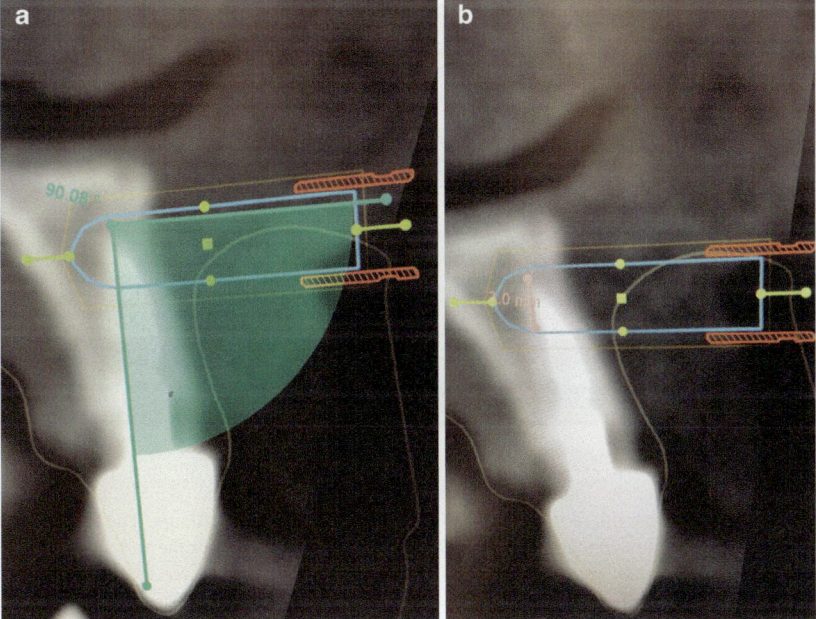

Fig. 8.23 Planning in a software designed for the purposes of implant dentistry (SMART Guide, dicomLAB Dental, Szeged, Hungary). (**a**) Setting the 90° angle; (**b**) Setting the 3 mm cut. Note that for this plan, model of a generic dental implant with the same diameter as that of the bone trephine (4.21 mm) was used, as at this time, the software had no endodontic option

8.3.5   Bone Trephine with a Stop

To prevent overpenetration of the drill, a bone trephine with a stop should be used. Such a trephine shall meet two critical criteria. First, the body and the cutting part shall have the same diameter in order to pass through the guide without friction, and second, they shall have a stop at the base. The function of this stop is to provide precisely calibrated drilling to prevent overpenetration. We have developed a trephine with 20 mm working length and integrated it in the implant planning software (SMART Guide, dicomLAB Dental, Hungary), thus extending the functionality of the software to include endodontic surgical planning. The diameter of the trephine (4.46 mm) was chosen to fit the existing guiding sleeves of the system (4.5 mm). The updated software contains the digital model of the trephine, so that the operator can plan the endodontic surgery just like an implant surgery and get a guide printed for it just as if an implant guide was printed. This innovation helps the operator to achieve 90° angled 3 mm root end resection as closely as possible, without the risk of overpenetration (Figs. 8.24 and 8.25).

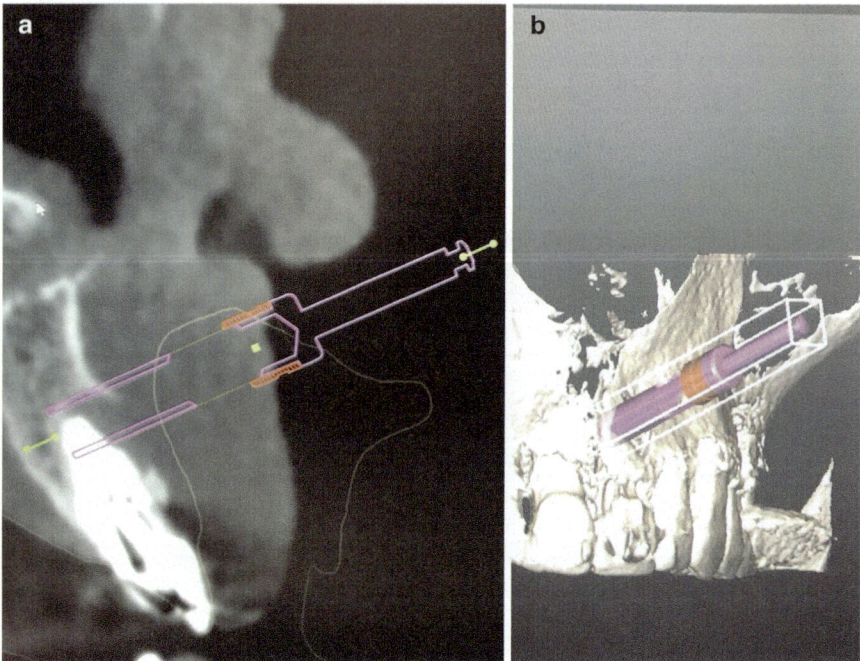

Fig. 8.24 (**a, b**) Trephine visualization in SMART Guide (dicomLAB Dental, Szeged, Hungary). The model exactly matches our custom-made endodontic bone trephine (see Fig. 8.25). The distance between the outer rim of the sleeve and the end of the trephine is 20 mm. The author and the developers are currently cooperating to develop an endodontic feature for the software

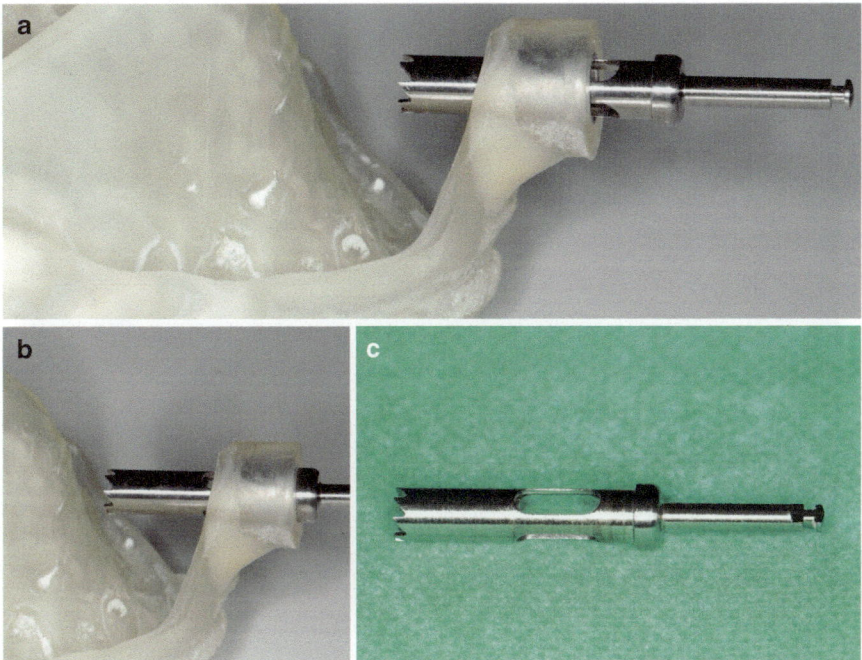

Fig. 8.25 (**a**) The custom-made endodontic bone trephine in the sleeve of the surgical template. (**b**) The stop prevents overpenetration. (**c**) The trephine. Note that the diameter is the same along the entire working length. This makes direct insertion possible, as shown in (**a**)

It is important to note that the diameter of our trephine is invariable, which makes orthograde (direct) insertion possible regardless of how much space is available between the body of the guide and the bone. With this method, the trephine is guided at full length, which certainly enhances accuracy [25].

As third party 3D printing offices charge per printed guide, it is a relevant question when to decide for preparing the guide. If an (nonsurgical) endodontic guide is printed, it is a good idea to plan it with an added periapical sleeve for the same tooth. This means only a small extra cost, and such a combiguide (Fig. 8.26) can be very useful if the nonsurgical endodontic treatment fails.

The latest development in the field is a prefabricated orientation grid, which is basically a visual aid whose aim is to help apex localization during planning and surgery [26]. The idea is that the patient has a prefabricated grid in his or her mouth, while the CBCT image is taken. This grid is then visible during the planning and will act as reference during the surgery as well (Fig. 8.27).

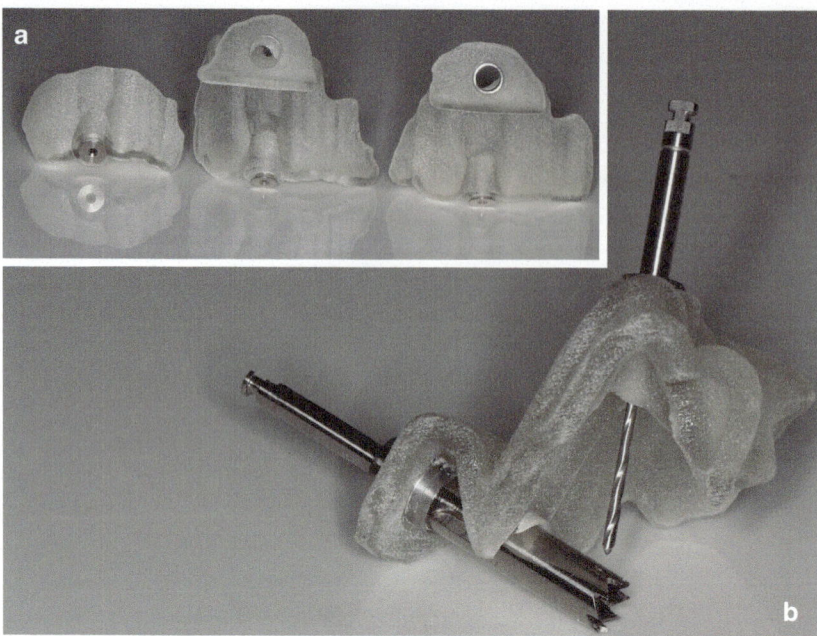

Fig. 8.26 Combiguides; (**a**) Different designs for the same case. From left-to right: Endodontic guide with StecoGuide drill sleeve (Steco, Hamburg, Germany), Endodontic guide + pilot surgical guide, Endodontic guide + full surgical guide. (**b**) A combiguide with a 1.0 mm drill (ATEC, Erbingen, Germany) and a stop trephine (Smile Dent, Szeged, Hungary)

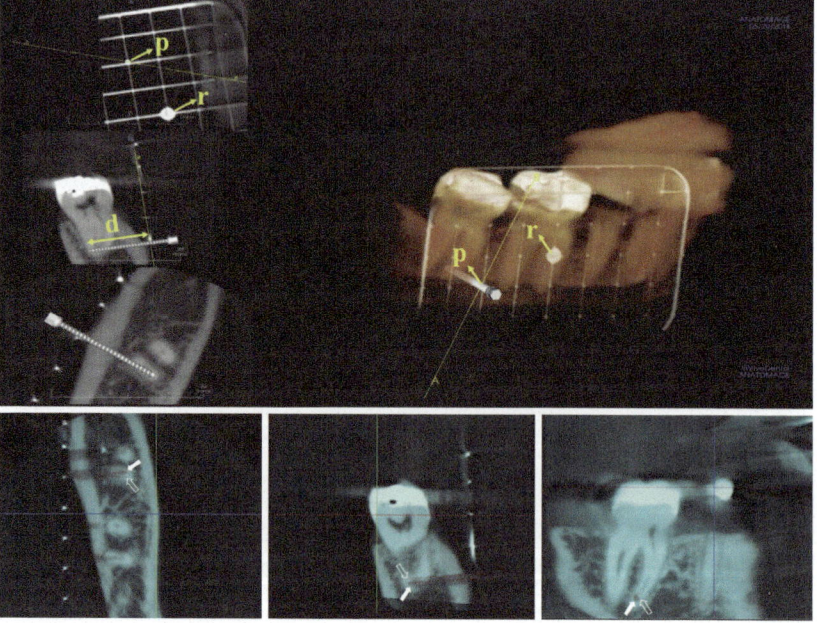

Fig. 8.27 Prefabricated grid for endodontic surgery by Fan et al. [26]

8.4 Recommended Workflow for Guided Endodontic Surgery

The first set of recommendations for a surgical endodontic workflow was given by Liu et al. in 2014 [18]. In the 5 years that has passed since then, the field has seen developments that justify revision. Here we recommend a simpler and more predictable workflow that is based on the new developments. While guided endodontic surgery could, in theory, be performed without microscopic magnification, our recommendations assume that a surgical microscope is certainly a necessity for such treatments (Fig. 8.28).

8.4.1 Case Assessment

First of all, the patient and the planned intervention must be assessed carefully and individually in each case. General medical assessment and risk analysis of the patient are essential even for a basic surgical intervention. Systemic diseases such as diabetes or cardiac conditions must be explored. Note that even if endodontic surgery is relatively minimally invasive, the healing period might be longer than for a simple extraction, and the complications are more varied. This underlines the importance of careful initial assessment. Case selection should be proper as majority of cases of poor root canal treatment can be resolved by nonsurgical re-treatment approach. Endodontic surgery may be considered in cases of canal blockage, irretrieved instrument separation or failed re-treatment cases.

If endodontic surgery is an option, it must be assessed if the anatomy of the tooth (with special attention to the target area) allows guided endodontic operation.

Anterior teeth are mostly easy to access even at the level of the apex, but in some cases, the vestibular area can be really tight or the lips of the patient do not allow retraction for 90° penetration at the root end.

Fig. 8.28 A suggested workflow for guided endodontic surgery. See text for details

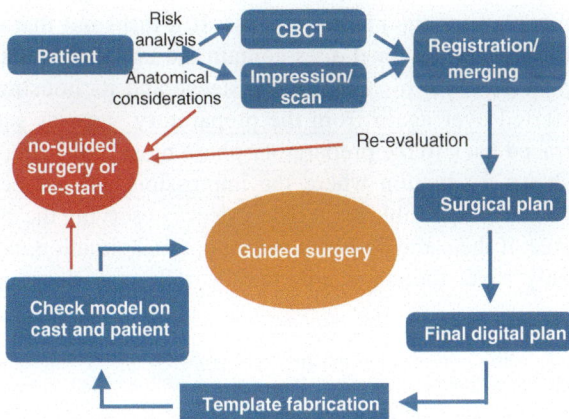

Premolars are a bit more difficult to access, but if the mobility of the vestibule is sufficient, guided surgery is definitely an option. The guided approach is especially advantageous in the lower premolar area, where the protection of the mental nerve is a concern. Minor spatial limitations can be overcome by slightly oblique planning toward the mesial so that the trephine will penetrate the bone not exactly at 90°. Note that this does not necessarily affect the angle formed by the axis of a given root and the axis of the trephine; that is, the penetration can be perpendicular to the root, even if it is not perpendicular to the surface of the bone. Such a plan is easily prepared in a dedicated software. Such an approach naturally comes at the expense of the removal of slightly more bone, but it is worth considering. Compared to conventional osteotomy, this approach will, still, preserve much more bone.

Molar teeth are always challenging. If the guided approach is chosen, molar roots are accessible almost only with a mesially oblique penetration from the buccal side. Still, the safety of the mandibular nerve or the sinuses might necessitate this. Straight access is possible to the palatal roots from the palatal side, but it has its own difficulties, which the guide cannot really solve. Flap elevation requires extreme care not to damage the palatine artery, while access preparation with a soft tissue trephine (which is possible through a guide) almost always results in excessive bleeding.

8.4.2   Image Acquisition and Registration

Having opted for guided surgery, the next step is to acquire the images that will serve as the input of the planning and manufacturing process. Any of the methods described earlier (Sect. 8.2) can be used, observing the needs of the actual case.

8.4.3   Planning Issues

First of all, assess if the outcome of the image registration (a three-dimensional model) suits the planning needs. If it turns out that the model does not contain the target area (or it does contain the target area but not extensively enough to provide room for the guiding sleeve and its housing), the procedure has to be started over again from the preparatory steps as such an insufficiency can be traced back to the preparatory phase most of the time.[2] The left side of Fig. 8.29 shows a situation where the impression had not been extended enough, so it became impossible to include a sleeve observing the 90° rule. In contrast, the right side of the same figure shows an optimal situation, where the extension does not only cover the target area but also allows a sleeve and housing to be inserted.

---

[2] If depth of vestibule is not recorded properly, it may lead to error during planning of surgical guide for root-end resection. Proper depth of vestibule can be recorded by modified impression trays or digital impressions.

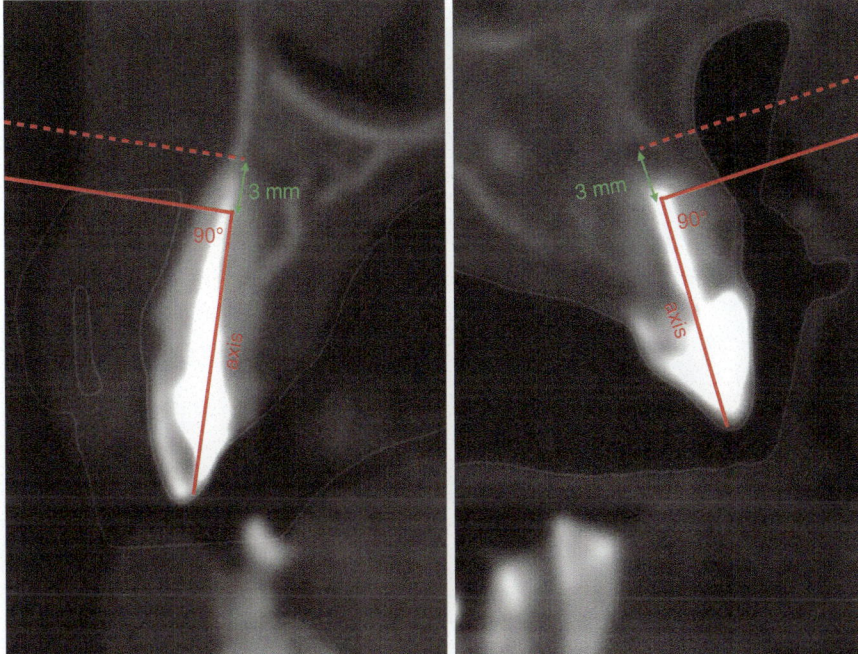

Fig. 8.29 Improper (left) and proper (right) vestibular extension of the model/impression. To determine the goodness of the extension, two lines are drawn. The first one is perpendicular to the apical endpoint of the tooth axis (dashed line). The second one is parallel to the first one, 3 mm below it (solid line). The extension is good if both lines fall within the impression or scan (the yellowish outline in the image). Depending on the system, extra extension for the sleeve might be necessary

Figure 8.30 shows a scenario with an almost good extension: only half of the guiding sleeve falls within the guide. One must remember that it is not enough to cover the target area, but it must be covered in such a way that it allows a sleeve to be inserted as per the rules. The importance of preparation and imaging cannot be overemphasized.

Another issue can be the access to the root apex with the trephine. Fortunately, this is an issue that can be addressed right in the planning phase if all relevant circumstances are considered. Most bone trephines have length of 10–20 mm, and, in most cases, it is not difficult to plan in a way that the apex is reached. However, if the soft tissue is thick above the apical area, it can increase the sleeve-apex distance enough to prevent a shorter trephine from reaching the apex, or allows the trephine to cut only part of it. Therefore, if the operator has a shorter trephine in mind, the thickness of the soft tissue must always be assessed. In contrast, planning with a long trephine carries the risk of overpenetration and suboptimal guidance (as the longer piece of the trephine is unguided, the more lateral movement within the bone becomes possible). Of course, overpenetration is not an issue if the trephine has a stop, or at least depth marks, as shown in Fig. 8.31.

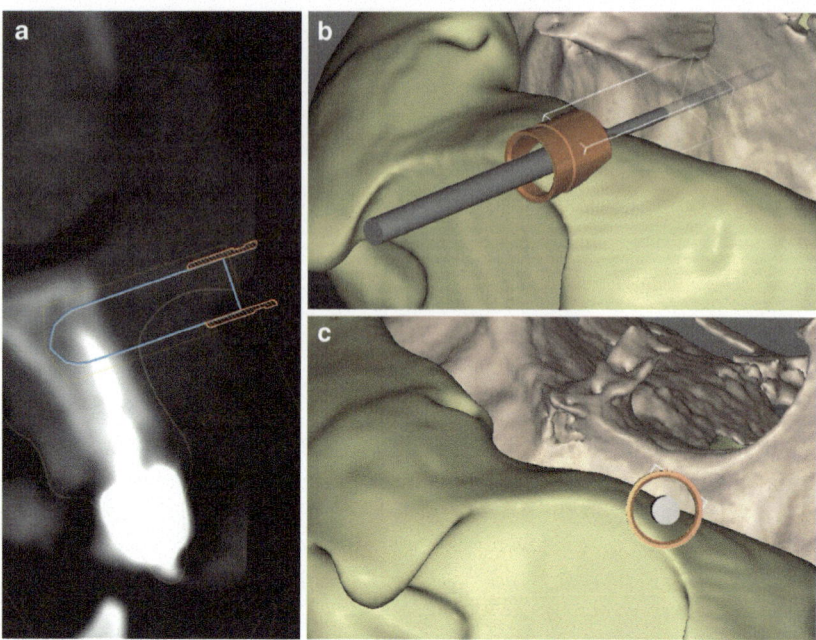

Fig. 8.30 (**a–c**) An "almost good" extension. Unfortunately, with all rules kept, only half of the sleeve would have been in the body of the template, so this plan had to be revised

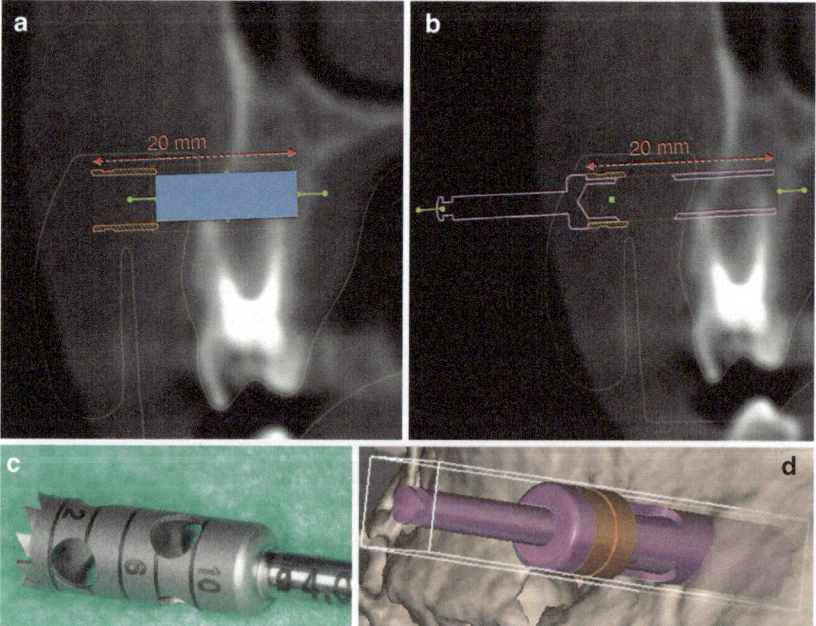

Fig. 8.31 Planning the surgical guide. (**a**) Planning with manual measurement of the distance from the outer margin of the sleeve until the tip of the planned trephine. (**b**) Planning with the stop trephine in SMART Guide (dicomLAB Dental, Szeged, Hungary). (**c**) Trephine with depth marks (Hager & Meisinger, Neuss, Germany); (**d**) Our custom-made stop trephine in 3D view

8.4.4 The Final Digital Plan

While some systems export three-dimensional data as an input for manufacturing automatically, few systems require manual data export to the printer. This means exporting the plan into an STL file, which can be used as an input for the printer. If one works with a system that offers all-around service, this is not an issue.

The drilling/osteotomy depth for any given sleeve is important parameter to be considered at this stage. This is calculated as the distance between the outer rim of the sleeve or guiding tunnel and the endpoint of the osteotomy as planned. If clinician works with an all-around system, this information comes with the surgical template, in the individual manual of the template (some systems call it a protocol). If, however, the system offers only planning and STL export, care must be taken that this information is noted.

Before going on to manufacturing, double check that the plan is compatible with the instruments at your disposal.

8.4.5 Template Fabrication/Manufacturing

There are few systems that offer all-around service including 3D printing, and there are ones that provide only the STL file for further use. In the former case, the dentist has to order the guide online and wait for delivery. In the latter case, however, the dentist must arrange 3D printing.

Although today more and more dental offices and dental laboratories have their own 3D printer, most of these are not suitable for the purposes of surgical guide printing. The reason for this is that a printer fit for such purposes must be one that works with a specific, biologically inert material that can be in direct contact with the tissues of the patient for ≥ 1 h (Fig. 8.32).

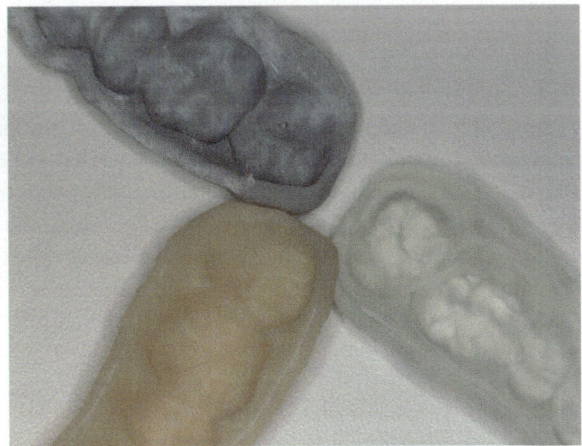

Fig. 8.32 Surgical guides printed form different materials. Only the transparent one is fit for actual medical use (VisiJet S300, 3DSystems, USA)

Fig. 8.33 A set of stop trephines for endodontic surgery (Endo-trephines, Smile Dent, Szeged, Hungary). From left to right (diameter/length): 3.46 mm/10 mm, 15 mm, 20 mm; 4.46 mm/10 mm, 15 mm, 20 mm

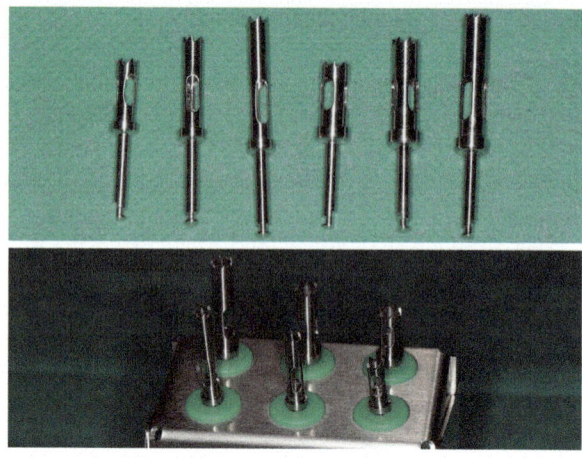

Some guides come with metal guiding sleeves, some without them. This is another important point to pay attention to when one starts working with a system, and especially when one starts planning, as the presence or absence of the sleeve determines the diameter of the trephine to be used. As said before, it is advisable to choose a diameter that is somewhat smaller than the inner diameter of the guiding tunnel (with or without the sleeve) to avoid friction. Alternatively, one may wish to have a set of endodontic trephines manufactured in a range of lengths and diameters (Fig. 8.33). Remember that a bone trephine for guided endodontic surgery is of the same diameter along its entire length.

8.4.6   Try-On

The optimal fit of the guide is a key to successful guided approach. First, try the guide on a stone model of the patient. The surgical template has to be checked first on a stone model of the patient (see Fig. 8.21). Check both fit and stability. If the guide fails to fit because of extra material (such as material in the interdental spaces), eliminate the excess and try the guide on again. If the guide still does not fit, repeat. Be careful, though, to progress in small steps and not to take away more than what is necessary. If the shape of any of the teeth of the patient is modified after the impression (e.g., by a new filling), it must be noted and that tooth must be cut out of the digital mesh, so that it cannot interfere with the fit of the guide. Physical elimination from the actual guide is an option, but only if the eliminated part is not close to the target area. Unfortunately, there are cases when the guide just will not fit. Sometimes, it is due to printing error and then reprinting solves the problem. Otherwise, the reason is probably a poorly taken impression or an overcorrected stone model.

If the fit is correct, the guide can be sterilized. Depending on the material, some guides can be heat sterilized, but some tolerate a cold sterilization solution only. Always consult the manufacturer's instructions before sterilization.

8.4.7   Preparations for the Surgery

For an endodontic surgical surgery, a surgical motor with sterile cooling and rpm control is necessary. For the retrograde preparation, it is also advisable to have a piezosurgical unit at hand. Apart from these, the same instruments are needed as for regular endodontic surgery (Figs. 8.34 and 8.35). In our experience, it is useful to have a CBCT image of the patient around, as well as the surgical plan, possibly projected on a screen in the operating theater. This helps orientation and the modification of the plan, if need be. Although retrograde preparation might be possible without a piezo unit, we do suggest that a piezo unit should be used, as working inside a bony housing indicates sterile irrigation. Before the start of any procedure (including anesthesia), the guide's fit must be checked in the patient's mouth. This is the last checkpoint where the operation can be cancelled if the guide does not fit as expected. It is also an option to perform free-hand surgery, but this shall be individually evaluated depending upon the operator's experience and the possible negative consequences. This shall be also communicated to the patient.

8.4.8   Endodontic Surgery

Apply local anesthesia in a dose that also helps to control bleeding during the operation. A minimum of 3–6 mL of epinephrine-containing anesthesia (depending upon patient's medical history) is recommended [27].

The incision will be determined by the anatomical considerations (such as local vascularization) and the accessibility of the apical area of the target tooth. The flap shall be designed so that the incision does not cross the osteotomy site. Before the flap is elevated, the guide shall be placed into its place to help determine the right incision. The base of the elevated flap shall be wide enough to allow tension-free retraction. A well-designed guide can double as a soft tissue retractor. After the flap

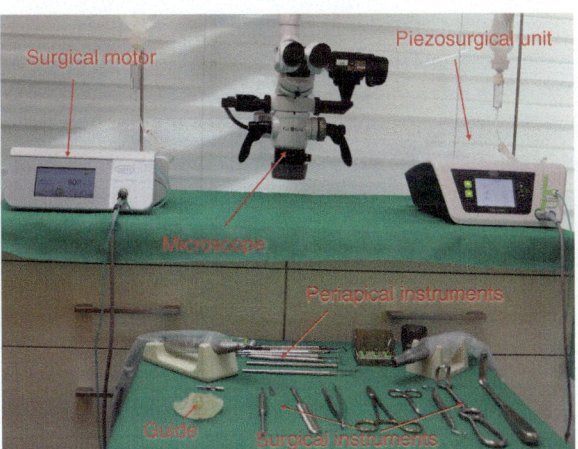

Fig. 8.34 Basic setup for guided endodontic microsurgery with surgical motor, piezosurgical unit (W&H, Bürmoos, Austria), and microscope (A6, Global, Saint Louis, USA)

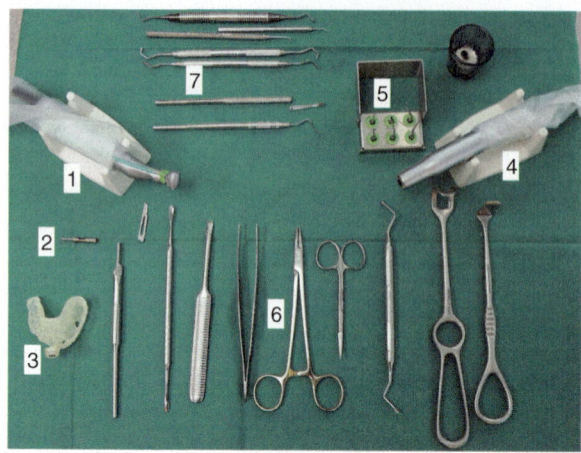

Fig. 8.35 Basic setup for guided endodontic microsurgery
1. Surgical motor with controllable rotational speed
2. Special bone trephine with stop
3. Endodontic surgical guide
4. Piezosurgery unit
5. Retrograde preparation tips for the piezo unit
6. Surgical instruments (left to right: scalpel, Freer elevator, raspatorium, surgical forceps, needle-holder, scissors, Volkmann bone curette, retractors)
7. Periapical instruments (top to bottom: ball burnisher, extra small burnishers, condenser, Heidemann spatula, micromirror, Williams probe)

has been elevated, the guide has to be placed in its place again, and fastened at least in three points. In most endodontic surgery situations, there are enough teeth to provide stable fit for the guide. Alternatively, it as an option to plan three anchor points on the guide and apply fastening (fixation) pins.

Once the flap has been elevated, osteotomy should be performed (Fig. 8.36). Its exact location and angulation is determined by the guide. If a bone trephine with a stop is used, the maximum depth is also predetermined. As for trephines without a stop, the actual depth of the osteotomy should be assessed continuously. If the trephine does not have depth marks, a periodontal probe should be used to gage the depth.

When a bone trephine is used, the apex is usually removed along with the bone. That is, two tasks are performed in one session. Should this not be the case (as it happens sometimes), a periotome can be utilized to remove the apex (Fig. 8.37).

Having removed the bone and the apex, retrograde preparation is performed with a piezosurgery unit under dental operating microscope. A retrograde preparation of at least 2–3 mm should be done [28]. If necessary, methylene blue can be used to visualize the accessory canal(s) and ramifications. This part of the surgery is not different from what has been described by Kim et al. [29]. The only difference may be the size and shape of the osteotomy, and the fact that along with the bone, trephine removes the apex and the surrounding bone and/or pathological tissues at the

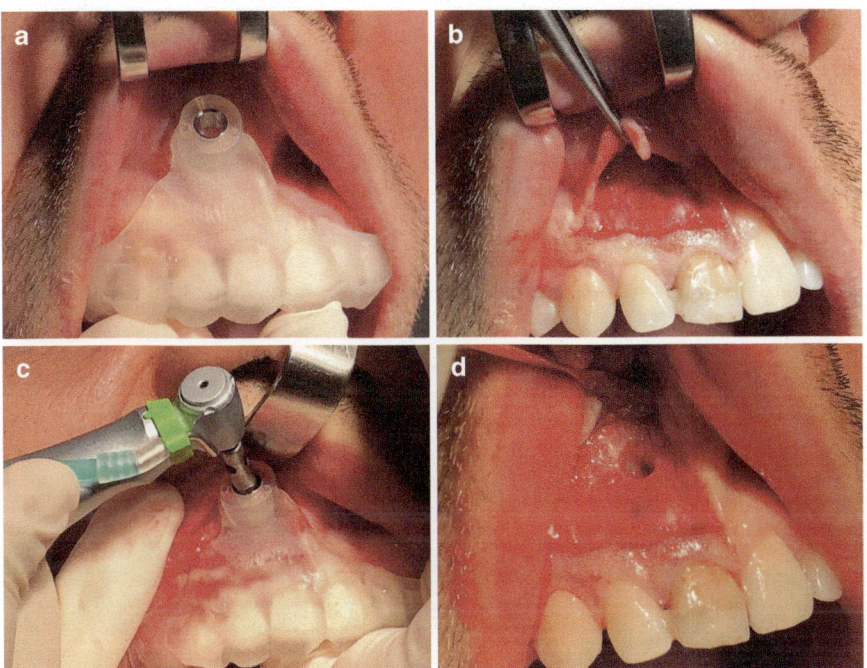

Fig. 8.36 The initial steps of the surgery. (**a**) Try-in for stability check flap design; (**b**) Elevation of the flap; (**c**) Osteotomy (the flap is kept retracted by the template); (**d**) The round osteotomy window

same time (Figs. 8.38 and 8.39). If one has to do retropreparation in a distal location, or the access is compromised because of short-length trephine, a keyhole extension of the osteotomy might become necessary, as described by Kim et al. [30] (Fig. 8.40).

Once the retrograde root-end preparation is finished, a retrograde filling shall be placed. In line with the current literature, we recommend MTA or bioceramic for this purpose [31, 32] (Fig. 8.41). To reduce the bleeding, epinephrine pellets, and, if indicated, ferric sulfate might be used inside and outside the osteotomy window [33] (Fig. 8.42).

To close the osteotomy site, fasten the flap with sutures (if the periosteum is intact). Another alternative is to perform either guided bone regeneration (GBR) or cover the lesion with collagen membrane. The detailed discussion of the advantages and disadvantages of different wound closure techniques after endodontic surgery is beyond the scope of this book, but ample literature is available on this question [30].

Right after the surgery, a periapical radiograph is recommended as a first control. For combined and complex lesions, though, small FOV CBCT might become necessary, but this should be avoided to keep patient irradiation as low as reasonably possible. In most cases, if the patient is clinically asymptomatic, periapical

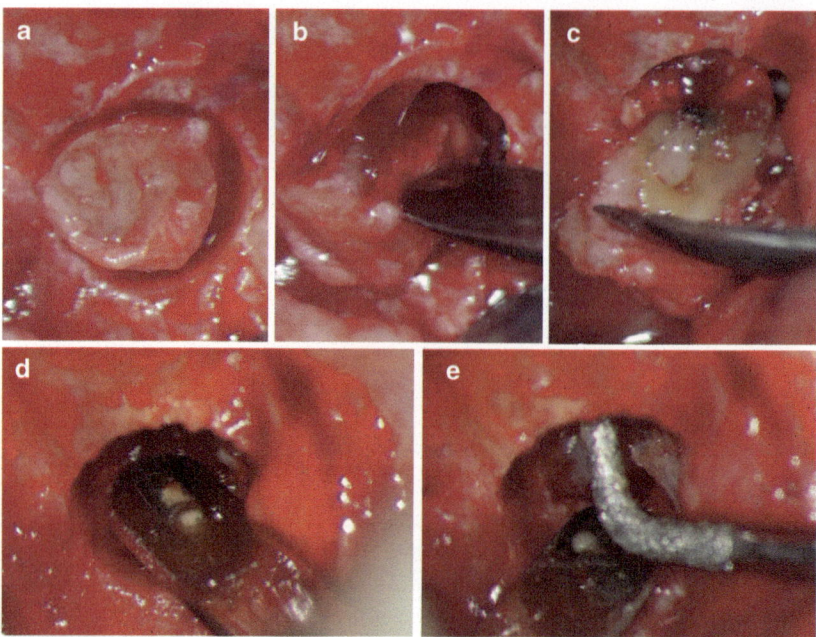

Fig. 8.37 Steps after osteotomy with the trephine. (**a**) Right after penetration. (**b**, **c**), Removing the bone with the apex with a periotome. (**d**) Locating the root canals. (**e**) Retropreparation with the piezosurgical instrument (Piezomed, W&H, Bürmoos, Austria)

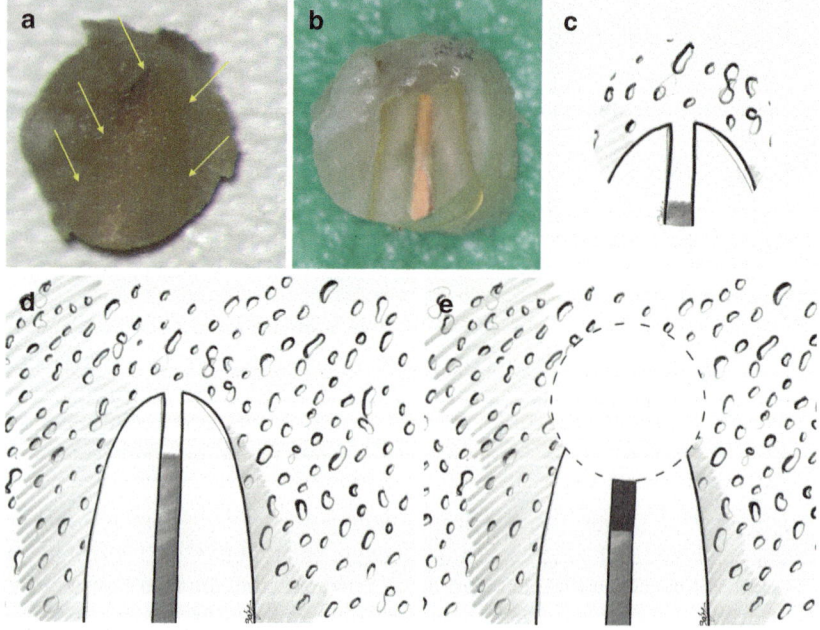

Fig. 8.38 The apex together with the removed bone. (**a**) The removed portion. The apex is slightly visible (yellow arrows) (**b**) The same portion, cut into half to show the root apex inside. Schematic drawings show the root before surgery (**d**) after (**e**) and the removed portion (**c**). (Drawings by Dr. Tekla Sáry)

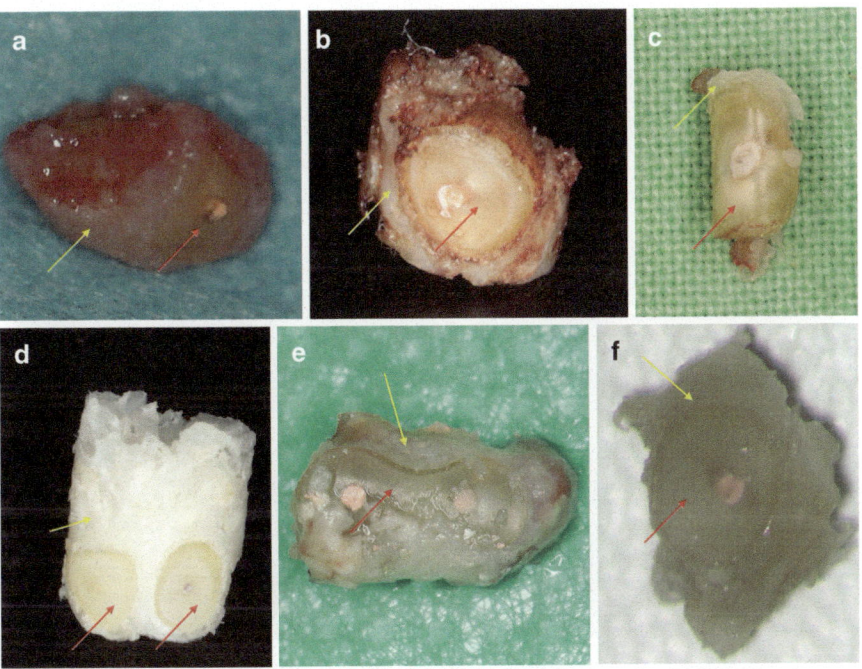

Fig. 8.39 (a–f) Apices removed with the surrounding bone and/or pathological tissues. Yellow arrow: bone; Red arrow: tooth

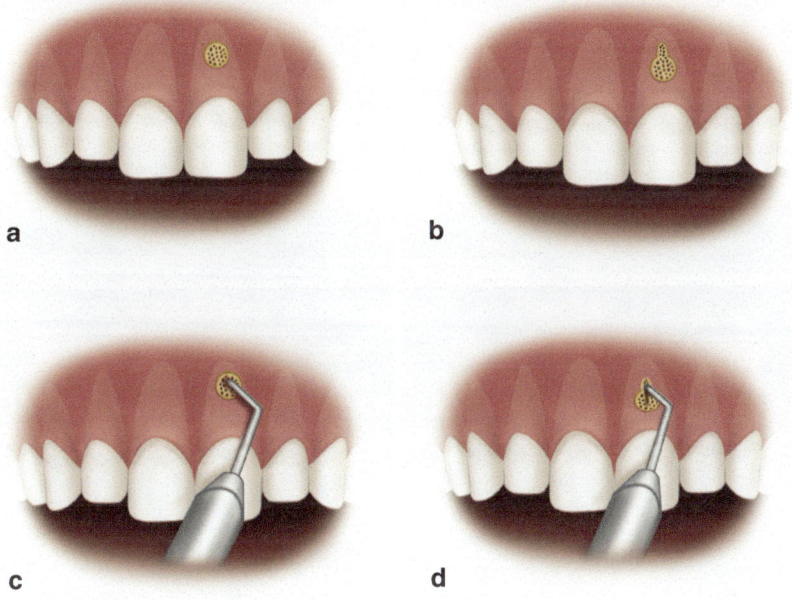

Fig. 8.40 Keyhole extension as described by Kim et al. [30], modified for the navigated endodontic surgery. (**a**) Osteotomy with the bone trephine; (**c**) The piezo instrument does not fit in; (**b**) Keyhole extension of the round osteotomy; (**d**) The piezo instrument fits. (Drawings by Dr. Tekla Sáry)

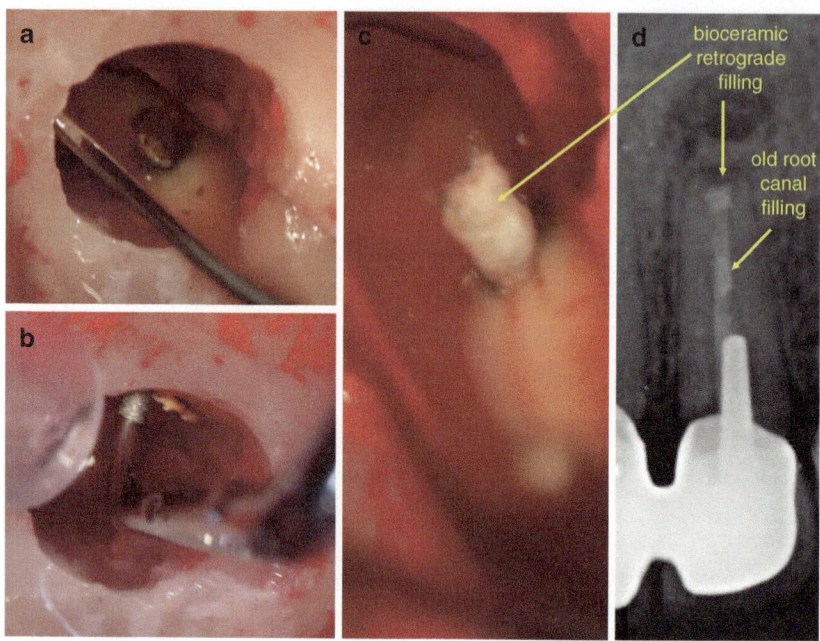

Fig. 8.41 Retrograde preparation and filling. (**a**) Cavity prepared with the piezo instrument through the round osteotomy; (**b**) Retrograde preparation. (**c**) Bioceramic filling in the cavity (TotalFill Fast Set Putty, FKG, La Chaux-de-Fonds, Switzerland); (**d**) Periapical control X-ray

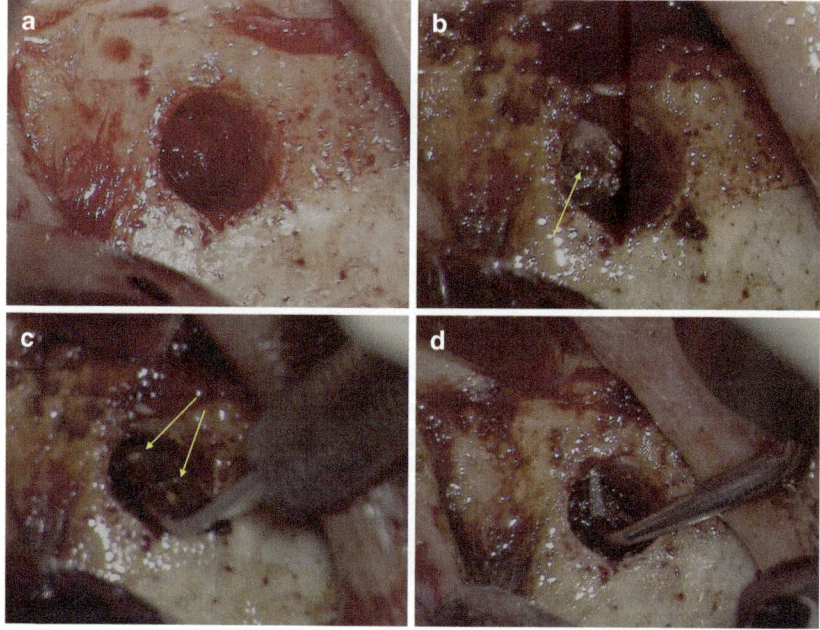

Fig. 8.42 Hemostasis during surgery. (**a**) Without hemostasis; (**b**) Hemostasis with ferric sulfate (the arrow shows a cotton pellet left in the cavity during retrograde preparation); (**c**) Root canals sealed with gutta-percha as reflected in the micromirror. (**d**) Retrograde preparation

radiographs can be taken every 6 month to follow the healing process [34]. Healing and success are evaluated as in any surgical endodontic case.

8.5 Unexplored Factors and Complications

One of the unexplored questions when performing guided endodontic microsurgery is the effect of the *crescent shape* of the apex (Fig. 8.43) after removal with a bone trephine (if any). Till date, no postoperative complication or failures have been documented following guided endodontic surgery. Ultrasonic tips can be used to round off the sharp margins of the root end and provide better periodontal attachments. Furthermore, as seen in Fig. 8.43b, d, after some time (in this specific case 2.5 years), the sharp edges go through resorption and healthy bone builds around the apex. It would be too early to draw a firm conclusion, though. Systematic observation is necessary to find out how this shape interacts with the surrounding tissues and if it has any effect on the elimination of the ramifications and lateral canals. It would be interesting to have long-term clinical trials for the same.

Different guide shapes and designs have been tested for endodontic surgery. In our experience, the most important factor in this respect is that the sleeve housing should have a firm support and that it should not be too distant from the body of the

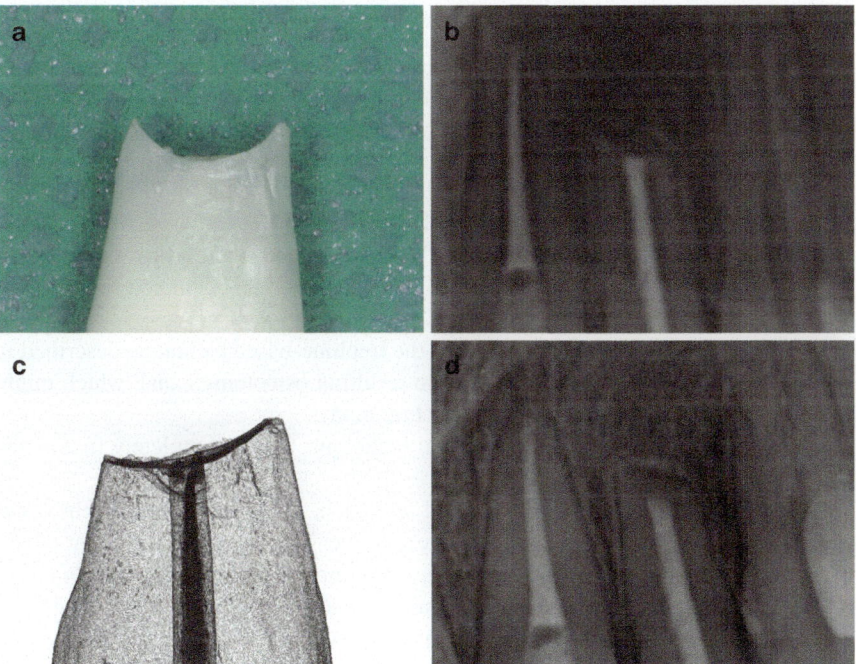

Fig. 8.43 The shape of the apex after guided endodontic surgery with bone trephine. (**a**) The crescent shape demonstrated on an extracted tooth. The tooth was cut with the trephine after extraction. (**b**) Six-month follow-up of an actual case. (**c**) The crescent shape visible on a micro-CT image. (**d**) The same case as above, 2 years after surgery

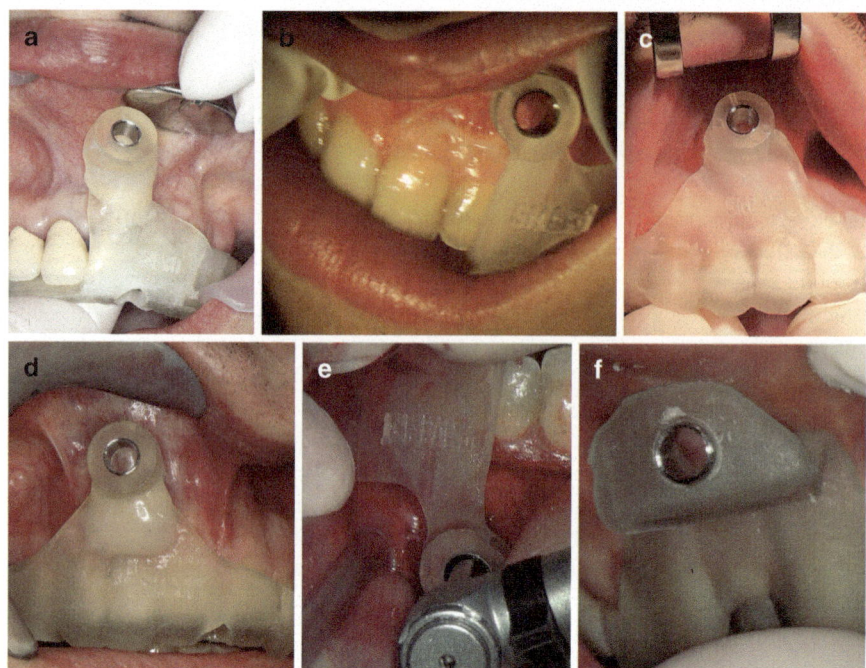

Fig. 8.44 (**a–f**). Different guide shapes for endodontic surgery. In our experience, shape c is the most practical and resilient, especially if it is reinforced at the sleeve housing, as shown in the image (**d**). In contrast, (**e**) is fragile and unstable, because the sleeve housing is distant from the bulk of the body and linked to it only by a relatively thin piece of material

template. We prefer a bulky template body with a thicker triangular support for the sleeve housing, as shown in Fig. 8.44. Note that this has a lot to do with how one shapes the extension in the preparatory phase.

Whether the guided approach is valid in cases where the cortical is not intact might well be a matter of debate. In our opinion, this should be judged in each individual case.

An obvious (relative) disadvantage of the trephine-based technique described in this chapter is the cylindrical shape of the resulting osteotomy canal, which might interfere with cleaning and debridement (Fig. 8.45).

This technique, like any other surgical technique, is not completely free of the possibility of complications.

As a major complication with guided approach, larger deviations might occur (especially with long trephines, see before). Studies indicate that the angular deviation of this technique is similar to that of guided implant surgery, ranging from 3° to 5° [35]. That is fairly good and clinically accurate and acceptable, but extreme deviations, for any reason, can never be completely excluded. The main problem with a large deviation is that it might result in the apex being only partially removed (Fig. 8.46). Therefore, we recommend that the site should always be inspected under magnification to see if the entire apex has been removed. For this reason, this approach should be renamed as guided endodontic microsurgery.

Fig. 8.45 Control X-ray of a guided endodontic procedure with some residual bioceramic (see text)

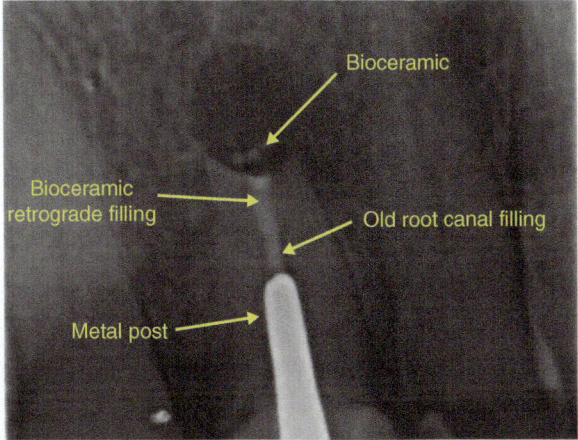

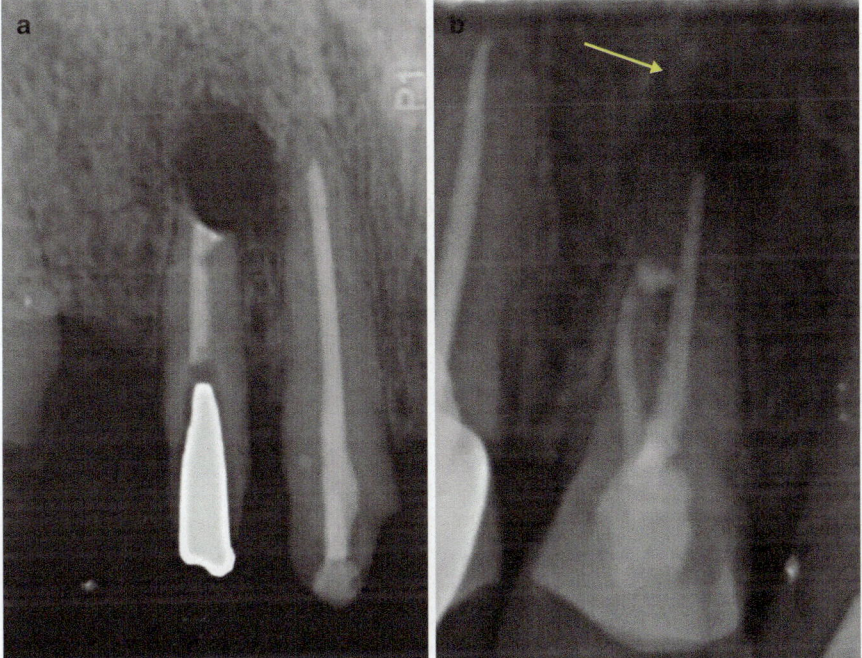

Fig. 8.46 Complications. (**a**) Angular deviation led to asymmetric apex removal, and the trephine almost damaged the neighboring root; (**b**) Palatal overpenetration. The mark of the trephine is clearly visible in the palatal cortical (arrow)

Another issue is the overpenetration, which can be overcome by use of trephines with stop.

Trephine fracture (Fig. 8.47) has been experienced only in in vitro studies, but the experience teaches us that this a real possibility. In fact, we do not know how durable a trephine is when used for this indication. Therefore, we

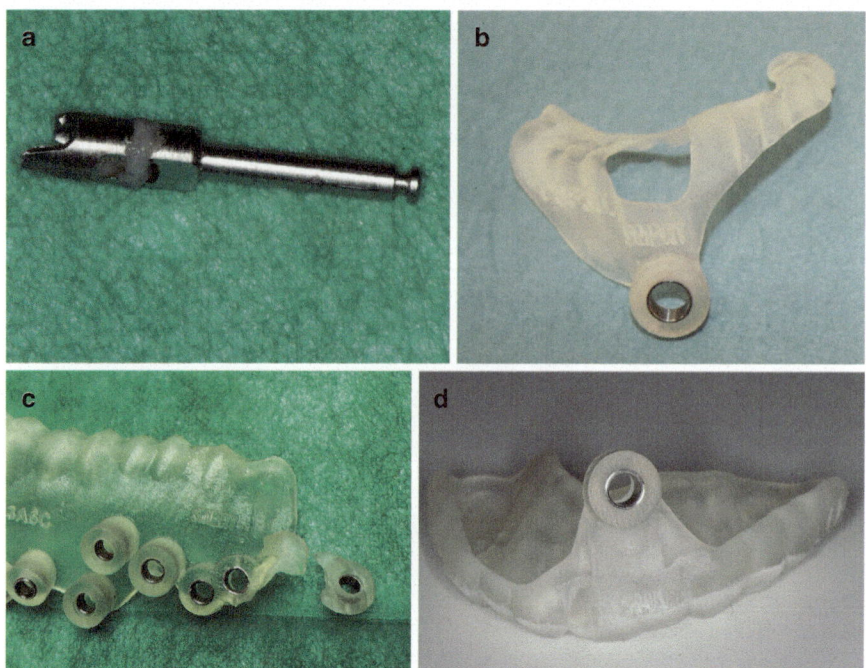

Fig. 8.47 Complications related to the applied materials and design. (**a**) A broken bone trephine from an in vitro study in porcine jaw. The rest of the instrument got stuck in the bone. (**b**). Bad guide design. The body of the template is not bulky enough, it is further weakened by the missing piece, and a weak, flexible piece of material is supposed to keep the sleeve housing stable during the surgery. Such a design is not stable enough and fractures easily. (**c**) Fracture due to bad design from an in vitro study. Guide fracture belongs to the most frequently seen complications. (**d**) Good design: the body is bulky, provides support all around, and the sleeve housing has a firm triangular support with a wide base

recommend that the surface of these instruments should be carefully inspected before each use for cracks and/or damage.

Finally, this approach is quite novel and reliable data on accuracy, complication rates, and long-term success are lacking. Furthermore, the endodontic indication is not an option in any major computer-assisted guide production system at this point. Naturally, for this to change, more researches are needed in this direction. Certainly, this approach is a valid and reliable option for everyday use.

Acknowledgments The author would like to express his gratitude to Dr. Gábor Braunitzer, chief researcher at dicomLAB Dental, for his critical comments on the chapter. The author is indebted to Dr. Tekla Sáry for the artistic illustrations. The author expresses his gratitude to Dr. Márk Fráter for his inspiration. This chapter would not have been possible without the support and love of my wife, Réka Antal-Szabó, and my children, Dávid, Bence, and Flóra.

References

1. Block RM, Bushell A, Grossman LI, Langeland K. Endodontic surgical retreatment--a clinical and histopathologic study. J Endod. 1979;5(4):101–15.
2. Molven O, Halse A, Grung B. Surgical management of endodontic failures: indications and treatment results. Int Dent J. 1991;41(1):33–42.
3. Rahbaran S, Gilthrope MS, Harrison SD, Gulabivala K. Comparison of clinical outcome of periapical surgery in endodontics and oral surgery units of a teaching dental hospital: a retrospective study. Oral Surg Oral Med Oral Pathol. 2001;91:700–9.
4. Christiansen R, Kirkevang LL, Hørsted-Bindslev P, Wenzel A. Randomized clinical trial of root-end resection followed by root-end filling with mineral trioxide aggregate or smoothing of the orthograde gutta-percha root filling–1-year follow-up. Int Endod J. 2009;42:105–14.
5. Tsesis I, Rosen E, Schwartz-Arad D, Fuss Z. Retrospective evaluation of surgical endodontic treatment: traditional versus modern technique. J Endod. 2006;32:412–6.
6. Kim E, Song JS, Jung IY, Lee SJ, Kim S. Prospective clinical study evaluating endodontic microsurgery outcomes for cases with lesions of endodontic origin compared with cases with lesions of combined periodontal-endodontic origin. J Endod. 2008;34:546–51.
7. Taschieri S, Del Fabbro M, Testori T, Weinstein R. Microscope versus endoscope in root-end management: a randomized controlled study. Int J Oral Maxillofac Surg. 2008;37:1022–6.
8. Tortorici S, Difalco P, Caradonna L, Tetè S. Traditional endodontic surgery versus modern technique: a 5-year controlled clinical trial. J Craniofac Surg. 2014;25(3):804–7. https://doi.org/10.1097/SCS.0000000000000398.
9. Gilheany PA, Figdor D, Tyas MJ. Apical dentin permeability and microleakage associated with root end resection and retrograde filling. J Endod. 1994;20(1):22–6.
10. Frater M, Antal M, Braunitzer G, Joob-Fancsaly A, Nagy K. An update on endodontic microsurgery – a literature review. FogorvSz. 2017;2:43–8.
11. Kim S, Kratchman S. Modern endodontic surgery concepts and practice: a review. J Endod. 2006;32:601–23.
12. vonArx T, Hänni S, Jensen SS. Correlation of bone defect dimensions with healing outcome one year after apical surgery. J Endod. 2007;33:1044–8.
13. Anderson J, Wealleans J, Ray J. Endodontic applications of 3D printing. Int Endod J. 2018;51(9):1005–18. https://doi.org/10.1111/iej.12917. Review.
14. Tsesis I, Rosen E, Taschieri S, Telishevsky Strauss Y, Ceresoli V, Del Fabbro M. Outcomes of surgical endodontic treatment performed by a modern technique: an updated meta-analysis of the literature. J Endod. 2013;39:332–9.
15. European Society of Endodontology, Patel S, Durack C, Abella F, Roig M, Shemesh H, Lambrechts P, Lemberg K. European Society of Endodontology position statement: the use of CBCT in endodontics. Int Endod J. 2014;47(6):502–4.
16. Pinsky HM, Champleboux G, Sarment DP. Periapical surgery using CAD/CAM guidance: preclinical results. J Endod. 2007;33:148.
17. Hawkins TK, Wealleans JA, Pratt AM, Ray JJ. Targeted endodontic microsurgery and endodontic microsurgery: a surgical simulation comparison. Int Endod J. 2020;53(5):715–22. https://doi.org/10.1111/iej.13243.
18. Liu Y, Liao W, Jin G, Yang Q, Peng W. Additive manufacturing and digital design assisted precise apicoectomy: a case study. Rapid Prototyp J. 2014;20(1):33–40. https://doi.org/10.1108/RPJ-06-2012-0056.
19. Patel S, Aldowaisan A, Dawood A. A novel method for soft tissue retraction during periapical surgery using 3D technology: a case report. Int Endod J. 2017;50(8):813–22. https://doi.org/10.1111/iej.12701.
20. Strbac GD, Schnappauf A, Giannis K, Moritz A, Ulm C. Guided modern endodontic surgery: a novel approach for guided osteotomy and root resection. J Endod. 2017;43:496.

21. Giacomino CM, Ray JJ, Wealleans JA. Targeted endodontic microsurgery: a novel approach to anatomically challenging scenarios using 3-dimensional-printed guides and trephine burs-a report of 3 cases. J Endod. 2018;44:671.
22. Ahn SY, Kim NH, Kim S, Karabucak B, Kim E. Computer-aided design/computer-aided manufacturing-guided endodontic surgery: guided osteotomy and apex localization in a mandibular molar with a thick buccal bone plate. J Endod. 2018;44(4):665–70. https://doi. org/10.1016/j.joen.2017.12.009.
23. Ye S, Zhao S, Wang W, Jiang Q, Yang X. A novel method for periapical microsurgery with the aid of 3D technology: a case report. BMC Oral Health. 2018;18(1):85.
24. Antal M, Nagy E, Braunitzer G, Fráter M, Piffkó J. Accuracy and clinical safety of guided root end resection with a trephine: a case series. Head Face Med. 2019;15(1):30. https://doi. org/10.1186/s13005-019-0214-8.
25. Antal M, Nagy E, Sanyó L, Braunitzer G. Digitally planned root end surgery with static guide and custom trephine burs: a case report. Int J Med Robot. 2020;16:e2115. https://doi. org/10.1002/rcs.2115.
26. Fan Y, Glickman GN, Umorin M, Nair MK, Jalali P. A novel prefabricated grid for guided endodontic microsurgery. J Endod. 2019;45(5):606–10. https://doi.org/10.1016/j. joen.2019.01.015.
27. Kim S, Rethnam S. Hemostasis in endodontic microsurgery. Dent Clin N Am. 1997;41(3):499–511.
28. Plotino G, Pameijer CH, Grande NM, Somma F. Ultrasonics in endodontics: a review of the literature. J Endod. 2007;33(2):81–95. Review.
29. Kim S, Kratchman S. Modern endodontic surgery concepts and practice: a review. J Endod. 2006;32(7):601–23. Review.
30. Kim S, Kratchman S, Karabucak B, Kohli M, Setzer F. Microsurgery in endodontics. 1st ed. New York, NY: John Wiley & Sons, Inc.; 2018. p. 61.
31. Abusrewil SM, McLean W, Scott JA. The use of Bioceramics as root-end filling materials in periradicular surgery: a literature review. Saudi Dent J. 2018;30(4):273–82. https://doi. org/10.1016/j.sdentj.2018.07.004. Review.
32. Nair U, Ghattas S, Saber M, Natera M, Walker C, Pileggi R. A comparative evaluation of the sealing ability of 2 root-end filling materials: an in vitro leakage study using enterococcus faecalis. Oral Surg Oral Med Oral Pathol Oral Radiol Endod. 2011;112(2):e74–7. https://doi. org/10.1016/j.tripleo.2011.01.030.
33. Bandi M, Mallineni SK, Nuvvula S. Clinical applications of ferric sulfate in dentistry: a narrative review. J Conserv Dent. 2017;20(4):278–81. https://doi.org/10.4103/JCD. JCD_259_16. Review.
34. Molven O, Halse A, Grung B. Observer strategy and the radiographic classification of healing after endodontic surgery. Int J Oral Maxillofac Surg. 1987;16:432–9.
35. Tahmaseb A, Wu V, Wismeijer D, Coucke W, Evans C. The accuracy of static computer-aided implant surgery: a systematic review and meta-analysis. Clin Oral Implants Res. 2018;29(Suppl 16):416.

Dynamic Navigation in Endodontics

Niraj Kinariwala, Mark Adam Antal,
and Ramóna Kiscsatári

In many different areas of medicine, there is an increasing tendency of using computer navigated surgical, and therapeutic methods in the daily practice. In dentistry, these technologies were first adopted in dental implant surgery. The technology originating from implantology has reached other areas of dentistry, in particular, endodontics. Its potential uses include endodontic procedures such as trephination and root canal localization.

What Is Dynamic Navigation?
Dynamic navigation is a promising technology designed to guide the placement of drills/implants in real time by a computer. It is based on information generated from the patient's computed tomography (CT). In dentistry, dynamic navigated surgery is placement of drill or implant, using real-time computer navigated system, based on the data generated from the patients' cone-beam computed tomography (CBCT).

N. Kinariwala (✉)
Karnavati School of Dentistry, Karnavati University, Gandhinagar, Gujarat, India
e-mail: niraj@ksd.ac.in

M. A. Antal
Department of Operative and Esthetic Dentistry, Faculty of Dentistry, University of Szeged, Szeged, Hungary
e-mail: antal.mark@szte.hu

R. Kiscsatári
Department of Oral- and Maxillofacial Surgery, Faculty of Medicine, University of Szeged, Szeged, Hungary

© Springer Nature Switzerland AG 2021
N. Kinariwala, L. Samaranayake (eds.), *Guided Endodontics*,
https://doi.org/10.1007/978-3-030-55281-7_9

9.1 Principles of Dynamic Navigation

Dynamic navigation system is in some way the same as a commonly used navigation system in a car. Both attempt to localize or determine a position in space in the context of its surroundings. The actual localization technology, however, differs as surgical navigation does not use triangulation like a global positioning system with the help of several geostationary satellites. Modern dynamic surgical navigation systems use a stereoscopic camera, with or without, emitting infrared light, which can determine a 3D position of prominent structures, like reflective marker spheres. This allows for real-time tracking of the marker spheres.

For the basic setup, the requirements are a stereoscopic camera, a computer platform with screen, and the respective navigation software. During the surgery, the marker spheres are attached to the patient and at surgical instruments (using reference arrays) to enable an exact localization in space and, hence, navigation in the operating room (OR).

With each reference array comprising of at least three marker spheres, the computer can calculate the position and orientation of each instrument. A correct localization and virtual display of the instrument on the computer screen is ensured by firmly attaching a reference array to the patient, for example, in the bone or via a head clamp. Movements of the camera intraoperatively are possible, because only the relative position of the tracked instruments to the tracked patient reference is relevant.

Dynamic navigation is usually "image based:" it requires patient's radiographic data for navigation. To understand the navigation process, there are three terminologies we need to know.

1. Image acquisition: It means obtaining patient's radiographic data. CBCT imaging data (DICOM file) is used for navigation in dental treatments.
2. Planning: Before surgery, objects and areas of interest may be planned within the images and hence enrich the data sets.
3. Registration: Before the first drill is used, the preoperative image data need to be matched to the current patient position via a registration process. This is the process to establish a relation between the "real" co-ordinate system as defined by the patient's reference array and the "virtual" co-ordinate system of the imaging data. Registration can be paired point-based or use surface matching routines. It is also known as Tracing or trace registration. The surgeon, then, virtually sees both the current situation and the imaging datasets overlapped. After proper registration process, dynamic navigated treatment can be initiated.

Modern orthopedic navigation systems are "model based" and work almost exclusively without information from external image sources. The patients do not need to be exposed to additional radiation, for example, through CT or X-ray. Instead the navigation software calculates an individual model of the patients' anatomy based on defined landmarks on the bone, which are acquired using a navigated instrument (registration). After an optional planning on the model (planning, e.g., virtual orientation and placement of the joint implant), the actual procedure follows where the surgeon gets supported by relevant information added through the

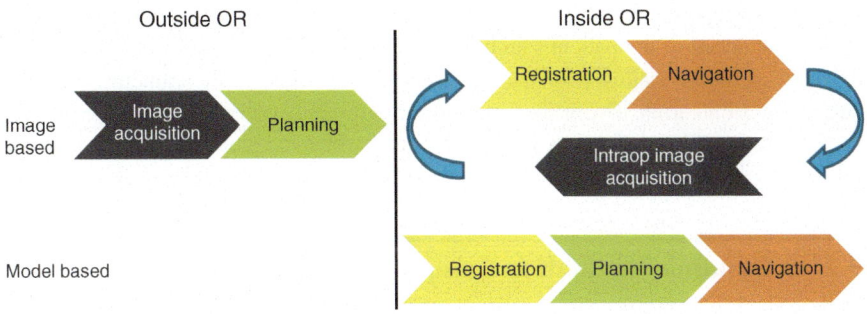

Fig. 9.1 Basic workflows of image-based and model-based navigation. Image-based navigation requires preoperative images, which need to be registered to the patient setup, typically employed for cranial or spinal surgery. Model-based navigation requires no imaging data and the process of registration matches the patient's anatomy to a virtual model, typically employed for orthopedic surgery. *OR* operating room. (Courtesy: Uli Mezger, Claudia Jendrewski)

navigation system (navigation). Figure 9.1 shows workflow of image-based and model-based navigation.

Each surgical discipline and each individual hospital and surgeon have different navigation requirements for their workflow, amount of flexibility, and needed functionality. A wide variety of navigation platforms are available to accommodate all surgical needs: The systems can be installed permanently mounted at the OR ceiling, require minimal OR footprint, or minimize cable clutter and be mobile platforms to be used in several ORs at different times or even be carried around between hospitals for maximum flexibility.

In dentistry, implant positions and root canal locations can be designed and correlated with reference points with preoperative CBCT data and the help of computer software programs. Dynamic navigation system is empowered by a motion tracking technology, which tracks the dental drill and patient position throughout the procedures by integrating surgical instruments, three-dimensional images, and optical positioning devices [1].

In this improved setup, an optical-motion-tracking system provides feedback during surgery, and therefore, the designed information is linked to the real-time clinical situation and the equipments used for the intervention. In summary, it facilitates the traceability of instrument position.

According to some publications, this method reduces the number of surgery-related errors and, considering the outcome of interventions, it is more accurate than manual (or freehand) placement [2]. Based on the observations of Bun San Chong et al. [3], the critical points of implant surgery, such as injury of critical anatomical structures (e.g., nerve canal, position of the adjacent tooth), can be minimized. This method also provides flexibility for the person performing the surgery, as in case of unexpected need of modifications, these can be done any time during the intervention.

The current dynamic navigation systems display the images on the monitor using optical technologies to track the patient and the handpiece. The optical systems use either active or passive tracking arrays. Active system arrays emit light, which is tracked by the stereocameras. Passive systems use tracking systems in which the light emitted from a light source is reflected back to the stereocameras.

A passive optical dynamic navigation system requires the use of fiducial markers securely attached to the patient's arch during CBCT scanning. The device attached to the fiducial markers allows for the registration of the arch to the cameras, with the attachment of an array. The array is positioned extraorally, which contains the fiducial markers. The implant handpiece also has an array, which in combination with the clip's fiducial markers, allows for triangulation, leading to accurate navigation [4].

9.2 Dynamic Navigation Components and Workflow

9.2.1 Components

The basic components of any dynamic navigation systems are as follows:

- Handpiece attachment
- Patient jaw attachment
- The system cart, which consists of the cameras, a computer with a navigation software
- Natural or fiducial markers that are used during the radiological scan as reference points for the instrument registration (Optional)

9.2.2 Workflow of Dynamic Navigation

To guide the drilling, navigation system must precisely map the drill tip to the CT image of the jaw used for planning the implantation. Sensors are attached on the body of the handpiece and the extraoral clip attached to the fiducial markers. It achieves this in three steps, performed in the following order:

1. Trace Registration: CBCT images are matched with the teeth, through the Jaw Tracker or Head Tracker mounted on the patient, by registering the CBCT scan to the teeth and/or bone. For trace registration, a calibrated tracer (like a stylus pen or ball burnisher) tracked by the Micron Tracker camera is slid along the tooth surface, in brushing motion, while the system samples point along its path. The collected "cloud of points" is then automatically matched in the best possible way with the outer surface of the teeth in the CBCT scan. Minimum 3 and maximum 6 teeth can be traced for better accuracy. An accuracy check should be performed in all 3 directions (anteroposterior, laterolateral, and occlusogingival) to verify registration accuracy in all 3 axes.
2. Calibration: Mapping the drill tip to the DrillTag. The drilling axis calibration is done once, prior to the start of the operation by placing the handpiece chuck over a pin in the JawTag. After each drill change, the drill tip location is calibrated by touching a dimple on the calibrator.
3. Tracking: Mapping the DrillTag (Handpiece attachment) to the JawTag (Jaw attachement). This is dynamic and is done throughout the operation by the optical tracking system (Fig. 9.2). Continuous tracking is very important to achieve

Fig. 9.2 Workflow for Nivident dynamic navigation system, which includes, registration, calibration and tracking

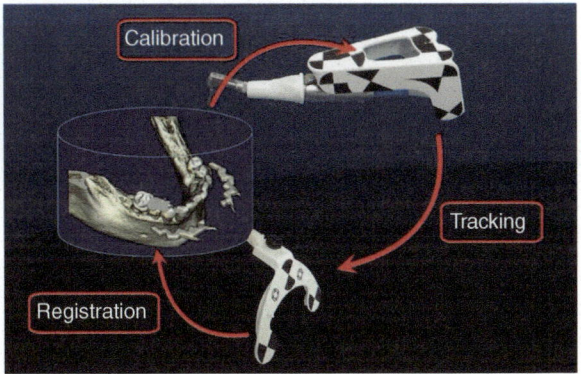

planned treatment outcomes. Tracking camera should be placed at position to provide broad operating field view during the treatment. Extension arm of navigation device may help to achieve broad view of operating field.

9.2.2.1 Step-by-Step Workflow

1. Take a CBCT scan of the entire arch with high resolution and small field of view (FOV). Import scan data to dynamic navigation system.
2. Plan endodontic treatment on CBCT file in the dynamic navigation software. Plan virtual drill path for non surgical treatment. Keep diameter of vitual path as minimal as possible (not more than 1.0 mm). For endodontic microsurgery, plan ostoeomy site and size. Level and angulation of root end resection can also be planned, simultaneously.
3. Install the patient tracker (JawTracker or HeadTracker). It should be placed within range of camera tracking system. Endodontic microscope should be used carefully to avoid any errors during use of dynamic navigation.
4. Register the CBCT scan to the patient using Trace registration in one of the following ways: (i) Tracing directly on the CBCT scan, (ii) Using an intra-oral scan superimposed or matched with the CBCT scan, (iii) Using the NaviBite (when the tooth and its neighbouring teeth have full coverage metallic restorations).
5. The patient tracker (JawTracker) placement and tracing should be completed prior to placement of the rubber dam. Rubber dam isolation should be performed and rubber dam and clamp should not exert any force on the patient tracker.
6. Calibrate handpiece (slow-speed, high-speed or piezoelectric handpiece) and bur (drill) with calibrator. Registration accuracy should be evaluated before drilling.
7. During drilling, follow the planned path and complete the treatment. If multiple drills have to be used, calibrate each drill before using it intraorally and perform accuracy check everytime.
8. For endodontic microsurgery, similar tracing and calibration has to be performed. Calibrate bone saw before use and also calibrate its dimensions for better accuracy. Usually, osteotomy and root-end resection are performed simultaneously with a precise bone saw cut. If accuracy check results are poor, re-trace the CBCT and perform the treatment.

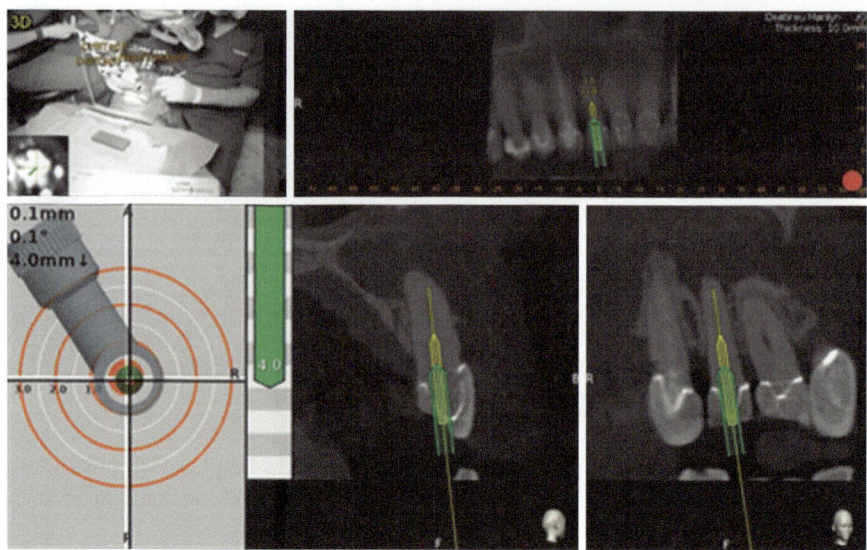

Fig. 9.3 Real-time navigation with dynamic navigation in nonsurgical endodontic treatment. Yellow color indicates planning. Green color indicates real-time navigation. (Courtesy: Dr. Yosef Nahmias)

9.3 Dynamic Navigation in Nonsurgical Endodontic Treatments

Several rules have been laid down for the correct implementation of nonsurgical endodontic treatments. In line with modern endodontic requirements, it should be kept in mind in every situation that during an intervention, as little as possible tooth material should be sacrificed. This is also called minimally invasive approach. The borders of the cavity as well as the access opening and orifice should be prepared with the most conservative method. Unfortunately, in real clinical situations, the person performing the surgery has to deal with several problems. Often, removal of excessive tooth material is required for successful exploration of a severely stenotic, calcified canal. However, this significantly weakens tooth tissue, threatens structural integrity, and carries the risk of perforation.

Therefore, in everyday practice, each effort, which facilitates the work of the person performing the surgery (i.e., makes preparation of a small cavity possible), decreases iatrogenic harm, preserves structural integrity, while at the same time meets all the expected access requirements.

To date, endodontists preferred static navigation. Relatively few publications are available concerning dynamic navigation [3, 5].

After taking CBCT of the patient, import the DICOM files to the Navident software and proceed to virtual drill path planning. Once registration and calibration are done, place the rubber dam and access into the tooth with a small diamond bur (Figs. 9.3 and 9.4). This technology allows smaller and more accurate access opening preserving pericervical dentin.

Fig. 9.4 This is the actual view the operator follows during active dynamic navigation. The operator aligns the head of the hand piece and the tip of the bur into the center circle ("Bulls eye"). The main center circle has a diameter of 1.0 mm. Each orange circle is separated by 1 mm orange intervals. The green bar on the right shows the distance (in millimeter) left to drill to the pointed tip of the planned trajectory (in yellow). Here, we are 4 mm away from the predetermined target. (Courtesy: Dr. Yosef Nahmias)

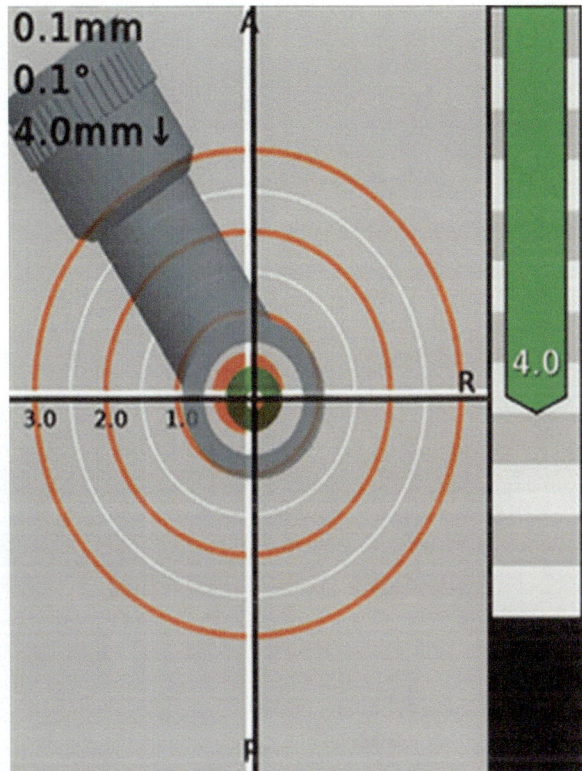

9.4 Dynamic Navigation in Surgical Endodontics

Dynamic navigation contributes to continuous development in the field of endodontic surgery. To date, only one case report is available in the literature, where Navident dynamic navigation system was used. In this case, dynamic navigation system made exact root apex localization and accurate apicoectomy possible in a minimally invasive manner. Improvement of targeted surgical navigation systems facilitates surgical maneuvers and decreases the risk of iatrogenic harm.

Gambarini et al. [6] presented dynamic navigation through the surgery of a 34-year-old patient. The patient refused removal of a crown on tooth 12. His tooth was sensitive to percussion, and periapical rarefaction was seen. His treating surgeon decided to perform root-end resection (Figs. 9.5 and 9.6). CBCT image made the accurate, step-by-step planning of the surgical intervention possible. The big advantage of the system is that during the operation, steps can be modified. The person performing the surgery can accurately check and correct any errors on the spot, since the instruments are calibrated and strictly observed during surgery. One of the challenges of root-end resection is to distinguish root apex from the surrounding bone. With the help of navigation, this problem can easily be solved with

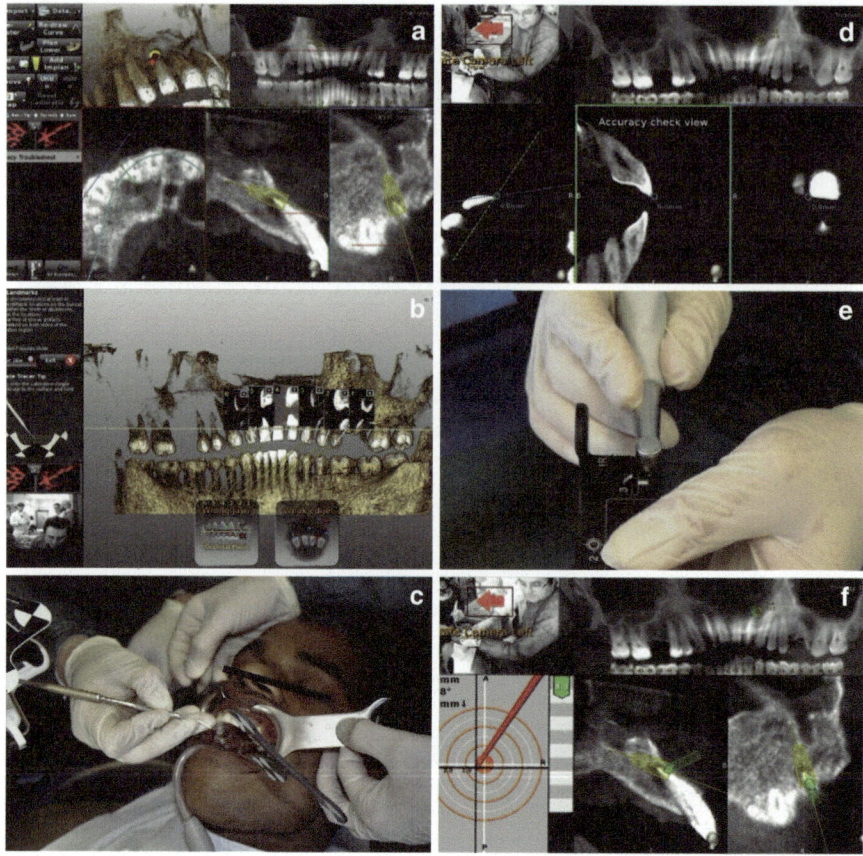

Fig. 9.5 (**a**) Treatment planning using patient's previous CBCT scan. (**b**) Tracing: the system cali-bration phase is performed by selecting six different points on software reconstructions. (**c**) A fixed support is mounted on the patient's mouth, which can be recognized by the Navident's cameras, after which the six preselected points are traced using a tool that presents a support that can be recognized by the Navident to create matching between the CBCT scan and the patient's jaw. (**d**) Tracing is completed by an accuracy check view. (**e**) Before use, the handpiece and burs must be calibrated. (**f**) Drilling under dynamic guidance: the direction and the angulation of the bur during the surgical procedure can be checked on three different CBCT views. (Courtesy: Gambarini et al., License no: 4797821243951)

minimum invasive approach. Another benefit of microsurgery is the minimization and eventual elimination of inclination of root end resection.

Endodontic surgical interventions performed with dynamic navigation are very forward-looking, as several sources of error such as radical osteotomy, inaccuracy of localization, and injury of critical anatomical structures can be eliminated. In addition to advance planning, errors detected during surgery can immediately be addressed. The posture of the person performing the surgery also improves as he/she concentrates on the display, and the learning curve is fast [6].

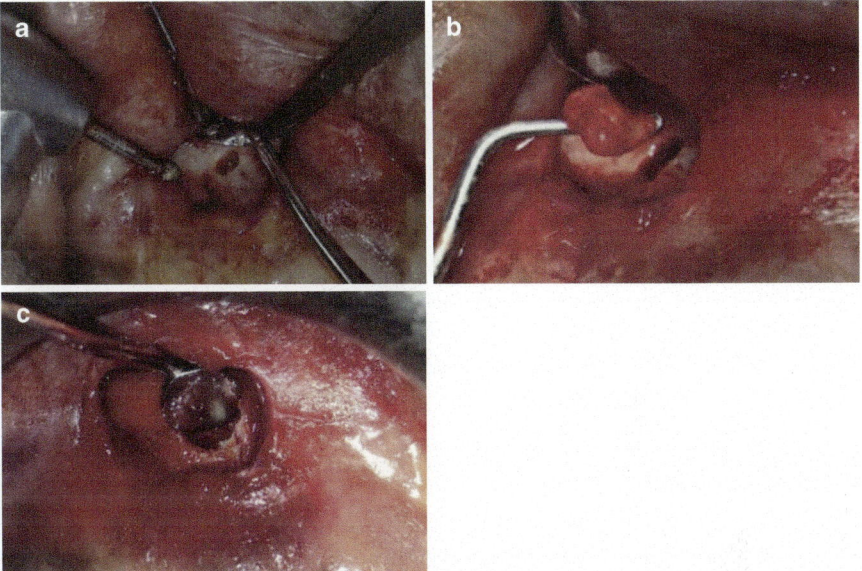

Fig. 9.6 (**a**) Minimally invasive surgical access with diameter of 3 mm was possible by the use of the dynamic navigation surgery system using a round surgical bur mounted on a high-speed hand-piece under 0.9% Nacl spray irrigation and visually checked on the Navident screen. (**b**) The removal of the lesion was performed very easily because of the precise access cavity. (**c**) The retrograde space was created using an ultrasonic tip for 3 mm in length; the minimal access cavity and the retrograde plug could be appreciated. (License no: 4797821243951)

9.5 Advantages and Limitations

The success of any surgery is dependent on the preoperative planning and preparation, which allow us to predict any difficulties that may arise during the surgery and may boost the surgeon's confidence. Dynamic navigation system forces the surgeon to plan the surgery and placement of a virtual implant in terms of angulation, depth, location, size, and depth, thus allowing for a well-planned surgery. Placement of implant using dynamic navigation is more accurate compared with implant placement with free-hand approach [7, 8].

9.5.1 Advantages of Dynamic Navigation System

1. CT scanning, planning, and surgery in a single appointment (when a CBCT is available on site)
2. Reduced harm to the patient: minimally invasive surgery, leading to reduced patient discomfort, reduced risk of infection, and faster recovery
3. Unintentional iatrogenic damage to nearby anatomical structures

4. Increased safety and predictability due to ability to verify guidance accuracy at any time
5. Simpler and faster planning (no plaster models, wax-ups, and guide fabrication)
6. Ability to view and modify the plan during the surgery, for example, to accommodate tactile feedback or unexpected complications
7. Cost-effective. (Lower per-procedure costs)
8. Improved irrigation, reducing risk of bone damage due to overheating
9. No need of specialized equipments. Works with any implant or drill system
10. Without sleeves, guidance is provided even when interocclusal or interdental space is limited
11. Elimination of guidance failures due to fractured or badly fitting guides
12. Improved ergonomics

9.5.2   Limitations

One of the main difficulties with the dynamic navigation system is the high cost of the navigation system, its updates, and maintenance of the system, which might not be financially feasible for the surgeon. Every system has its own planning software; thus, one might not be able to use any other advanced software. Adequate learning is expected from the clinician as a learning curve is associated with it [9].

References

1. Bordin TB, Refahi P, Karimbux N, et al. Dynamic navigation in implant dentistry. Trends in clinical periodontology and implant dentistry. http://www.trendsperioimplantresourcecenter. com/content/dynamic-navigation-implant-dentistry.
2. Block MS, Emery RW, Cullum DR, Sheikh A. Implant placement is more accurate using dynamic navigation. J Oral Maxillofac Surg. 2017;75(7):1377–86. https://doi.org/10.1016/j. joms.2017.02.026. PubMed PMID: 28384461.
3. Chong BS, Dhesi M, Makdissi J. Computer-aided dynamic navigation: a novel method for guided endodontics. Quintessence Int. 2019;50(3):196–202. https://doi.org/10.3290/j. qi.a41921.
4. Block MS, Emery RW. Static or dynamic navigation for implant placement—choosing the method of guidance. J Oral Maxillofac Surg. 2016;74(2):269–77.
5. Sukegawa S, Kanno T, Shibata A, Matsumoto K, Sukegawa-Takahashi Y, Sakaida K, Furuki Y. Use of an intraoperative navigation system for retrieving a broken dental instrument in the mandible: a case report. J Med Case Rep. 2017;11(1):14. https://doi.org/10.1186/ s13256-016-1182-2. PubMed PMID: 28088226; PubMed Central PMCID: PMC5237551.
6. Gambarini G, Galli M, Stefanelli LV, Di Nardo D, Morese A, Seracchiani M, De Angelis F, Di Carlo S, Testarelli L. Endodontic microsurgery using dynamic navigation system: a case report. J Endod. 2019;45:1397. https://doi.org/10.1016/j.joen.2019.07.010. pii: S0099-2399(19)30544-8. PubMed PMID: 31515047.
7. Block MS, Emery RW, Cullum DR, Sheikh A. Implant placement is more accurate using dynamic navigation. J Oral Maxillofac Surg. 2017;75(7):1377–86.
8. Block MS, Emery RW, Lank K, Ryan J. Implant placement accuracy using dynamic navigation. Int J Oral Maxillofac Implants. 2017;32(1):92.
9. Sun TM, Lan TH, Pan CY, Lee HE. Dental implant navigation system guide the surgery future. Kaohsiung J Med Sci. 2018;34(1):56–64.

Future Trends of 3D Guidance in Dentistry

10

Niraj Kinariwala, Lakshman Samaranayake,
Gunpreet Oberoi, and Hermann Agis

10.1 3D Printing in Autotransplantation

Use of 3D-printed template makes the procedure faster, predictable, and more convenient. Autotransplantation is the transplantation of organs, tissues, or even particular proteins from one part of the body to another in the same person (Word "auto" means "self" in Greek). It is an extremely successful, but underrated, treatment form, which saves significant time and cost compared to implants. From the patient's perspective, the dentition is preserved using a natural tooth rather than a mechanical prosthesis. The dental practitioner should definitely have the knowledge to recommend and perform this procedure to the appropriate patient.

Hard tissue transplantation such as teeth requires a procedure for contouring the recipient bone in order for the donor tooth to sit properly in the recipient site. The tooth root is covered with a thin layer of connective tissue, which is known as the periodontal ligament. The presence of intact and viable periodontal ligament cells on the root surface of a donor tooth is most important for the healing of transplanted teeth [1]. Several factors affecting the periodontal ligament healing include the extraoral time of the donor tooth, the storage method until transplant, surgical trauma, and contamination of the root surface and/or root canal. Among those, the extraoral time of the donor tooth prior to transplantation has the most significant

N. Kinariwala (✉)
Karnavati School of Dentistry, Karnavati University, Gandhinagar, Gujarat, India
e-mail: niraj@ksd.ac.in

L. Samaranayake
Faculty of Dentistry, University of Hong Kong, Hong Kong, China
e-mail: lakshman@hku.hk

G. Oberoi · H. Agis
Department of Conservative Dentistry and Periodontology, University Clinic of Dentistry,
Medical University of Vienna, Vienna, Austria
e-mail: gunpreet.oberoi@meduniwien.ac.at; hermann.agis@meduniwien.ac.at

© Springer Nature Switzerland AG 2021
N. Kinariwala, L. Samaranayake (eds.), *Guided Endodontics*,
https://doi.org/10.1007/978-3-030-55281-7_10

effect on the success rate [2]. In clinics, it is frequently found that the extended extraoral time of the donor tooth causes severe root resorption.

Another important factor in tooth transplantation is the distance between the recipient bone tissue and the root surface of the transplanted tooth. Optimal contact with the recipient site can improve the level of blood supply and nutrients to the periodontal ligament cells, which can improve the success rate of the tooth transplantation [3, 4].

The major problem in tooth transplantation is how to precisely contour the recipient alveolar bone to fit the donor tooth in such a limited time so as to prevent the cell death of the root surface. Previously, most of the donor teeth were extracted first, and then used as templates for contouring of the recipient bone, which involved a process of trial and error for fitting. Multiple insertions of the extracted donor tooth in a prepared socket would not only result in an extended extraoral time but damage the root cells of the donor tooth, which can lead to failure. If a duplicated tooth model that has exactly the same shape and size as the donor tooth can be obtained, the recipient bone cavity can be prepared using this model tooth prior to extraction, which can avoid the complications arising from multiple trials of real donor tooth.

Rapid prototyping technology, better known as 3-dimensional (3D) printing, is widely used for preoperative planning, procedure rehearsal, and custom prosthetic design in clinical practice as well as an educational tool for teaching and to enhance communication between the patient and doctor.

The computer-aided rapid prototyping (CARP) technique was first introduced in mechanical engineering and has been used mainly to pre-evaluate the procedures for assembling and manufacturing designed products ahead of actual production. The clinical application of a computer-aided rapid prototyping (CARP) model for autotransplantation was first introduced in 2001 using 3D computed tomographic (CT) image acquisition followed by fabrication of a 3D printing copy model [5]. This technique allowed surgeons to simulate the contour of the recipient bone using the actual-sized CARP models of donor teeth and recipient alveolar bones preoperatively. Using CARP models for autotransplantation has an advantage of minimized extra-alveolar time and trauma to the donor tooth, thereby increasing the success rate of the surgery [6]. The survival rates for the conventional autotransplantation technique using teeth with mature roots vary from 59% to 81% at 4 years and 59.6% at 10 years [7–9]. CARP models improve survival rates for teeth with mature roots to 88.1% and 68.2% at 3 years and 12 years, respectively [6]. This improvement is more pronounced when donor teeth with immature roots are used [10].

Figures 10.1, 10.2, and 10.3 describe a case report using a CARP model and a computer-aided design (CAD) program for autotransplantation of an immature third molar [11].

A compromised left mandibular second molar (#18) was extracted and replaced by autotransplantation using an immature left mandibular third molar (#17). In order to minimize the surgical time and injury to the donor tooth, a virtual 3-dimensional (3D) rehearsal surgery was planned. Cone-beam computed tomographic images were taken to fabricate the 3D printing CARP model of the donor tooth and tentative extraction socket. Subsequently, both CARP models were scanned with an intraoral scanner (CEREC Omnicam; Dentsply Sirona, Bensheim, Germany) followed by superimposition and virtual simulation of osteotomy preparation of the recipient alveolus using the CAD analysis program (Fig. 10.2). During the surgery, the extraction socket was precisely prepared according to the

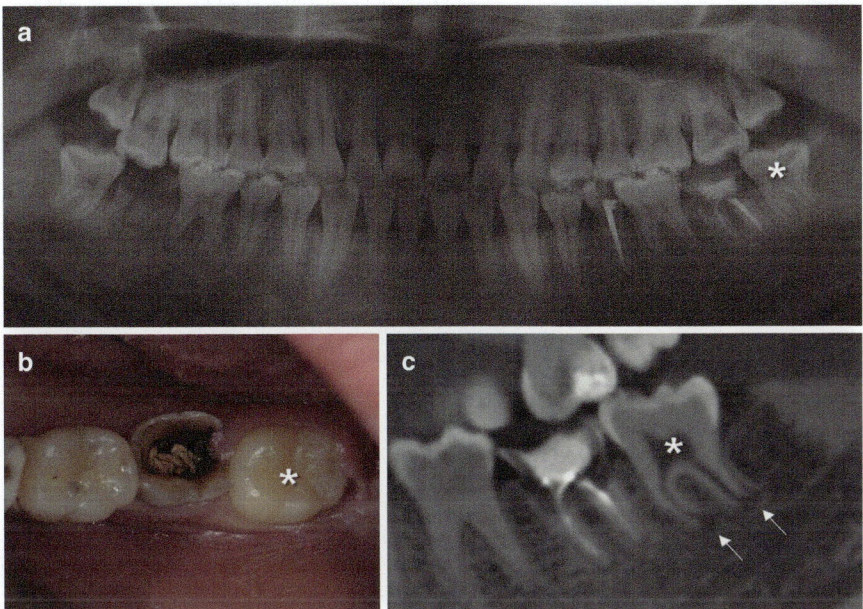

Fig. 10.1 Preoperative examination. (**a**) A panoramic radiograph and (**b**) a clinical photograph showing tooth #18, which received root canal treatment for extensive caries, and tooth #17 with sound appearance and an immature root (asterisk). (**c**) CBCT image showing the difference in root morphology of tooth #17 (asterisk) and #18 and the divergent apex of tooth #17 (arrows). (Courtesy: Oh S Et al. License no: 4793540387916)

predetermined location and dimensions via virtual simulation rehearsal surgery using CAD analysis. The donor tooth was atraumatically transplanted into the prepared socket. The follow-up examination revealed that the root developed with a normal periodontal ligament and lamina dura (Fig. 10.3). Virtual simulation using a 3D printing CARP model and a CAD program could be clinically useful in autotransplantation of an immature third molar by ensuring an atraumatic and predictable surgery. Many clinicians and researchers have started adopting dynamic navigation technology for predictable autotransplantation treatments. Combining 3d printing and dynamic navigation proposes exciting treatment strategies for cases of autotransplantation.

10.2   Bioprinting

3D printing has become a promising technology allowing the design of anatomically correctly designed scaffolds, which can be populated with cells. These cells include bone marrow stem cells, adipose tissue stem cells (ATSCs), cells from oral tissues, and many more (Fig. 10.4). Stem cells can also be isolated from oral tissues (Table 10.1). These cells include dental pulp stem cells (DPSCs), stem cells from human exfoliated deciduous teeth (SHEDs), immature dental pulp stem cells (IDPSCs), stem cells from apical papilla (SCAPs), periodontal ligament stem cells (PDLSCs), gingiva stem cells (GSCs), and dental follicle stem cells (DFSCs) (Table 10.2).

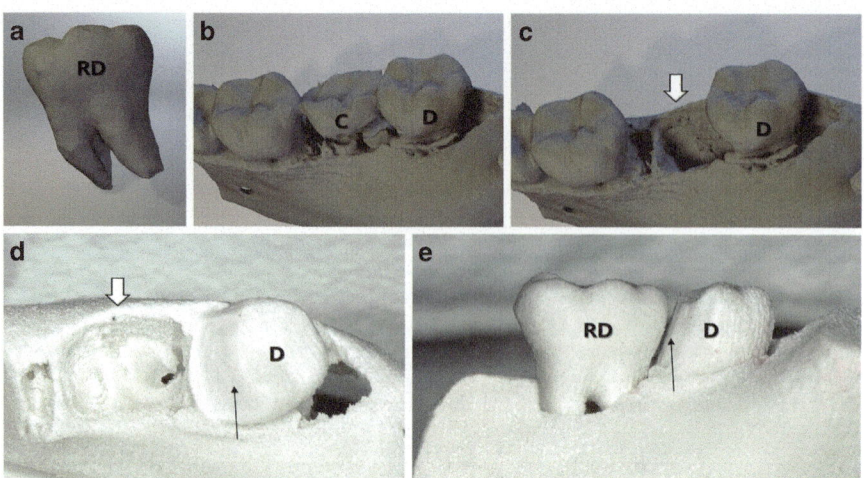

Fig. 10.2 Virtual construction and 3D-printed CARP models of the donor tooth and extraction socket. Digital Imaging and Communications in Medicine format files were created using CBCT radiographs followed by the construction of 3D virtual images using surgical planning software (OnDemand 3D). (**a**) Constructed replica of donor tooth #17 (RD). (**b**) The recipient alveolar bone before extraction of the compromised tooth (#18) (**c**). (**c**) The virtually constructed tentative extraction socket of the recipient alveolar bone (white arrow). (**d**) The CARP model of the tentative extraction socket (white arrow). (**e**) The replica of donor tooth #17 (RD) was inserted into the virtually constructed extraction socket of the alveolar bone. The constructed extraction socket model with the donor tooth, which will be extracted in the real procedure. The donor tooth (**d**) was trimmed (black arrow) to avoid premature contact between RD and D. (Courtesy: Oh S Et al. License no: 4793540387916)

Novel technologies allow also the generation of induced pluripotent stem cells based on reprogramming using the Yamanaka factors [13]. The isolation and the extension of the specific cells however require specialized facilities, which are accredited and follow the required guidelines for good manufacturing practice. A variety of cultivation systems have been developed, which allow the expansion of these stem cells. These systems include open cultivation systems and closed, automated, and intelligent cultivation systems. Changing the culture conditions either with regard to oxygen levels, dynamic settings, or cultivation in 3D settings can modulate the properties of the stem cells [14]. 3D printed scaffolds can have benefits compared to the applications of hydrogels with regard to their impact on dental pulp cells [15]. When Alg-Gel scaffolds were compared to 3D-printed Alg-Gel scaffolds, the 3D printed scaffolds showed better properties and induced cell proliferation and promoted differentiation. The 3D printed scaffolds can be further functionalized to improve cell seeding efficiency and scaffold performance. By modifying the surface architecture and introducing cell guiding structures, cells can be steered to develop more in-vivo-like structures [16].

For pulp regeneration, injectable hydrogels based on collagen or fibrin have been the focus of research as carriers for cells, growth factors, and differentiation factors [17–20]. Due to their properties, they allow application via a syringe by the dentist.

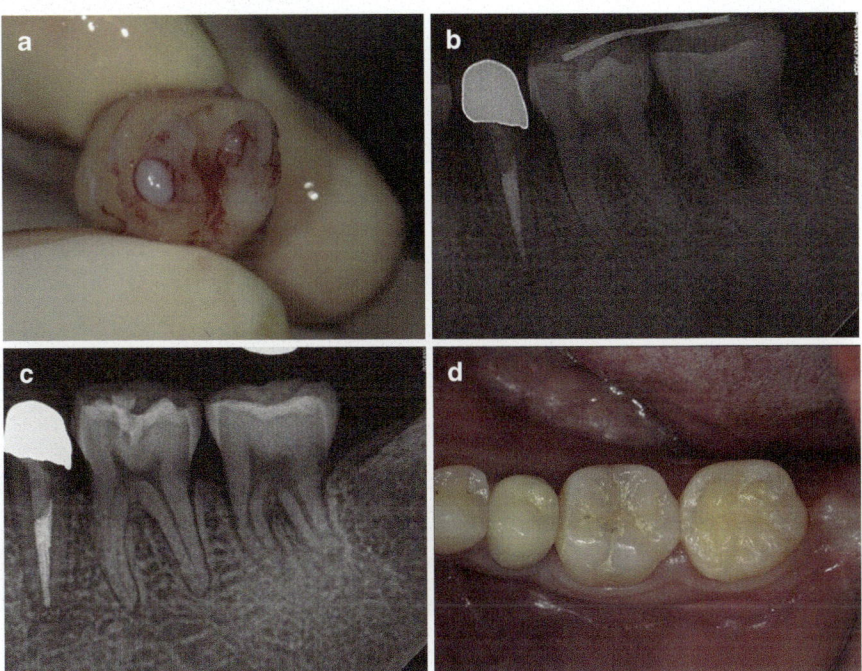

Fig. 10.3 Autotransplantation of tooth #17 into the extraction socket of tooth #18. (**a**) The apical papilla was observed at the root apex of tooth #17 after extraction. (**b**) Immediately after autotransplantation. (**c**) The 8-month follow-up radiograph showing closure of the root apex and further development of the root. (**d**) A clinical photograph at 8 months showing normal functioning of the transplanted tooth. (Courtesy: Oh S Et al. License no: 4793540387916)

Platelet-rich plasma was also suggested as a carrier. However, while these approaches seem to have the capacity to induce tissue repair, full regeneration was not achieved. Additionally, the formation of nonpulp tissue was observed. Noninjectable scaffolds were also assessed, including PLGA/TCP-nanofabric scaffolds, which contained silver to induce antibacterial effects. Interestingly, this combination induced cytotoxic effects in dental pulp cells and increased their pro-inflammatory capacity [21].

The development of bioprinters has given further inspiration and tools to the field of endodontics, allowing cell printing either in bioink or as spheroids. This bioprinting approach gives the opportunity to print more than one cell type with control over the spatial distribution of the cells within the construct. For endodontics, 3D printing can be applied to deliver stem cells, pulp scaffolds, injectable calcium phosphates, growth factors, and for gene therapy with the aim to maintain or regenerate the dental pulp [22]. Commercially available cellulose-based hydrogels have also shown to allow cell application (Unpublished data). Additionally, using the culturing model of single cell cultures or spheroid cultures can modulate the cellular response with regard to the specific hydrogels (unpublished observation). Some cellulose-based gels such as carboxyl methyl cellulose have also been shown to

Fig. 10.4 Stem cells for tissue engineering purposes

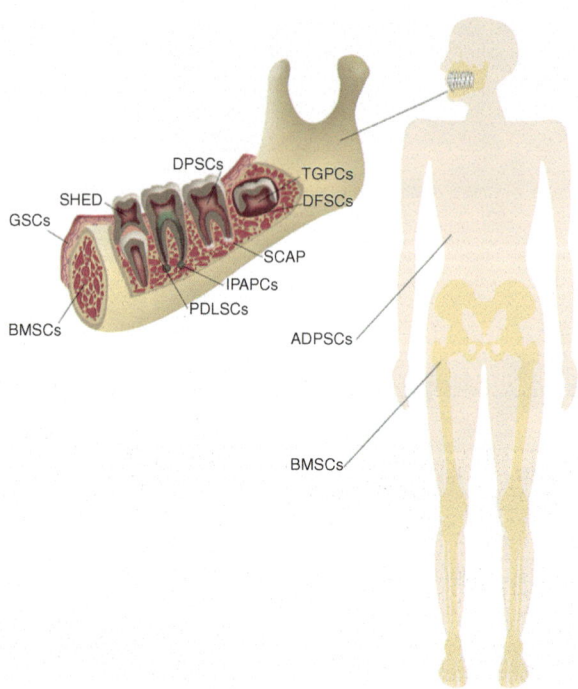

Table 10.1 Stem cells for tissue engineering purposes

Source	Stem cells
Oral tissue	Apical papilla stem cells (SCAPs)
	Dental follicle stem cells (DFSCs)
	Dental pulp stem cells (DPSCs)
	Exfoliated deciduous teeth stem cells (SHEDs)
	Gingiva stem cells (GSCs)
	Inflamed periapical progenitor cells (IPAPCs)
	Periodontal ligament stem cells (PDLSCs)
	Tooth germ progenitor cells (TGPCs)
Non-oral tissue	Adipose tissue stem cells (ATSCs)
	Bone mesenchymal stem cells (BMSCs)
	Inducible pluripotent stem cells (iPSs)

have antiresorptive effects via the inhibition of osteoclast formation [23]. Recently, a novel approach based on dentin extract has been established in which dentin-derived matrix components were combined with alginate (56). This supported cell viability and enhanced odontogenic differentiation of stem cell. Whether or not this novel bioink is beneficial with regard to collagen- or fibrin-based hydrogels with regard to pulp regeneration or dentin formation is yet to be determined. Several calcium phosphate cements have been established which allow the production of porous scaffolds for regeneration of the pulp-dentin complex [24]. Polycaprolactone coated with freeze-dried platelet-rich plasma in combination with dental pulp cells

Table 10.2 A selection of biomaterials used for dental pulp tissue engineering

Materials	Cells
Collagen I and dentin matrix acidic phosphoprotein (DMP)1	DPSC
Collagen I, Collagen III, chitosan, gelatin	Dental pulp cells
Fibrin	Without cells
Hydroxyapatite (HA), tricalcium phosphate (TCP)	SHED, DPSC
PEGylated fibrin	DPSC
Platelet-rich fibrin (PRF)	DPSC
Platelet-rich plasma (PRP)	DPSC
Poly lactic-co-glycolic acid (PLGA)	SCAP, DPCS
Polyglycolic acid (PGA), collagen I, alginate	Pulp fibroblasts
Polylactic acid (PLA)	SHED
Puramatrix	Apical Papilla Cells, DPCS, endothelial cells

Adopted with modifications from [12]

has positive effects in vitro [25]. This new technology also inspired researchers to follow the vision of building a new tooth from scratch [26]. The anatomically shaped "bio-tooth" is a tooth-like structure, which was produced by printing poly-epsilon-caprolactone and hydroxyapatite-based scaffolds in combination with stromal-derived factor-1 and bone morphogenetic protein-7 [27]. This approach did not require cell loading of the scaffold but rather relied on the homing of the required cells. In both ectopical and in situ animal models, the approach was promising [27].

While these approaches require the application of a biomaterial, it is still unclear what the optimal scaffold in this context is. Therefore, scaffold and carrier-free approaches were developed. These include the formation of microtissues called spheroids [28–30]. Spheroids and more complex microtissues can be generated using the hanging droplet approach, rotating wall vessels, ultralow attachment wells, prelabeling with magnetic beads, and the application of magnetic fields or the use of stenting weaves. The use of agarose molds for the generation of spheroids and more complex microtissues has also shown promising results. The application of spheroids of dental pulp cells for regenerative strategies led to positive results. The cells remain vital and attach to the dentin surface [28, 30–33]. To improve vascularization, the addition of endothelial cells leading to prevascularized microtissues has shown promising results [32]. Bioprinting systems have been developed to apply these spheroids and microtissues instead of using single cells. These systems include syringe-like applicators or needle arrays as well as applicators, which can handle more complex structures such as the pick, place, perfuse approach [34]. Currently, these printing systems have not been applied for endodontic approaches.

FDM printing was also used to print microfluidic devices easily and cost-effectively. These devices have been successfully applied to embed dental pulp stem cells into alginate droplets. Such approaches make the application of microfluidic devices easier and open for a wider field of researchers [35].

While it is unknown when bioprinting can lead to the clinical application of vital pulp implants, engineered tooth buds, or full bioteeth, the development of novel in vitro models for the evaluation of biomaterials and therapeutics on the dental pulp, such as in organs, can be expected in the near future. These models would lead to more reproducible results and be less complicated than current in vitro pulp models, which are based on tooth-slice or full-tooth models. Through the development of novel 3D pulp models, 3D printing can help to reduce the number of animal experiments required, following the 3R guidelines (Replace, Reduce, Refine) first described by Russel and Burch in 1959. This will not only lead to a better understanding of the biology of dental pulp but also boost the development of novel approaches for regenerative endodontics and conservative dentistry. Thus, even if, bioprinting does not become a direct clinical tool for endodontics in the near future, it will shape the clinical practice for the benefits of the clinician and the patients.

10.3   3D Printing in Smile Designing

The anterior teeth play an important role in facial beauty, and fully recovering a fractured anterior tooth requires restoration of the color, dental anatomy, and translucency of the tooth in addition to the curvature of the smile line and harmony with the other teeth in the arc [36]. The restored maxillary central incisors must also be well adapted, aesthetic, functional, and accepted by the patient. Wong et al. [37] used 3D dental models and visualization techniques to analyze different parameters in smile arcs. Rosati et al. [38] used 3D morphological facial and dental analyses to aid practitioners during diagnosis and treatment planning.

Figure 10.5 presents a case report of a 61-year-old female patient, referred to the clinic, with dental caries of her left maxillary central incisor [39]. The patient had no clinical symptoms (Fig. 10.7a). A clinical examination revealed that the left maxillary central incisor had caries involving incisal edge, which involved the enamel and dentin with no pulp exposure. A routine cold vitality test revealed that the tooth was sensitive. Finally, the relationship between the anterior teeth overbite and overjet was normal. A radiographic examination of the central incisors was conducted, and a radiographic analysis of the maxillary left central incisor revealed that there

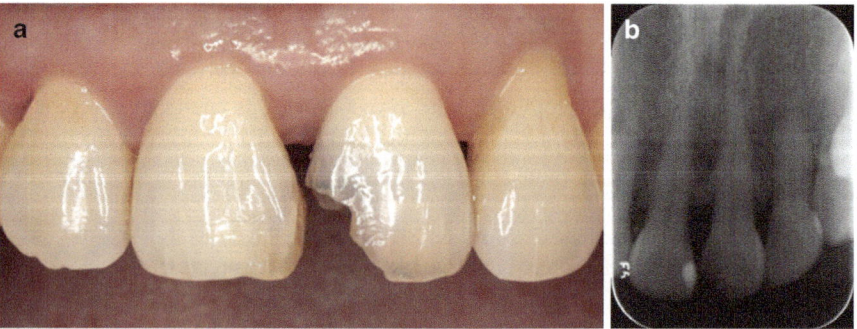

Fig. 10.5 (**a**) Preoperative view of dental caries in maxillary left central incisor. (**b**) Initial radiographic view of anterior teeth. (Courtesy: Xia J et al. [39])

was caries in the middle third of the crown. A 3D-printed template was fabricated using intraoral scanning, CAD, virtual modeling, and 3D printing as in the first case. Finally, the 3D-printed template was fabricated (Fig. 10.6).

Before treatment, the 3D-printed template was detached and soaked in disinfectant. Then, the template was positioned on the patient's dentition, and a correct and reproducible fit was verified. Initially, the anterior teeth were isolated using a rubber dam. The teeth were subjected to minimal tooth preparation using a diamond bur (Mani SF-41, Japan) to produce an improved alignment for the bond (Fig. 10.7a). Both surfaces of the connection were etched using acid gel (Ultra-Etch® 35% Phosphoric Acid, Ultradent, USA), rinsed, and gently dried. Single bond (Adper™ Single Bond 2, 3 M ESPE, USA) was applied first. The surface was then air-dried for 5 s and exposed to light activation for 10 s before the appropriate enamel composite (E3, Ceram*X duo, DENTSPLY, Germany) was placed on the defect area of the 3D template. Subsequently, the 3D template was positioned on the back of the anterior teeth (Fig. 10.7b) and exposed to light activation for 20 s (Fig. 10.7c). The palatal surface was then constructed. After polymerization, the palatal wall was sufficiently strong to support the next stratification steps (Fig. 10.7d). The integration of A2 (Ceram*X duo, DENTSPLY, Germany) was used to match the functional aesthetic bevel. Reconstruction was performed using an opaque dentin shade (D2, Ceram*X duo, DENTSPLY, Germany) to construct the dentin body (Fig. 10.7e). The enamel shade E3 was used to match the superficial enamel, and each composite

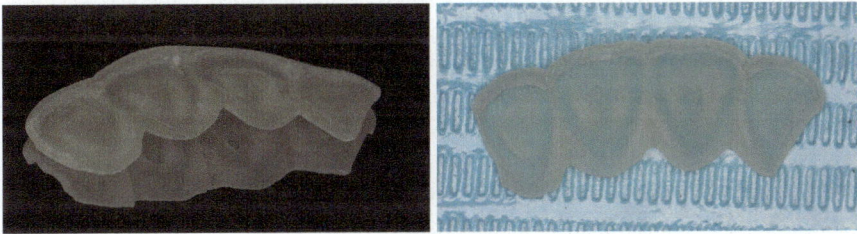

Fig. 10.6 The three-dimensional (3D) printed template

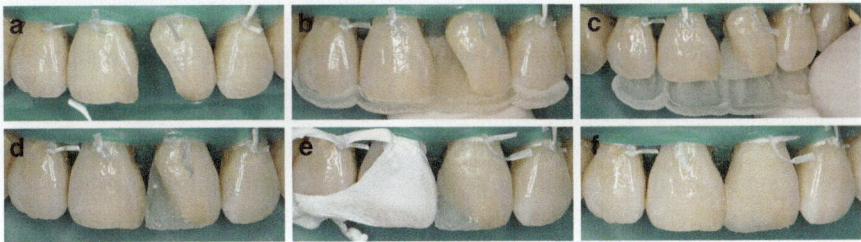

Fig. 10.7 (a) Functional esthetic bevel. (b) The 3D printing template was placed on the anterior teeth. (c) The palatal surface was augmented with template. (d) The palatal surface was constructed after polishing. (e) The dentin core. (f) The restoration was completed before polishing

increment was light-cured for 20 s. The final step consisted of performing an additional 20 s of polymerization at each site. After excess composite material was removed, an occlusion test was performed using carbon paper, and the restorations were shaped to the proper anatomic morphology (Fig. 10.7f). Next, finishing and polishing procedures were performed using fine-diamond-coated burs and a polishing system.

10.4   Haptic Virtual Reality in Endodontics

Haptic virtual reality (VR) has revolutionized the skill acquisition in dentistry. Virtual reality (VR) is a computer graphic technique for realizing an experience by supplying variable three-dimensional images [40]. The strength of the haptic VR system is that it can automatically record the outcome and associated kinematic data on how each step of the task is performed, which are not available in the conventional skill training environments. In particular, the haptic interface is the cutting-edge technology. The word "haptic" means relating to or proceeding from the sense of touch [41]. Haptic interface is a device that allows a user to interact with a computer by means of tactile feedback. This feedback is derived by using a manipulator to apply a degree of opposing force to the user along the x, y, and z axes. Haptic interfaces can be used to simulate operations and actions such as deformation and cutting. Three-dimensional haptic devices can be used for applications such as surgical simulation of complex procedures and training unskilled surgeons. Recently, the haptic VR simulators have been introduced into the dental curriculum as training devices for clinical skill acquisition in several tasks [42].

Endodontic procedures require an operator to have sound anatomical knowledge, correctly interpret radiographs and CBCT scans, be highly organized, exhibit manual competency, have good hand-eye co-ordination, correctly handle endodontic and surgical armamentarium, and be familiar with visual, acoustic, and tactile feedback sensations during treatment. Thus, for the teaching of endodontic treatments, haptic simulators should ideally provide realistic simulation of a wide variety of nonsurgical and surgical treatment procedures, alongside relevant armamentarium, and consideration of anatomical complexities. Haptic simulators can be useful as a teaching tool for endodontic procedures (Fig. 10.8). However, only access cavity preparation, osteotomies, and root-end resections are possible with commercially available haptic simulators. These include VirTeaSy Dental (HRV, Laval cedex, France) and Simodont® Dental Trainer [43].

With continuous improvements in 3D imaging, 3D printing, and 3D virtual planning, combined with the need for skill development, to optimize treatment outcomes and to improve patient comfort, there are potential benefits for teaching and management of nonsurgical and surgical endodontic procedures using these technologies. Further research on the various applications of 3D printed models, 3D printed guides, and haptic simulators in endodontics is required.

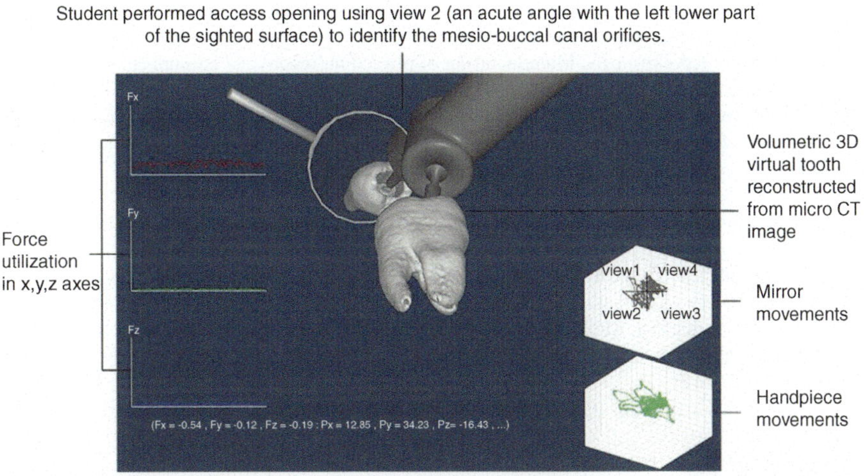

Student performed access opening using view 2 (an acute angle with the left lower part
of the sighted surface) to identify the mesio-buccal canal orifices.

Fig. 10.8 A student performing endodontic access opening with haptic virtual reality system

References

1. Andreasen JO. Interrelation between alveolar bon and periodontal ligament repair after replantation of mature permanent incisors in monkeys. J Periodontal Res. 1981;16:228–35.
2. Hupp JG, Mesaros SV, Aukhil I, Trope M. Periodontal ligament vitality and histologic healing of teeth stored for extended periods before transplantation. Endod Dent Traumatol. 1998;14:79–83.
3. Andreasen JO. Periodontal healing after replantation and autotransplantation of incisors in monkeys. Int J Oral Surg. 1981;10:54–61.
4. Lee SJ, Kim E. Minimizing the extra-oral time in autogeneous tooth transplantation: use of computer-aided rapid prototyping (CARP) as a duplicate model tooth. Restor Dent Endod. 2012;37(3):136–41.
5. Lee SJ, Jung IY, Lee CY, et al. Clinical application of computer-aided rapid prototyping for tooth transplantation. Dent Traumatol. 2001;17:114–9.
6. Jang Y, Choi YJ, Lee SJ, et al. Prognostic factors for clinical outcomes in autotransplantation of teeth with complete root formation: survival analysis for up to 12 years. J Endod. 2016;42:198–205.
7. Mejàre B, Wannfors K, Jansson L. A prospective study on transplantation of third molars with complete root formation. Oral Surg Oral Med Oral Pathol Oral Radiol Endod. 2004;97:231–8.
8. Nethander G, Andersson JE, Hirsch JM. Autogenous free tooth transplantation in man by a 2-stage operation technique. A longitudinal intra-individual radiographic assessment. Int J Oral Maxillofac Surg. 1988;17:330–6.
9. Schwartz O, Bergmann P, Klausen B. Autotransplantation of human teeth. A life-table analysis of prognostic factors. Int J Oral Surg. 1985;14:245–58.
10. Jang JH, Lee SJ, Kim E. Autotransplantation of immature third molars using a computer-aided rapid prototyping model: a report of 4 cases. J Endod. 2013;39:1461–6.
11. Oh S, Kim S, et al. Virtual simulation of autotransplantation using 3-dimensional printing prototyping model and computer-assisted design program. J Endod. 2018;44:1883–8.
12. Goldberg M, editor. The dental pulp: biology, pathology, and regenerative therapies. New York, NY: Springer; 2014.

13. Shi Y, Inoue H, Wu JC, Yamanaka S. Induced pluripotent stem cell technology: a decade of progress. Nat Rev Drug Discov. 2017;16(2):115–30.
14. Yin JQ, Zhu J, Ankrum JA. Manufacturing of primed mesenchymal stromal cells for therapy. Nat Biomed Eng. 2019;3(2):90–104.
15. Yu H, Zhang X, Song W, Pan T, Wang H, Ning T, et al. Effects of 3-dimensional bioprinting alginate/gelatin hydrogel scaffold extract on proliferation and differentiation of human dental pulp stem cells. J Endod. 2019;45(6):706–15.
16. Pilipchuk SP, Monje A, Jiao Y, Hao J, Kruger L, Flanagan CL, et al. Integration of 3D printed and micropatterned polycaprolactone scaffolds for guidance of oriented collagenous tissue formation in vivo. Adv Healthc Mater. 2016;5(6):676–87.
17. Ruangsawasdi N, Zehnder M, Weber FE. Fibrin gel improves tissue ingrowth and cell differentiation in human immature premolars implanted in rats. J Endod. 2014;40(2):246–50.
18. Kakarla P, Avula JSS, Mellela GM, Bandi S, Anche S. Dental pulp response to collagen and pulpotec cement as pulpotomy agents in primary dentition: a histological study. J Conserv Dent. 2013;16(5):434–8.
19. Kikuchi N, Kitamura C, Morotomi T, Inuyama Y, Ishimatsu H, Tabata Y, et al. Formation of dentin-like particles in dentin defects above exposed pulp by controlled release of fibroblast growth factor 2 from gelatin hydrogels. J Endod. 2007;33(10):1198–202.
20. Suzuki T, Lee CH, Chen M, Zhao W, Fu SY, Qi JJ, et al. Induced migration of dental pulp stem cells for in vivo pulp regeneration. J Dent Res. 2011;90(8):1013–8.
21. Cvikl B, Hess SC, Miron RJ, Agis H, Bosshardt D, Attin T, et al. Response of human dental pulp cells to a silver-containing PLGA/TCP-nanofabric as a potential antibacterial regenerative pulp-capping material. BMC Oral Health. 2017;17(1):57.
22. Murray PE, Garcia-Godoy F, Hargreaves KM. Regenerative endodontics: a review of current status and a call for action. J Endod. 2007;33(4):377–90.
23. Agis H, Beirer B, Watzek G, Gruber R. Effects of carboxymethylcellulose and hydroxypropylmethylcellulose on the differentiation and activity of osteoclasts and osteoblasts. J Biomed Mater Res A. 2010;95(2):504–9.
24. Xu HH, Wang P, Wang L, Bao C, Chen Q, Weir MD, et al. Calcium phosphate cements for bone engineering and their biological properties. Bone Res. 2017;5:17056.
25. Li J, Chen M, Wei X, Hao Y, Wang J. Evaluation of 3D-printed polycaprolactone scaffolds coated with freeze-dried platelet-rich plasma for bone regeneration. Materials (Basel). 2017;10(7):e831.
26. Yan M, Yu Y, Zhang G, Tang C, Yu J. A journey from dental pulp stem cells to a bio-tooth. Stem Cell Rev. 2011;7(1):161–71.
27. Redwood B, Schöffer F, Garret B. The 3d printing handbook: technologies, design and applications. 1st ed. Amsterdam: 3d Hubs; 2017.
28. Ozbolat IT, Moncal KK, Gudapati H. Evaluation of bioprinter technologies. Addit Manufac. 2017;13:179–200.
29. Ozbolat IT, Peng W, Ozbolat V. Application areas of 3D bioprinting. Drug Discov Today. 2016;21(8):1257–71.
30. Mironov V, Visconti RP, Kasyanov V, Forgacs G, Drake CJ, Markwald RR. Organ printing: tissue spheroids as building blocks. Biomaterials. 2009;30(12):2164–74.
31. Oberoi G, Janjić K, Müller AS, Schädl B, Andrukhov O, Moritz A, et al. Contraction dynamics of rod microtissues of gingiva-derived and periodontal ligament-derived cells. Front Physiol. 2018;9:1683.
32. Oberoi G, Janjić K, Müller AS, Schädl B, Moritz A, Agis H. Contraction dynamics of dental pulp cell rod microtissues. Clin Oral Investig. 2020;24:631.
33. Ji S, Guvendiren M. Recent advances in bioink design for 3D bioprinting of tissues and organs. Front Bioeng Biotechnol. 2017;5:23.
34. Blakely AM, Manning KL, Tripathi A, Morgan JR. Bio-pick, place, and perfuse: a new instrument for three-dimensional tissue engineering. Tissue Eng Part C Methods. 2015;21(7):737–46.

35. Morgan AJL, Hidalgo San Jose L, Jamieson WD, Wymant JM, Song B, Stephens P, et al. Simple and versatile 3D printed microfluidics using fused filament fabrication. PLoS One. 2016;11(4):e0152023.
36. Pontons-Melo JC, Furuse AY, Mondelli J. A direct composite resin stratification technique for restoration of the smile. Quintessence Int. 2011;42(3):205–11.
37. Wong NK, Kassim AA, Foong KW. Analysis of esthetic smiles by using computer vision techniques. Am J Orthod Dentofac Orthop. 2005;128(3):404–11.
38. Rosati R, De Menezes M, Rossetti A, Sforza C, Ferrario VF. Digital dental cast placement in 3-dimensional, full-face reconstruction: a technical evaluation. Am J Orthod Dentofac Orthop. 2010;138(1):84–8.
39. Xia J, Li Y, Cai D, et al. Direct resin composite restoration of maxillary central incisors using a 3D-printed template: two clinical cases. BMC Oral Health. 2018;18:158.
40. Maass H, Chantier BB, Cakmak HK, et al. Fundamentals of force feedback and application to a surgery simulator. Comput Aid Surg. 2003;8:283–91.
41. Cosman PH, Cregan PC, Martin CJ, et al. Virtual reality simulators: current status in acquisition and assessment of surgical skills. ANZ J Surg. 2002;72:30–4.
42. Shah P, Chong BS. 3D imaging, 3D printing and 3D virtual planning in endodontics. Clin Oral Investig. 2018;22(2):641–54.
43. Suebnukarn S, Haddawy P, Rhienmora P, Gajananan K. Haptic virtual reality for skill acquisition in endodontics. J Endod. 2010;36(1):53–5.

Printed by Printforce, the Netherlands